HOME SAFE HOME

HOME SAFE HOME

*Protecting Yourself and Your Family
from Everyday Toxics and
Harmful Household Products*

DEBRA LYNN DADD

JEREMY P. TARCHER/PUTNAM

a member of PENGUIN PUTNAM INC. *New York*

Most Tarcher/Putnam books are available at special quantity discounts for bulk
purchases for sales promotions, premiums, fund-raising, and educational needs.
Special books or book excerpts also can be created to fit specific needs.
For details, write or telephone Putnam Special Markets, 200 Madison Avenue,
New York, NY 10016; (212) 951-8891.

Jeremy P. Tarcher/Putnam
a member of
Penguin Putnam Inc.
200 Madison Avenue
New York, NY 10016
http://www.putnam.com

Library of Congress Cataloging-in-Publication Data

Dadd, Debra Lynn.
    Home safe home : protecting yourself and your family from everyday toxics and harmful
household products / Debra Lynn Dadd.
        p.   cm.
    Includes bibliographical references and index.
    ISBN 0-87477-859-X
    1. Housing and health.   2. Household supplies—Toxicology.   3. Indoor air pollution.
I. Title.
RA770.5.D27   1997   96-36714   CIP
615.9'02—dc20

Design by Mauna Eichner
Cover design by Susan Shankin
Cover illustration inspired by a needlework design by Ursula Michael

Printed in the United States of America
1   2   3   4   5   6   7   8   9   10

This book is printed on acid-free paper. ∞

For my literary agent,
Martha Casselman,
who has represented me
since my very first book,
Nontoxic & Natural.
It was she
who tended the seedling
that has flowered
into this book.

ACKNOWLEDGMENTS

WHILE THE IDEA of writing about safe alternatives to household toxics was my own, I have to give credit for the book in its current form to others.

I would like to thank Janice Gallagher, former executive director at Jeremy P. Tarcher, Inc., for originally coming up with the idea and asking me to write *The Nontoxic Home,* on which this book was based, and Suzanne Lipsett, editor of that book, who greatly helped me to become a better writer.

I also want to thank Rick Benzel, former senior editor at Jeremy P. Tarcher, Inc., for expanding the idea of the original book and asking me to write *The Nontoxic Home & Office.*

My appreciation, too, goes to Irene Prokop, editor-in-chief at Jeremy P. Tarcher/Putnam, for seeing the continued value of my work and envisioning a new format that better serves today's consumer, and to assistant editor Jennifer Greene, who competently carried the book through all the phases of production.

And thanks to you, Jeremy, for continuing to publish my books all these many years.

Finally, my acknowledgments would not be complete if I did not mention my patient and understanding husband, who cheerfully fixes my dinner and rubs my shoulders as deadlines draw near. Thank you, Larry!

CONTENTS

CHAPTER 7: BEAUTY AND HYGIENE — 167

CHAPTER 8: FOOD — 214

AUTHOR'S NOTE

PLEASE THINK OF the recommendations you find here as guidelines—not gospel. Like a map, they point the way to new things you might wish to explore for yourself, with *you* being a responsible explorer. Follow the suggestions given here with the same care you would use on a hike through a forest. Although a map allows you to choose your course with confidence regarding the general terrain, as you walk you still need to watch out for boulders, the weather, poisonous snakes, and other hazards that the map cannot portray or prepare you for. (Certainly you'll also unexpectedly find such delights as wildflowers, deer, or a fallen tree bridging a creek.) Similarly, because of space limitations, I cannot possibly mention every item you might find in a store or mail-order catalog, so you are in for some wonderful surprises. In this book, as in the forest, only you can decide which path to take.

In order to help you choose products and to learn more about safe alternatives, I have included information about brand-name products, mail-order businesses, books, publications, and organizations. Buying these products, encouraging your friends and family members to buy them, and asking for them by name at your local stores will help guarantee their continued and increased availability. No advertising or promotional fees were accepted, and the inclusion of any product, business, book, publication, or organization here is not intended as an endorsement. If I occasionally mention that I use a product personally, this indicates only my preference; that item is not necessarily superior to other products mentioned.

To be an effective user or consumer of products means to take responsibility for the choices you make. Be as wary of blindly accepting the information presented here as you would of assuming that all products on the market are safe. Despite heroic efforts on my and the publisher's parts to assure accuracy, we cannot guarantee *everything* to be absolutely correct, though we both have worked hard toward that goal. Specifically, we can make no representations about, and therefore cannot be responsible for:

> incorrect or incomplete information regarding products;
>
> changes in product ingredients or production methods;
>
> substances or processes with toxicity yet undiscovered;
>
> the continued availability of any item;
>
> the effectiveness of any product or process listed; or
>
> any adverse health effects caused by any product or process listed.

All the information I used to evaluate the safety of products mentioned in this book has come from written materials supplied by the manufacturer or retailer, or from personal conversations with people who make and sell these products. The assessments were made according to information available to all consumers; no independent testing was done by me. It is possible that the products selected may contain as-yet-undisclosed harmful or environmentally destructive substances. Nevertheless, one can be fairly certain that these products are safer than those revealing contents known to be dangerous. It is my belief that products produced and sold by conscientious people truly are purer than those produced and sold by manufacturers unconcerned with the issues addressed here.

Throughout these pages, suggestions are made for using products in ways other than those for which those products were originally intended. Because government regulations do not allow manufacturers to recommend their products for certain uses without laboratory proof that they are indeed safe and effective for such uses (and then procuring government approval of the results), these alternate uses are not necessarily approved by the manufacturer. Not all of the suggestions given are tried and true, but all have been found to work for many people.

This book is designed to serve people with different interests, budgets, medical conditions, and lifestyles, and as such it may occasionally mention products or processes that are not appropriate for you personally. At these times, simply make an individual choice, and remember that the primary purpose of this book is to report on the availability of products that generally are safe to our health.

And last but not least, the omission of a product from these pages should not imply that it isn't safe. My intention was to help consumers learn to choose safe products and to give practical information, not to catalog every item in every store. It is my hope that, based upon the information you find here, you will make your own wise choices.

INTRODUCTION

THIS BOOK IS THE COMBINED revised and expanded edition of two books that were published back in the mid-1980s as *Nontoxic & Natural* and *The Nontoxic Home*. Both titles were updated at the beginning of this decade as *Nontoxic, Natural & Earthwise* and *The Nontoxic Home & Office*. Now, in this single volume, I bring you the best of both books.* *Home Safe Home* will both explain the hazards found in household products and their safe alternatives—as did *The Nontoxic Home*—and give the resource listings and do-it-yourself formulas *Nontoxic & Natural* was valued for.

As in my other books, I speak to you not as a doctor, scientist, or toxicologist, but as an educated consumer. You will benefit from what I have learned in seventeen years of firsthand experience living in a safe home, and from my investigation of the subject as a full-time profession.

Researching toxic substances in everyday products, as well as safe substitutes for them, has been of vital interest to me since 1980, when I was diagnosed as having a severe breakdown of my immune system, caused, I was told, by the combination of a high-stress lifestyle and heavy chemical exposure. I was shocked, for I thought my chemical exposure was no worse than that of anyone else living in our modern world. I worked as a classical musician

---

*Those of you familiar with my previous books know that *Nontoxic, Natural & Earthwise* had a strong environmental focus. I expanded on the environmental effects of products in *Sustaining the Earth: Choosing Consumer Products That Are Safe for You, Your Family, and the Earth* (New York: William Morrow, 1994), so *Home Safe Home* focuses only on health effects. I recommend both books as complementary volumes. (See my Website—www.worldwise.com/debra—for *Sustaining the Earth*.)

and lived an urban existence in a major metropolitan city. I had no occupational exposure to chemicals. Ironically, the chemicals that disabled me were all in my home.

Because my illness caused violent reactions to all man-made products, I began to look for products I could use that did not contain toxic substances or any petrochemical derivatives. After much trial and error, I finally came up with a small list. But my search was difficult because most toxic substances generally found in the home are hidden in products—that is, the law does not require that they be listed on product labels. For example, a canned food might contain remainders of the detergent used to wash the food, traces of lead from the solder used to hold the can together, artificial additives that could have been used in any of the ingredients, and pesticide residues. All the law requires of food manufacturers is that they list on the label the ingredients and additives mixed together in the final stage of processing, and not the additives and contaminants in the ingredients themselves. Ferreting out this information is no mean task of detection: Most of my information about toxic chemicals in products has come from materials written for poison-control centers, toxicology books, federal regulations, and trade journals—not from the product labels themselves.

My list of products and their nontoxic alternatives steadily grew, through personal experience and contributions from friends, until finally, in 1982, I self-published a small directory of safe brand-name products, local stores where they could be purchased, and mail-order sources for some hard-to-obtain items. Soon my mailbox was filled with orders from all over the country, as news of my directory (a stapled packet of photocopies) spread by word of mouth. Meanwhile, my health improved drastically— thanks primarily to my new nontoxic lifestyle—and within a few months I was totally free of my formerly disabling symptoms.

The media picked up my story, and I began receiving orders for my directory from people who weren't ill, but who were concerned about the environment or the health of their children, and from those who were concerned about the possible long-term health effects of unknown substances. In 1984, an expanded directory of safe products was published by Jeremy P. Tarcher, Inc., *Nontoxic & Natural,* which now has grown to become *Home Safe Home.*

Much has changed since that first book was written. Among other things, the EPA discovered indoor air pollution, household hazardous-waste collection programs have sprung up all over the country, and there's been a steady increase in the production and purchasing of organically grown food ever since Meryl Streep appeared on television and alerted the country to the danger of Alar on apples. We now have more safe products than ever to choose from—and also we know more about the dangers of those that cause harm. In 1984, I had few scientific studies on which I could base my recommendations. It's been heartening to see my logic substantiated by scientific tests on more consumer products in recent years.

In 1984, everything I could find about dangerous products and safe alternatives filled a book. Now it could fill a library. So this book—instead of being the definitive guide—serves as an introduction and overview with enough "take action" information to get you started. It is not exhaustive—no one book on the subject could be today—but it covers the basics and provides plenty of resources at the back of the book, for your continued explorations.

Like its predecessors, *Home Safe Home* is a response to the question I am asked most frequently about household toxics: *Where do I begin?* This book will discuss, in easy-to-understand language, toxic chemicals and other health hazards found everywhere in your home and home office, and give you information that will help you determine which pose greater risks, and which are easier (and less expensive) to change. It is full of helpful hints and suggestions that will lead you to safe solutions you can make yourself, and to safe products you can purchase in local stores or through mail-order catalogs.

There are many reasons why you might be interested in creating a safe home and work space. The most obvious, of course, is that it is better for your own health and the health of those who visit or live with you. Exposure to toxic chemicals can aggravate symptoms of allergy and compromise the immune system to the point where disabling sensitivities to certain chemicals can develop. Over a long period of time, toxic products can contribute to the development of cancer, birth defects, genetic changes, and other illnesses. Some estimates suggest that nationally, the indirect costs of what is now called "indoor pollution" exceed $6 billion per year—more than $1 billion in medical bills and $5 billion from sick leave and reduced worker productivity. Radon alone is suspected of causing between 5,000 and 20,000 deaths per year, while exposure to indoor chemicals and tobacco smoke may add up to 10,000 more.

Many of the products mentioned in this book can also affect the environment, releasing toxic substances either in their manufacture, use, or disposal. A large majority of the products that are toxic to humans are synthesized from petrochemicals, which cause pollution ranging from oil spills to toxic waste. If you've been taking household hazardous waste to a community collection event, you'll find this book to be full of suggestions that will help you reduce the amount of household hazardous waste you produce. When I was working on *Nontoxic, Natural & Earthwise,* I did some research into the *eco*toxic effects of products—that is, how products are toxic to other species in the environment and to the functioning of the earth as a whole living organism. What may be safe for humans can kill or harm more delicate species and ultimately disrupt the balance of our ecosystem. However, toxic chemicals in the environment affect us directly too, through the air we breathe, the water we drink, and the food we eat.

Ecotoxicity of a substance generally is determined by evaluating the inherent toxicity of the substance to a particular species, how long it persists in the environment, and its tendency to bioaccumulate up the food chain. Currently, there is little information on the ecotoxicity of chemicals, and because of the complexity and cost of testing, we may not see these tests even in the future. For now, I'm assuming that if a product contains a known toxic substance, its manufacture and disposal probably produce toxic waste in the environment. Even though I won't be mentioning this repeatedly throughout the book, keep in mind that virtually every product mentioned as being harmful to our health is probably not good for the earth either.

Because these substances have molecular structures that do not appear in the natural world, ecologist Barry Commoner calls them "inherently antagonistic to life." Natural systems have evolved without them, and no one knows what ultimate effects the massive quantities we produce, use, and eventually return to the air, water, and soil will have on our health or other species. It's much easier and less expensive to simply use safer alternatives.

Making changes in your home can be difficult, I know, especially when the amount of information to consider seems overwhelming. When I sat down to write the original version of *The Nontoxic Home*, I thought I would simply list alternatives for the hundred more-toxic products. A worker at my local poison-control center laughed when I told her what I was trying to do. I quickly discovered it was an impossible task. So many factors determine toxicity that to say one thing is more toxic than another is like saying New York–style pizza is better than Chicago-style.

The best we can do is assess each product individually, learn the risks, weigh the risks against the benefits (and the low-risk and risk-free alternatives), and decide whether or not we personally want to take these risks and to subject those we love and our earth to them. The choice is in our hands.

HOW TO USE THIS BOOK

While many products and ideas might be considered for use in a safe home, I have suggested only those that I have found, in my personal experience, to be the easiest and most effective. Also, this book does not cover every toxic product that might be in your home, only the most common and most dangerous, and those for which there are safer alternatives.

I have kept my comments simple, hoping to inspire you to seek more information. Since it is impossible to give a complete listing of nontoxic products in today's market, brand-name products and mail-order sources given in this book are meant only to be *examples* of what is available, and not an exhaustive listing.

Relative Toxicity of Products

The arrangement of the chapters within *Home Safe Home* and the items within them reflect the relative toxicity to humans of the items discussed, with the *more immediate* hazards first. Ironically, some of the simpler and more inexpensive to change are also among the more important to change (e.g., cleaning products, pesticides, personal-care products), as they are recognized poisons and major contributors to the toxicity of your home.

Manufacturers' Warning Labels

Throughout the book I have included information from manufacturers' warning labels, which summarize the warnings I have found on different products of the same type. Although no single manufacturer prints the warnings exactly as they are found in this book, I have combined the information found on various labels to show you more clearly the overall danger.

Route of Exposure

When assessing the risk of a product, it is very important to consider how the chemical is entering your body. Some substances do not give off fumes, but can be deadly if swallowed. Others may cause skin irritation and also cause reactions if they are inhaled. To help you quickly assess the danger, I have used four simple symbols to indicate the modes of exposure by which the product may be harmful. In many cases there are secondary exposures that are not often recognized.

  Ingested by mouth

  Splashed in eyes

  Absorbed through skin

  Inhaled through nose or mouth

Typefaces

Toxic substances are set in **lowercase boldface** type.
Brand-Name Products are set in **Uppercase and Lowercase Boldface** type.
Mail-Order Catalogs are set in *Uppercase and Lowercase Boldface Italic* type.

Manufacturers' warning labels are set in this font.

Chapter **1**

How Safe Is Your Home?

IF THERE IS ONE WORD we universally associate with home, it is *safe*. Home is the one place we can always go to feel loved, secure, and that all is well. No harm can come to us at home.

The dictionary sitting next to my desk defines *safe* as "that which we can depend on to be secure from harm, injury, danger, or risk." Unfortunately, too often today our homes are not safe—they are filled with common everyday consumer products that are associated with harm, injury, danger, and risk. But the good news is that there are many things each of us can do to create a home where we *can* feel safe, knowing we are free from exposures to substances and materials that may be hazardous to our health.

There are many different kinds of safety issues, ranging from how to handle knives so you don't cut yourself to securing your valuables against loss. This book specifically focuses on safe-guarding your health from dangers found in consumer products in and around your home. It will both reveal the hidden hazards and offer safe solutions, giving you the information you need to make choices and changes for a toxic-free home environment. The changes aren't going to be radical, the choices aren't going to be difficult—but simple as it is, in the long run *and* the short run, this book could save your life, or the life of someone you love.

Why should you care about household toxics? Simple. Because your greatest exposure to toxic substances is right in your home, and every toxic product used at home ultimately ends up in the environment, from which it can return to harm us. Your house or apartment probably is full of everyday products made from materials and substances that cause cancer, birth defects, and changes in genetic structure, and that weaken the immune system, leaving your body vulnerable to many kinds of diseases and infections. A multitude of common symptoms can be related to exposure to household toxics—headaches, depression, even ordinary flu symptoms might not be flu at all, but a pesticide poisoning or a reaction to your furniture polish.

Sometimes it's hardest to see what's closest to you, what you see every day. But let's take a quick mental tour of the typical American home, where you consider yourself and other members of your household to be safe from the dangers of the outside world. The list below includes items you may be surprised to learn pose potential safety problems. Check those items you might find in each room to see how safe you *really* are from household health hazards.

Living Room

- alcoholic beverages
- artificial light
- carpet/upholstery shampoo
- electromagnetic fields
- ionization-type smoke detectors
- fireplace
- furniture/floor polish
- gas heater
- houseplants
- kerosene heater
- particleboard furniture
- spot remover
- synthetic wall-to-wall carpet
- tobacco smoke
- urea-formaldehyde foam insulation
- wood stove

Kitchen

- ❏ aluminum cookware
- ❏ ammonia/all-purpose cleaners
- ❏ artificial sweeteners
- ❏ asbestos-vinyl floor tiles
- ❏ canned food
- ❏ chlorinated scouring powder
- ❏ chocolate and coffee
- ❏ dishwasher detergent
- ❏ dishwashing liquid
- ❏ drain cleaners
- ❏ dried fruits
- ❏ fish and seafood
- ❏ gas appliances
- ❏ insecticides
- ❏ microwave ovens
- ❏ nonstick cookware
- ❏ oven cleaner
- ❏ particleboard cabinets
- ❏ plastic clock
- ❏ plastic drinking glasses
- ❏ plastic food wrap and storage containers
- ❏ plastic lighting fixtures
- ❏ plastic telephone
- ❏ processed foods
- ❏ rat and mouse killers
- ❏ silver polish and other metal cleaners
- ❏ store-bought water in plastic bottles
- ❏ supermarket eggs
- ❏ supermarket meat
- ❏ supermarket milk
- ❏ supermarket produce
- ❏ tap water
- ❏ vitamin and mineral supplements

Bathroom

- ❏ aerosol hair spray
- ❏ air fresheners
- ❏ antiperspirants
- ❏ astringents
- ❏ bubble bath
- ❏ contact lenses
- ❏ cosmetics
- ❏ dandruff shampoo
- ❏ denture cleaners
- ❏ deodorant soap
- ❏ drugs and medication
- ❏ feminine deodorant spray
- ❏ feminine douches
- ❏ fluoride mouthwash
- ❏ fluoride toothpaste
- ❏ germ-killing disinfectants
- ❏ glass cleaner
- ❏ hair color

- ❏ hair-removal products
- ❏ hairstyling mousse
- ❏ mold and mildew cleaners
- ❏ nail polish/nail-polish remover
- ❏ perfume and aftershave
- ❏ permanent-wave solutions
- ❏ scented toilet paper
- ❏ superabsorbent tampons
- ❏ talcum powder
- ❏ vinyl shower curtain

Bedroom

- ❏ children's sleepwear
- ❏ contraceptives
- ❏ disposable diapers
- ❏ dry-cleaned fabrics
- ❏ fireproofed synthetic mattresses
- ❏ mothballs
- ❏ no-iron bed linens
- ❏ nylon stockings
- ❏ permanent-press clothing
- ❏ plastic baby pants
- ❏ plastic baby toys
- ❏ plastic raincoat and umbrella
- ❏ vinyl shoes and handbags

Laundry Room

- ❏ chlorine bleach
- ❏ do-it-yourself dyes
- ❏ fabric softeners
- ❏ laundry detergents
- ❏ spray starch

Home Office

- ❏ artificial lighting
- ❏ computers
- ❏ copy machines and computer printers
- ❏ paper
- ❏ permanent-ink pens and markers
- ❏ typewriter correction fluid

How did you do? Are there lots of check marks? Every one of the items on this list poses a health hazard—either by immediate poisoning or by slowly breaking down your health over a long period of time. Fortunately, *there is a safe, nontoxic alternative* for each of these products. And remember, using these alternatives also will help improve the environment.

Don't expect to change your whole house overnight; the very nature of change is a gradual process. It begins with a decision, a commitment to change. Next, you have to take action. Simply reading this book will not protect you from common health hazards. You will need to act on the information you find here.

Deciding to make the changes is the hardest part. Finding safe products is easy and can be fun, and you'll love the simplicity of the safe alternatives you can make at home. Following the suggestions outlined in this book just may save your child from an accidental poisoning or keep you from getting cancer. I know it seems like such a small thing to do, given the enormity of the problem of toxics in our world, but fortunately even the smallest steps you take can have an enormous beneficial effect. Remember, it's your *home,* your oasis of warmth and safety, and you alone are responsible for what you choose to put in it. There is an environmental slogan: "Think globally, act locally." And remember that old saying "Charity begins at home"? That's just where we have to begin with toxics, too.

HOW TO DETERMINE IF A PRODUCT IS TOXIC TO YOU

Over the years, I've learned that to most people, *safe* and *toxic* are polar opposites—a product is either all right to use or it is harmful to health, in their minds. In fact, the safety or toxicity of a product is not so cut-and-dried. There are many variations and gradations of inherent toxicity among products, and a number of factors that can affect whether or not the product will cause harm to you individually.

While it sounds complex, the basics of toxicology aren't really so hard, and the differences are worth learning if you are concerned about your exposure. In fact, while learning about the different degrees of toxicity, you'll be relieved to find that many products aren't so toxic after all, if used occasionally and with care.

Types of Toxicity

Toxicity of chemicals is of two types: acute and chronic.

Acute toxicity refers to poisoning as the result of a one-time exposure to a relatively large amount of a chemical. Acute toxicity is a concern for most consumer products that have warning labels, and is the reason we have poison-control centers. Every year, 5 to 10 million household poisonings are reported as the result of accidental exposure to toxic products in the home. Some are fatal, and most of the victims are children. These poisonings are the result of accidental ingestion of common household products that, despite warning labels, are not kept out of children's reach.

Chronic toxicity refers to illness as the result of many repeated exposures to small amounts of a chemical over a long period of time, and this is what makes it so difficult to identify some toxics. We can easily see the effects when drain cleaner is spilled on someone's hand and the skin burns. The effects of chronic toxicity may not show up for years. Numerous common household products can cause cancer—not an immediate effect, because carcinogenic substances take twenty years or more to act. Other household chemicals are mutagenic: they can change genetic material and lead to health problems. Still others are known to be teratogenic, and the high incidence of birth defects continues to remind us that not all household substances have been tested for this danger.

Toxic chemicals are made biologically by nature, and in the laboratory by humans. Just because something is "natural" doesn't mean it's not toxic. Some of the more toxic substances in the world are made by plant and animal species and used for protection against predators. We don't generally encounter natural toxins in our everyday world, but we are exposed to many man-made substances in everyday products that have potentially toxic effects.

The basic problem is that nowadays most of our products are made from petrochemical derivatives of nonrenewable crude oil. Often these compounds are not otherwise found in nature, and our bodies have not developed the means to identify or assimilate them. These chemicals are used in nearly every industry and every type of consumer product.

In 1987 the United States produced almost 400 billion pounds of synthetic organic chemicals, more than four pounds of man-made substances for every person in this country each day. Worldwide, about 70,000 synthetic chemicals are in use, with nearly 1,000 new ones added every year. Some of these chemicals are considered safe for human use, but the vast majority have not been fully tested.

Next to nothing is currently known about the toxic effects to humans of almost 80 percent of the more than 48,000 chemicals listed by the EPA. Fewer than 1,000 have been tested for immediate acute effects, and only about 500 have been tested for their ability to cause long-term chronic health problems such as cancer, birth defects, and genetic changes. A National Research Council study found that complete health-hazard evaluations were available for only 10 percent of pesticides and 18 percent of drugs used in this country.

Almost no tests have been undertaken to evaluate the possible synergistic reactions that occur when chemicals are combined in food, water, or air, or when chemicals interact with other chemicals in our bodies. The few studies that have been done indicate that such combinations increase risks dramatically. Because scientists do not understand the ultimate effects of these chemicals, the government cannot begin to regulate their use sufficiently.

The average American home is literally filled with products made from these inadequately tested synthetic substances; we use more chemicals in our homes today than were found in a typical chemistry lab at the turn of the century. When professionals use chemicals in industrial settings, they are subject to strict health and safety codes, yet we use some of these same chemicals at home without guidance or restriction.

As further research is done, scientists are finding that many household products we assumed to be safe are actually toxic to some degree or another. A multitude of common symptoms such as headaches and depression can be related to exposure to household toxics. Insomnia, for example, is listed in toxicology books as a common symptom from exposure to the formaldehyde resin used on your bedsheets to keep them wrinkle-free.

How to Decide If a Product Is Toxic

Determining the toxicity of any product can be difficult because there are so many factors to consider. It's easy to identify some substances that are inherently unsafe, such as the bacteria that cause botulism, or benzene, which has known harmful effects, but tracking down the toxicity of other substances can be a much more complex process.

Toxicity of a substance is scientifically determined primarily through the use of animal studies in controlled laboratory experiments, although studies sometimes are made on human subjects if the effect of the substance is thought to be reversible. An experiment to find acute effects (known as the LD_{50}) determines the dose that causes the immediate death of 50 percent of the animals. Experiments on chronic effects might look for changes in blood chemistry, enzyme activity, tissue damage, and cancer induction over a period of a few months or even years. Some experiments require several generations of animals. Though animal rights activists may object, the government requires these animal tests by law to assess the potential hazards of compounds before they are released for use by the general population.

Epidemiological studies are also used. They show a statistical correlation between the occurrence of disease in a population and the factors suspected of causing that disease. These studies often begin with a clinical observation, such as an unusually high frequency of cancer among those who smoke. They are valuable because they are based on the actual occurrences of real diseases in humans.

Whether or not a particular substance creates a toxic effect *in you* depends on:

- the quantity of the substance you are exposed to;
- the strength of the substance (a small amount of one substance might be much more harmful than a large amount of another);
- the method of exposure (ingestion, inhalation, or skin absorption)—some substances are safe to inhale, but not to eat or rub on your skin; others are dangerous regardless of how you are exposed;

- how frequently you are exposed—many substances have a cumulative effect in the body and do not cause harm until a certain concentration is reached over repeated exposure; and

- your own individual tolerance for a substance.

WHY **YOU** SHOULD BE CONCERNED ABOUT HOUSEHOLD TOXICS

I hear many people say, "I'm not sick. Why should I worry?" If you are a young adult in good health who is emotionally well balanced and not under stress, if you do not drink, smoke, or take drugs, if you get adequate nutrition, exercise regularly, and get enough rest, you probably are in good shape to withstand the barrage of toxic substances that assault you daily. But most household toxics are universally injurious and harmful even to otherwise healthy people. Remember, the long-term health effects of many chemicals are unknown. We do not know the possible synergistic reactions that occur when chemicals are combined in food, water, or air, or when the chemicals are in your body interacting with other chemicals.

When you have an illness of any type, even a minor cold, your tolerance for household pollutants decreases. In fact, if you or a family member gets sick often, it may be an indicator that your home is highly toxic. Many subtle poisonings show up as flu symptoms and often go undetected by doctors. Even the amount of stress you are under affects your body's ability to process toxic chemicals, and in today's high-stress society, we all qualify, even the young and healthy.

While there are certainly some people who are more sensitive to household pollutants than others, it is important to remember that these substances are poisoning all of us, whether or not we feel the effects immediately. Some toxics poison instantly; others show their devastating effects only after years of everyday exposure. How many times have we said we would have done something to prevent a tragedy "if only I had known . . ."?

We tend to think of toxic substances as something "out there," separate from us. Yet in reality, once we breathe or ingest or absorb toxic chemicals through our skin, they tend to stay inside our bodies, particularly in our adipose fat tissue. The following table, compiled by the National Adipose Tissue Survey of the National Public Health Service (a department of the Environmental Protection Agency), shows how frequently chemicals are retained by our bodies and how common the exposures are. This is only a partial list; the actual list includes 100 chemicals and is still growing.

COMPOUND	POSSIBLE SOURCES OF EXPOSURE	FREQUENCY OF OBSERVATION IN TEST SUBJECTS
Styrene	disposable plastic foam cups, carpet backing	100% of people tested had this chemical in their fat
1,4-Dichlorobenzene	mothballs, house deodorizers	100%
Xylene	gasoline, paints	100%
Ethylphenol	drinking water	100%
OCDD (dioxin)	wood treatment, herbicides, auto exhaust	100%
HxCDD (dioxin)	wood treatment, herbicides, auto exhaust	98%
Benzene	gasoline	96%
Chlorobenzene	drinking water	96%
Ethylbenzene	gasoline	96%
DDE	pesticide in produce	93%
Toluene	gasoline	91%
PCBs	air, water, food pollution	83%
Chloroform	drinking water	76%
Butylbenzylphthalate	plastics	69%
Heptachlor	termite control	67%
DDT	food and air pollution (pesticide banned for use in the US in 1972)	55%

NEW STUDIES SHOW HOUSEHOLD TOXICS
REALLY ARE TOXIC

In the last seventeen years of studying this subject, I've watched the evidence against household toxics steadily mount. I was one of the first to sound the alarm, an action prompted by my own personal experience with and recovery from chemical sensitivities. At the time, my claims were viewed with some trepidation by the medical community, but now, almost twenty years later, science is catching up with anecdotal evidence.

In 1987, the EPA embarked on an ambitious program to identify and compare the severities of environmental problems, with the idea that, in a world of limited resources, the agency should be focusing on those pollutants that pose greater dangers to society. The task force of agency managers and outside experts were surprised to find, right up at the top of the list, indoor air pollution from radon, space heaters, gas ranges, pesticides, cleaning solvents, and drinking-water contamination—all exposures we have right at home.

Multiple chemical sensitivities (MCS) is now fairly widely known and accepted by at least part of the medical community. A person becomes sensitive through immune system damage caused by either a one-time dangerously high-level exposure (such as an industrial chemical spill or pesticide spraying) or continuous low-level exposure, such as is found in modern homes and office buildings. Once the damage is done, all sorts of low-level exposures, such as to perfume or cleaning products, can cause symptoms. All sorts of symptoms are possible, including dizziness, fainting, itchy or burning eyes, runny or congested nose, dry throat, shortness of breath, asthma, upset stomach, diarrhea, menstrual problems, extreme fatigue, insomnia, memory lapses, poor concentration, depression, and behavioral changes. Though the medical community is still divided, in 1988 the Social Security Administration added MCS to their list of determinations for disability, and in 1990 the Department of Housing and Urban Development also recognized MCS as a disability under the 1973 Fair Housing Act. The National Academy of Sciences estimates that about 15 percent of the population in this country suffer from some degree of "increased sensitivity to chemicals."

It is also becoming more accepted that cancer is caused by exposure to toxic chemicals. At the time of this writing, eight million Americans have cancer. The odds of developing cancer are currently one in three and climbing. My mother died of cancer. Both my grandmothers died of cancer. This afternoon I took time off from writing this book to go to the funeral of a friend who died of cancer. Dr. Samuel Epstein, professor of occupational and environmental medicine at the University of Illinois School of Public Health, says that cancer rates are escalating to epidemic proportions. Despite the fact that many Americans have stopped smoking and lowered their dietary fat intake, since 1950 overall cancer incidence has increased by 44 percent. Clearly, the carcinogens still are out there, and we need to protect ourselves from them.

Since my books were first published, the neurotoxic effects of common household chemicals have become more widely known. Neurotoxins are so called because they are toxic to your nervous system. The core of your nervous system is your brain, which not only affects thinking and feeling but regulates every system in your body. When your nervous system is damaged, your entire body can be affected. The more common symptoms caused by neurotoxins are fatigue, memory loss, personality changes, headaches, sleep disturbances, muscle incoordination, visual disturbances, aches and pains, and sexual dysfunction. And what are these neurotoxic substances? Many of the same petrochemicals that cause MCS and cancer.

The latest research on household chemicals shows that they can act as endocrine disruptors. Most of the functions of the body are triggered by the interaction between hormones, neurotransmitters, or other molecules naturally present in the body and their receptors. Receptors are like locks; hormones and other molecules are like keys. The "keys" circulate through the body until they find the right "locks." When a hormone key is inserted into its correct receptor lock, this hormone/receptor complex binds to specific parts of DNA in the cell. Keys target genes, then send messages that direct the cell's function. The problem is that *certain toxic substances fit the receptors,* interfering with the body's ability to make its own natural connections, which can lead to disruption of normal cell functions. A whole new branch of toxicology is emerging—called "functional toxicology"—to study this effect. Although research in this field still is very new, scientists suspect that it takes a very small amount of these chemicals—even a single exposure—to disrupt normal functioning. The immune, nervous, endocrine, and reproductive systems can be affected, leading to a variety of illnesses that may not seem to be chemically related at all. The culprits? You guessed it—pesticides, plastics, preservatives (including BHA, widely used because it doesn't have many known acute toxic effects), dioxin, lead, and others.

My intent here is not to alarm or overwhelm you, but to point you in a direction toward constructive change. We are grappling with a new problem here, for which there is no precedent. We have reached the point at which we *must* be informed consumers—we can no longer rely on our instincts, upbringings, personal tastes, or what is easily available in stores to guide us as we shop. We must learn the risks and how to minimize them. If we ignore the toxic problems in our world, they won't go away—they will only get worse.

After years of studying all the complexities of the toxicity of consumer products, the best advice I can give is that rather than trying to figure out if something that is inherently toxic is safe for you, just use as many safe alternatives as you can. The more we stay away from toxics, the better off we will be, for our health and the environment.

On the other hand, don't get overly frantic about trying to avoid every possible exposure. As you read through this book, be aware of the different degrees of toxicity of products and their ingredients, then use your own common sense to evaluate what you want or need to avoid.

READING PRODUCT LABELS

It would be nice if every safe product had a little sticker on it that said "safe," but they don't. And I'm not even sure they could. I think if you were to ask a manufacturer, an industry spokesperson, a government regulator, an average consumer, and me if a specific product were safe, you would get five different answers. And because of your own individual degree of tolerance, personal taste, and budget, only you can decide how to choose safe products that are right for you.

My first book on this subject was called *Nontoxic & Natural* because those were the qualities I was looking for in safe alternatives to more toxic products. Still today, I look for products that are either made from petrochemicals that have no known acute or chronic effects, or natural materials—plants, animals and minerals—that are present on the surface of the earth. We can look for these two buzzwords—"nontoxic" and "natural"—to find safe products, but it's important to know what they mean.

Defining Nontoxic

When we read the word *nontoxic* on a product label, our first impression is that the product is "not toxic." The word *nontoxic* is generally used only on those types of products that typically have significant known toxicity—such as cleaning products and pest controls—to indicate that the product is a safer alternative to a more toxic formulation. To identify products that do not contain toxic ingredients, the word *nontoxic* is frequently used on the labels.

It is often easier to determine that a product is toxic than to find products that actually are nontoxic. Choosing nontoxic products can be a matter of looking for labels that indicate toxicity rather than looking for the word *nontoxic*.

Scientifically, there is no experiment that can prove something is nontoxic (or safe, for that matter). In an article in the October/November 1992 issue of *Garbage* magazine, toxicologist Dr. Alice Ottoboni, formerly of the California State Department of Public Health, explained why: "It is not possible to prove a negative . . . Many of the questions asked about the effects of environmental chemicals . . . are unanswerable by science because science cannot conduct the experiments necessary . . . Toxicologists can answer all questions about what quantities of exposure would be harmful, but they cannot answer many questions about what quantities of exposure would be absolutely harmless."

With regard to "tolerances" set for substances such as food additives and pesticide residues, "acceptable daily intakes" for all sorts of environmental chemicals, and "threshold limit values" set for workplace exposures, Dr. Ottoboni says, "There is no absolute proof that these standards are totally protective for all people . . . Toxicologists are fully aware of the deficiency of such standards, but consider that they are protective for the great majority of people because they are set using large margins of safety."

Ironically, toxic products are not required by law to completely list their ingredients. One way to find out what's in a product that does not list ingredients is to contact the manufacturer and ask for their Material Safety Data Sheet (MSDS) for the product. An MSDS lists the ingredients, the manufacturer, hazards to safety and health, and precautions to follow when using it. The Household Hazardous Waste Project has an MSDS Fact Sheet if you need help deciphering the form.

Sometimes the information on an MSDS can be very revealing. I once requested the MSDS on a well-known cleaning product that advertises itself as nontoxic, socially responsible, and otherwise committed to the environment, and found glycol ether as the main ingredient. After I couldn't find this in my chemical dictionary, I called and was told that glycol ether was a class of substances and the specific glycol ether used was butyl cellosolve. This I did find in my dictionary as ethylene glycol monobutyl ether, a chemical so toxic that a major chemical company decided no longer to manufacture it. Butyl cellosolve is neurotoxic and rapidly penetrates the skin. Once they diluted it down to 2 percent (98 percent of the product's plastic bottle is filled with water) the toxicity studies came out relatively harmless, but I had to ask myself if a product made from a diluted toxic chemical ethically should be called nontoxic. Not surprisingly, in 1994, a front-page story in my local newspaper reported that this company was being sued for misrepresentation of environmental claims.

One limitation to MSDS sheets is that manufacturers are required to report hazardous ingredients present only in concentrations greater than 1 percent, or .1 of 1 percent for carcinogens. Thus they are not a complete listing of ingredients or even a complete listing of hazardous ingredients.

In addition to labels and MSDSs, federal and local "right-to-know" programs also can teach us about toxic wastes that companies put into the environment. Title III of the Superfund

MATERIAL SAFETY DATA SHEET
(Prepared according to OSHA 29CFR 1010, 1200)

PRODUCT NAME

SECTION 1. MANUFACTURER/DISTRIBUTOR INFORMATION

PREPARED BY:_____ ON DATE:_____ FOR: (COMPANY NAME) _____
ADDRESS:_____ EMERGENCY PHONE:_____
_____
_____

SECTION 2. INGREDIENT INFORMATION

_____
_____

SECTION 3. PHYSICAL AND CHEMICAL CHARACTERISTICS

BOILING POINT:_____ SPECIFIC GRAVITY:_____ VAPOR PRESSURE:_____
SOLUBILITY IN WATER:_____ APPEARANCE:_____ ODOR:_____

SECTION 4. FIRE AND EXPLOSION HAZARD DATA

FLASH POINT:_____ FLAMMABLE LIMITS:_____
EXTINGUISHING MEDIA:_____
SPECIAL FIRE FIGHTING PROCEDURES:_____
_____
UNUSUAL FIRE AND EXPLOSION HAZARDS:_____
_____
D.O.T. CLASSIFICATION:_____

SECTION 5. REACTIVITY DATA

STABILITY:_____ INCOMPATIBILITY (MATERIALS TO AVOID):_____
_____
HAZARDOUS PRODUCTS OF DECOMPOSITION:_____
HAZARDOUS POLYMERIZATION:_____

SECTION 6. HAZARD DATA

PRIMARY ROUTES OF ENTRY: (INHALATION, SKIN ABSORPTION, ETC.)_____
_____
HEALTH HAZARDS:_____ ORAL TOXICITY:_____ INHALATION:_____
EYE IRRITATION:_____ PRIMARY SKIN IRRITATION:_____
CARCINOGENICITY:_____ SIGNS AND SYMPTOMS OF EXPOSURE:_____
_____
EMERGENCY AND FIRST AID PROCEDURES: EYES_____ SKIN_____
INGESTION_____

SECTION 7. SPECIAL PROTECTION INFORMATION

RESPIRATORY PROTECTION:_____ PROTECTIVE GLOVES:_____
EYE PROTECTION:_____ PROTECTIVE CLOTHING:_____
VENTILATION:_____

SECTION 8. SPECIAL PRECAUTIONS AND SPILL/LEAK PROCEDURES

STEPS TO BE TAKEN IF SPILLED OR RELEASED:_____
WASTE DISPOSAL:_____
PRECAUTIONS TO BE TAKEN IN HANDLING AND STORAGE:_____
_____

Amendment and Reauthorization Act (SARA) requires 4 million businesses to provide hazardous-chemical inventory data to a hierarchy of local, regional, and state public committees. These data include information on hazardous chemical usage and storage, emergency response plans, and routine, permissible discharges of toxics into air and water. Basic information on toxic discharges is compiled by the EPA and can be found in your local county library through the Toxics Release Inventory database. If companies are discharging toxics into the environment, we should question which toxics might be present in their finished products, too.

I have been unable to find any legal or regulatory definition of nontoxic, though manufacturers tend to use nontoxic if a product does not meet the legal definition of toxic. According to Part 1500 of the 1960 Federal Hazardous Substances Act:

> "Toxic" shall apply to any substance (other than a radioactive substance) which has the capacity to produce personal injury or illness to man through ingestion, inhalation, or absorption through any body surface.
>
> "Highly toxic" means any substance which falls within any of the following categories:
>
> A. Produces death within 14 days in half or more than half of a group of 10 or more laboratory white rats each weighing between 200 and 300 grams, at a single dose of 50 milligrams or less per kilogram of body weight, when orally administered; or
>
> B. Produces death within 14 days in half or more than half of a group of 10 or more laboratory white rats each weighing between 200 and 300 grams, when inhaled continuously for a period of 1 hour or less at an atmospheric concentration of 200 parts per million by volume or less of gas or vapor or 2 milligrams per liter by volume or less of mist or dust, provided such concentration is likely to be encountered by man when the substance is used in any reasonably foreseeable manner; or
>
> C. Produces death within 14 days in half or more than half of a group of 10 or more rabbits tested in a dosage

of 200 milligrams or less per kilogram of body weight, when administered by continuous contact with the bare skin for 24 hours or less.

Later in the document, the Hazardous Substances Act notes that "highly toxic" also could refer to "a substance determined by the [Consumer Product Safety Commission] to be highly toxic on the basis of human experience."

With these definitions, one could assume that a nontoxic substance does not have the capacity to produce personal injury or illness to humans through ingestion, inhalation, or skin absorption. The scientific measure for toxicity depends on animal studies. If half or more than half of the animals die, then the test substance is highly toxic; if less than half die, it's not. So *up to half of the test animals can die and the product can be called "nontoxic."* This certainly isn't the same as the mere negation or absence of the capacity to produce personal injury or illness, nor does it mean that a nontoxic product is completely safe.

Based on these animal tests, the EPA has defined four categories of immediate acute toxicity that correspond to different dose levels received through ingestion, inhalation, and skin contact (see chart on p. 26). At one time, these signal words accurately indicated the dose required to cause a toxic effect, but because of poor labeling practices, these words now suggest only a general degree of danger. While I was writing this book, I found it interesting to compare the label warnings with the *actual* dangers of the products, especially after my local poison-control center had told me that about 85 percent of household items on the market are mislabeled! Some products are labeled as poison that really aren't; some are poisons not labeled as such; some labels warn of dangers but don't list the poison; and many contain incorrect first-aid information. Also, label warnings are required only on products that are harmful or fatal if accidentally swallowed or inhaled in extreme concentrations. No warnings are given on products that affect health when used long-term. In many cases these effects are suspected, but currently unknown.

To indicate long-term chronic hazards, the EPA has a classification scheme for cancer-causing agents (see chart on p. 25), based on animal tests and epidemiological studies. Based on an assessment of the weight of evidence, these classifications are similar to those developed by the World Health Organization and the International Agency for Research on Cancer. Classification of a substance may change as new evidence, improved testing methods, or better analytical techniques become available, which also may affect regulations.

EPA CLASSIFICATION SYSTEM FOR CARCINOGENS

Group A Human Carcinogen	There is sufficient evidence from epidemiological studies to support a cause-effect relationship between the substance and cancer.
Group B Probable Human Carcinogen	B_1. There is sufficient evidence from animal studies and limited evidence from epidemiological studies.
	B_2. There is sufficient evidence from animal studies, but epidemiological data are inadequate or nonexistent.
	B_3. There is limited evidence from animal studies and no epidemiological data.
Group C Possible Human Carcinogen	Data are inadequate or completely lacking, so no assessment can be made (does not mean it is not carcinogenic).
Group D Not Classifiable as to Human Carcinogenicity	Substance has tested negative in at least two EPA-defined animal cancer tests in different species and in adequate epidemiological and animal studies.
Group E Evidence of Noncarcinogenicity for Humans	Classification is based on available evidence, and substances may prove to be carcinogenic under certain unknown conditions.

Defining Natural

The word *natural,* as it relates to consumer products, is meaningless, since every consumer product is made from the natural resources of the earth. Because there is no legal definition, natural has been both overused and misused on many product labels.

Natural is commonly used to mean that a product is made primarily of renewable resources, as opposed to man-made ingredients derived from nonrenewable resources. The basic sub-

SIGNAL WORDS FOR TOXIC PRODUCTS

			PRECAUTIONARY STATEMENT	
CATEGORY	SIGNAL WORD(S)	APPROXIMATE AMOUNT NEEDED TO KILL AN AVERAGE PERSON	ORAL, INHALATION, OR DERMAL TOXICITY	SKIN AND EYE LOCAL EFFECTS
I. Highly toxic	DANGER POISON	A few drops to 1 teaspoon	Fatal if swallowed (inhaled or absorbed through skin). Do not breathe vapor (dust or spray mist). Do not get in eyes, on skin, or on clothing. (Front panel statement of treatment required.)	Corrosive, causes eye and skin damage (or skin irritation). Do not get in eyes, on skin, or on clothing. Wear goggles or face shield and rubber gloves when handling. Harmful or fatal if swallowed. (Appropriate first-aid statement required.)
II. Moderately toxic	WARNING	1 teaspoon to 1 ounce	May be fatal if swallowed (inhaled or absorbed through skin). Do not breathe vapor (dust or spray mist). Do not get in eyes, on skin, or on clothing. (Appropriate first-aid statement required.)	Causes eye and skin irritation. Do not get in eyes, on skin, or on clothing. Harmful if swallowed. (Appropriate first-aid statement required.)
III. Slightly toxic	CAUTION	More than 1 ounce	Harmful if swallowed (inhaled or absorbed through skin). Avoid breathing vapors (dust or spray mist). Avoid contact with skin, eyes, or clothing. (Appropriate first-aid statement required.)	Avoid contact with skin, eyes, or clothing. In case of contact, immediately flush eyes or skin with plenty of water. Get medical attention if irritation persists.
IV. Not toxic or nontoxic	(none required)		(none required)	(none required)

stance or material used to make the product is found in nature (instead of being manufactured from petroleum) and is therefore thought to be more compatible with the human body and the entire ecological system. Materials generally thought of as being natural are those plants, animals, and minerals that appear wholly formed in nature (such as cotton, wool, or salt), or ingredients derived from plants, animals, and minerals (such as lavender oil, gelatin, and baking soda).

The main drawback to the term *natural* is that it gives the illusion that the product is "of nature," and therefore absolutely acceptable and harmless to our health. In fact, most "natural" products are natural only in the respect that *some* part of the product exists in nature, that it is not *completely* made from petrochemicals.

Natural products are rarely completely natural—in our modern world of processing, petrochemicals are almost always used with the natural materials when making a "natural ingredient." More accurately, most "natural" substances and materials might be called (I'm coining a new term here) "hybrid-natural"—basically of nature, but grown or processed by industry with added petrochemicals. Virtually all products being currently marketed as natural are really hybrid-natural.

One excellent example of a hybrid-natural ingredient was described by Philip Dickey of the Washington Toxics Coalition in an article for *Green Alternatives* magazine (May/June 1992). He specifically wrote of a coconut oil surfactant used in natural cleaning products, but the same principle applies to all so-called natural ingredients.

> This detergent is called linear alcohol ethoxylate . . . The alcohol from which this surfactant is made is similar to the ethyl alcohol we know from beer and wine except it has more carbon atoms . . . They are arranged in a straight line, hence the term *linear alcohol*. This alcohol (called lauryl alcohol) can be manufactured from either coconut oil or petroleum. Let's pretend that our alcohol came originally from coconuts. . . .
>
> Lauryl alcohol is not a surfactant. To make it function as a surfactant, we have to build on a hydrophilic, or water-soluble, structure . . . In an ethoxylated alcohol it is done

through a chemical reaction with a highly toxic (and carcinogenic) compound called ethylene oxide, distilled from
crude oil. During this process, called ethoxylation, carbon
atoms from ethylene oxide are progressively added to one
end of the coconut-based structure until a hydrophilic
chain of the desired length is reached. At this point *the surfactant can be thought of as part vegetable, part petroleum . . .
a hybrid* [italics mine]. The ratio varies, but is often near
50:50.

In the chapters that follow, I'll be giving you specific advice
on the kinds of products and labeling information to look for so
that you can choose the safest products from among those available to you.

HOUSEHOLD HAZARDOUS WASTE: THE FIRST STEP

If you are like I was, once you're convinced of the dangers of certain products, you're going to want to throw everything away and
start using safe alternatives immediately. But when you do, you
face the dilemma of proper disposal.

Why is disposal of household toxics a problem? Because
when we dispose of our household products, we generate hazardous waste. When we throw a half-used can of pesticide into
the garbage, it will ultimately end up in a municipal landfill,
which is designed for refuse, not toxic waste. According to an article in *National Geographic,* we throw away 4 million tons of hazardous waste each year. Disposal is becoming such a problem that
many communities are setting up special disposal programs to
keep their city dumps from becoming toxic-waste dumps.

Unfortunately, the answer isn't to flush hazardous waste
down the drain, either. If your house is hooked to a sanitary or
municipal treatment facility, the contaminated wastewater will go
to a local sewage-treatment plant before it is discharged into your
local rivers, lakes, and streams. These sewage-treatment plants
aren't designed to remove hazardous waste any more than landfills are, so the toxic substances go right on through. And if you
have a septic tank, hazardous waste can slow down or destroy the
microorganisms that make the system work properly.

If you think you don't have any household hazardous waste in your home, think again. Here's a list of hazardous household products from the San Francisco Household Hazardous Waste Program. **Do not dispose of these products in your household garbage:**

Housecleaning Supplies

Ammonia cleaners
Chlorine bleach
Cleansers
Disinfectants
Drain openers
Furniture and floor polish
Lye
Metal polish
Oven cleaner
Rug cleaners
Tub, tile, and shower-stall cleaners

Laundry Supplies

Dry-cleaning solvent
Mothballs and flakes
Spot remover

Cosmetics

Cuticle remover
Depilatory cream
Hair-permanent solutions
Hair-straightener solutions
Nail polish
Nail-polish remover

Medicines

Chemotherapy drugs
Liquid medicine
Mercury from a broken thermometer
Prescription medicine
Rubbing alcohol
Shampoo for lice

Other Household Products

Aerosol cans containing *any* pressure
  or fluid
Butane lighters
Flea powder
Lighter fluid
Pet shampoo
Shoe dye and polish

Automotive Supplies

Aluminum cleaner
Auto-body filler
Automatic-transmission fluid
Brake fluid
Carburetor cleaner
Car wax
Chrome polish
Diesel fuel
Engine degreaser
Gasoline
Kerosene or lamp oil
Lubricating oil
Motor oil, used (see if you can find
  a place that will accept this for
  recycling)

Building and Woodworking Supplies

Asbestos
Fluorescent lamp with ballasts
   and tubes
Glues and cements
Wood preservatives

Garden Supplies

Fungicides
Herbicides
Insecticides
Rat, mouse, and gopher poison
Snail and slug poison
Soil fumigants
Weed killers

Hobby and Pet Supplies

Acrylic paint
Artist's mediums, thinners, and
   fixatives
Chemistry sets
Oil paint
Photographic chemicals/solutions
Resins, fiberglass, and epoxy
Rubber-cement thinner

Painting Supplies

Latex-based paint
Model-airplane paint
Oil-based paint
Paint stripper
Paint thinner, turpentine, and
   mineral spirits

SAFE SOLUTIONS

The very best thing we can do to reduce household hazardous waste is simply to stop using these dangerous products and re-place them with safer alternatives. That is what this book is all about. Throughout the chapters that follow, you'll find out just how easy it is. You'll never have to buy products that produce household hazardous waste again.

However, you are still faced with the problem of what to do with the household hazardous waste you already have. Here are some suggestions.

USE IT UP

When products are fully used up as intended, there is no haz-ardous waste to dispose of. If you only need a small amount of paint, pesticide, or other hazardous product, check with friends, relatives, or neighbors to see if they have any they want to use up. Or, if you have leftovers, offer it around instead of throwing it away.

TAKE IT TO A HOUSEHOLD HAZARDOUS
WASTE COLLECTION PICKUP DAY

Call your local public health department, environmental health department, department of health services, or sanitation department to see if you have a hazardous-waste disposal program in your community. They will generally accept such items as pesticides, household cleaners, paints and paint products, automotive products, solvents, pharmaceuticals, aerosol products, pool chemicals, hobby supplies, acids, and waste oil. If you don't have a local program, ask your local authorities how best to dispose of your toxics. It may even be illegal to dispose of certain products with your normal household garbage.

While you're waiting for the pickup day, follow these safety guidelines for storing household hazardous waste.

- Keep products out of reach of children and animals.
- Protect the label. Store in the original container and make sure the product is clearly labeled with the product name and date. Place the word "danger" on the container.
- Never store hazardous products in food or beverage containers.
- Store products away from sparks, flame, or intense heat. Electrical appliances, light switches, light bulbs, electric garage door openers, etc., all can generate a spark, which can become a source of ignition.
- Make sure lids are sealed tightly and are childproof.
- Make sure containers are kept dry to prevent them from corroding.

Chapter 2

INDOOR AIR POLLUTION

T HOUGH INDOOR AIR POLLUTANTS are not easy to deal with, I have to begin our rundown of household toxics with them, because they pose the greatest hazards to health. If your home contains one of these pollutants, changing anything else won't make much difference, because these override everything both in their degree of harm and their quantity of exposure.

Indoor air pollution has become a problem in the past two decades because of the combination of sealing up our homes for energy efficiency without appropriate air-exchange equipment and filling them with more and more toxic products. Particleboard furniture and cabinets, cleaning products, pesticides, plastics and synthetic fibers used in furnishing and construction, carpeting, drapes, scented items, gas appliances and heaters, and many other common items made from petrochemicals all contribute to an increase in indoor air pollution. The level of toxic pollutants inside many houses is often higher than that of the air outside—sometimes even higher than the maximum allowable outdoor standards.

At present, many government agencies and private firms are studying indoor air pollution, its effects, and what to do about it.

In one study in New Jersey, researchers outfitted 350 people with special test monitors that would continuously sample the surrounding air and measure their exposure to 20 separate organic chemicals. At the same time, they also monitored 100 backyards for outdoor levels of pollutant. When they looked at the test data, they found that people living farther away from polluting industries did not show any less personal exposure than people who lived closer. The most important factor was *indoor* air pollution. In some homes, pollutant levels were *100 times higher* than outdoors.

This study also pointed out another important fact: What we breathe travels throughout our bodies. Samples showed residues of gasoline on the breath of some people hours after they had filled their gas tanks, while a short visit to the dry cleaner resulted in tetrachloroethylene on the breath. Even taking a hot shower elevated breath levels of chloroform, which is released in the stream of chlorinated water.

Often indoor air problems go undetected by those exposed because of a phenomenon known as "olfactory fatigue." You might remember a time when you noticed a strong odor when you first walked into a room, but then a few minutes later, you completely forgot about it and, in fact, couldn't smell it at all. This is olfactory fatigue. A few sniffs of the same smell, and the ability of your nose to perceive odor is dulled. Gas leaks, for example, frequently go undetected until someone else visits the house and smells gas upon entering.

Your nose is the first tool you can use to identify indoor pollutants.

To get a fresh sniff of your house, spend the day outdoors in the cleanest air you can to "cleanse" the olfactory sense in your nose. Then come home and sniff the minute you open the door. Keeping windows closed while you're away will help intensify the smells. If there are odors present, you should be able to smell them in the first few sniffs, and then less and less as you continue to breathe. If you need another round of sniffs, go back outside and breathe some "clean" air, then go inside again and notice what you smell in the first few sniffs.

If you don't notice any odors, have a friend or two come over and sniff. After breathing the same odors day in and day out, it may take some time to restore your sense of smell.

Once you determine there is a problem, the air quality in your home can be professionally tested, if necessary, and you can take steps to remove sources of pollution.

SAFE SOLUTIONS

The most effective way to reduce indoor air pollution is to eliminate pollutants at their source. This book describes many products that emit toxic fumes that can be inhaled. All of them are contributing to the toxic cloud of indoor air pollution in your home. The more of them you replace with nontoxic products, the cleaner—and safer—the air inside your home will be. In particular, try to remove:

- plastics (see chapter 2)
- scented beauty and hygiene products (see chapter 7)
- cleaning products made from synthetic chemicals (see chapter 3)
- pesticides (see chapter 4)
- synthetic fibers and fabrics (see chapter 9)
- office supplies with volatile ingredients (see chapter 10)
- household furnishings made from synthetic materials (see chapter 11)
- gas appliances and heaters (see chapter 2)
- building materials made from formaldehyde (see chapter 14)

A second option is to increase ventilation. Keep your windows open as much as the weather allows and, even better, invest in a window fan. If you need more ventilation but don't want to lose heat, consider an air-to-air heat exchanger (for more information, contact a local HVAC contractor—look in the Yellow Pages of your telephone book under Heating, Ventilation, and Air Conditioning).

Houseplants can also help clean the air. Tests done by NASA

have shown that common houseplants remove pollutants as they go through their natural process of photosynthesis—while plants draw in carbon monoxide, they also pick up airborne pollutants through small openings called stomates in the leaves. They are very effective at removing gases such as formaldehyde, carbon monoxide, carbon dioxide, benzene, cigarette smoke, and ozone, which are harmful for us to breathe, but a gourmet meal for a plant (such is the mutualism of nature). Aloe vera (which is a good plant to have around to treat burns and skin irritations), bamboo palm, common chrysanthemums, dracaena palms, philo-dendrons, golden pothos, spider plants, and scheffleras are among the better air filters.

HOUSE PLANTS THAT REMOVE TOXINS

Wolverton Environmental Services studied indoor plants for NASA and found the following percentages of toxins removed by one plant in a 12-cubic-foot area, during a 24-hour period*:

COMMON NAME	TOXINS REMOVED
Aloe vera	Formaldehyde: 90%
Elephant ear philodendron	Formaldehyde: 86%
English ivy	Benzene: 90%
Ficus (weeping fig)	Formaldehyde: 47%
Golden pothos	Carbon monoxide: 75%; benzen: 67%; formaldehyde: 67%
Janet Craig (corn plant)	Benzene: 79%
Peace lily	Benzene: 80%; trichloroethylene: 50%
Spider plant	Carbon monoxide: 96%

*A 9 x 12–foot room with an 8-foot ceiling is 864 cubic feet, so you would need 72 plants to duplicate these results— a virtual jungle! However, a few plants can do a lot to freshen the air, depending on the level of pollutants present.
Source: Wolverton Environmental Services.

If you can't solve your indoor air pollution problem by removing pollutants at their source or diluting them with added ventilation, then air filters are necessary.

AIR FILTERS

I don't usually recommend air filters because the air produced by them is no match for nature's finest clean air. But there are times when we need to protect our health, and using an air filter makes good sense. Air filters are best used:

- When you are driving or riding in an automobile (this is probably the best use of an air filter)
- When all major sources of indoor air pollution have been removed and significant levels of pollutants still are present because of outdoor air pollution or materials used inside the building (if this is the case, you might consider moving)
- When you absolutely have to use a toxic chemical and you want to give yourself some measure of protection
- When you are very sensitive to all sorts of air pollutants (from chemicals to pollen) and cannot move someplace where there is outdoor air free from these contaminants

Air filters can be purchased as portable models, or you can have them built into your central heating/air-conditioning system. An important point to remember is that the cleaning capabilities of any portable unit are generally limited to the air in the room in which it is being used. And as with air-conditioners, air cleaners are most effective if no outside air is entering from adjacent rooms, open windows, or a central air system.

There is no one "best" air filter that is most appropriate for every person and every use. When evaluating air filters, you will want to consider the following.

- Which pollutants you want to remove from the air, and the effectiveness of pollutant removal
- The area you want to remove the pollutants from
- The cost of the filter

- The aesthetics of how the filter looks, and how much noise it makes
- What you need to do to maintain the filter

Air pollutants fall into two classes: gases or misty vapors of volatile chemicals such as formaldehyde, plastics, paints, solvents, pesticides, and perfumes; and particulates such as bits of pollen, dust, mold, and animal dander. If you need to remove particles from the air, you'll probably know it because you'll be sneezing or you'll have other allergic symptoms. You'll need to remove gases if you have any of the products mentioned in this book that emit volatile toxic chemicals.

If you want to have the air in your home tested, look in the Yellow Pages under "Laboratories—Analytical." Ask these places what testing they do and get estimates from several of them, because prices and services vary considerably.

To remove pollutants, air-cleaning devices use one or more of four types of cleaning methods: activated carbon, mechanical filtration (HEPA), electrostatic filtration (precipitators, electret), and negative-ion generation. Each method works in a different way, and each removes different pollutants.

ACTIVATED CARBON

Activated carbon used in filters works by *adsorption,* a process by which pollutant gases are attracted by and stick to the carbon. There are several types of activated carbon; generally, coconut-shell carbon is considered to be the highest quality.

In addition to plain activated carbon, filters can contain other filter media that have special qualities. Some coconut-shell carbon is impregnated to increase efficiency in removing formaldehyde. CI-impregnated carbon, also known as Formaldezorb, uses a copper-nickel salt; Formaldepure uses nonmetal salts. These special carbons can increase formaldehyde adsorption 90 percent and beyond.

Most filter manufacturers recommend that carbon beds be at least one inch thick; anything less than that is practically useless. The small air cleaners found in most department, drug, and discount stores are inexpensive and convenient, but do not contain sufficient carbon to effectively clean the amount of air that passes through.

When choosing a carbon filter, also take into consideration the placement of the motor, which can produce objectionable fumes of its own. Some filters have the motor placed on top; others are inside. Motors can be lubricated, if necessary, with jojoba oil, available in natural-food stores.

In some activated-carbon units, the carbon is combined with Purafil, a nontoxic odoroxidant made of activated alumina impregnated with potassium permanganate. Purafil works by both absorbing and adsorbing gases and then destroying them by oxidation. This combination is more effective than carbon alone, but not as effective as nonmetal-impregnated carbon.

MECHANICAL FILTRATION

Mechanical filters work by trapping particles. High-Efficiency Particulate Arrestance (HEPA) filters are rated at 99.99 percent efficient for particles .3 microns in size (dust, pollen, and plant and mold spores). Developed by the Atomic Energy Commission during World War II to remove radioactive dust from industrial exhausts, they are paperlike filters made of randomly positioned fibers that create narrow passages with many twists and turns. As the air passes through, particles are trapped, clogging holes and making the grid smaller, which enables the filter to be even more efficient with ongoing use. One disadvantage is that HEPA filters generally are bonded with polyvinyl acetate plastic, although non-petrochemical HEPA filters are also available.

ELECTROSTATIC FILTRATION

Electrostatic filters attract particles by static electricity. There are two types:

Electronic air cleaners (electrostatic precipitators) are not recommended. They are rarely more than 80 percent efficient and can quickly drop to 20 percent efficiency. They also produce ozone and positive ions and must be cleaned often with volatile petrochemical solvents.

Electronically charged plastic panel filters (electret) that can be inserted into your central heating system are extremely efficient for removing dust particles as well as the chemicals that cling to the dust. In addition, some are available with added carbon to enhance chemical removal. Because these are made from plastic, some may give off a strong odor, so be cautious about using these.

NEGATIVE-ION GENERATION

The biological advantages of negative ions are well known, but because negative-ion generators and ionizers cannot be sold to promote these health effects, they are often advertised as air cleaners.

As air cleaners, however, they are quite limited. The negative ions produced by the generator will precipitate only certain small particles. While practically useless for dust or pollen, these generators are very effective at removing the particles found in cigarette smoke and smog, cleaning the air so that it becomes clear and odorless. What they cannot remove are the invisible, odorless toxic gases that also are present in cigarette smoke and smog.

Negative-ion generators and ionizers should be purchased for their health benefits or for use with activated-carbon filters for removal of cigarette smoke, but not as broad-spectrum air cleaners. One problem with ion generators in the past has been a buildup of black particles on the walls and furniture around the generator. Newer ionizers have built-in collection systems to trap these particles.

ROOM SIZE

Each unit is designed to effectively remove pollutants from the air contained in a certain measured space. The amount of filter media the unit contains, the rate at which the air flows through the media, the size of the motor, and all other aspects of the unit's design are geared to the designated room size. You may need several filters to continuously clean the air throughout the house, or a unit portable enough to be easily moved from room to room.

PRICE

In general, prices correspond to room sizes and the amount of filter media used. The more you get, the more you pay. But bigger is not necessarily better if it's more than you need. Expect to pay around $200 to clean the air in your car or a small room, and perhaps $1,000 or more to have a unit built into your central air system.

COMPARISON OF POLLUTANTS REMOVED BY AIR FILTERS

	ACTIVATED CARBON	MECHANICAL FILTRATION (HEPA)	ELECTROSTATIC FILTRATION	NEGATIVE-ION GENERATION
Particles (larger than .01 microns), e.g., asbestos dust, pollen, mold, animal hair, tobacco-smoke particles	No	Yes	Yes	Some
Gases (smaller than .001 microns)				
Ammonia	Some	No	No	No
Carbon monoxide	No	No	No	No
Formaldehyde	Some	No	No	No
Lead	Yes	No	No	No
Nitrogen oxides	Some	No	No	No
Pesticides	Yes	No	No	No
Phenol	Yes	No	No	No
Plastic emissions	Yes	No	No	No
Sulfur dioxide	Some	No	No	No
Tobacco-smoke gases	Yes	No	No	No
Other organic chemicals	Yes	No	No	No

AESTHETICS

Style is an important factor in choosing an air filter, because all portable units have to be sitting out in the room in order to be effective. Most filters are nondescript painted metal boxes or cylinders, but manufacturers are beginning to make them more aesthetically pleasing.

Metal housings are preferable and are standard on the units listed in this book. I don't recommend plastic housings because these often release a plastic smell of their own into the air.

The level of noise the motor makes is also a consideration. It's useless to have a filter if you don't run it because it's too loud. A filter with variable speeds will allow you to adjust noise levels as well as air flow.

MAINTENANCE

Activated carbon and other filter materials must be changed regularly. How often you'll need to change them depends on how many hours a day the filter is used and how polluted the air is, so it is impossible to predict how long filter media will last. Manufacturers estimate that activated carbon will last about two thousand hours, or twelve hours per day for six months; under normal use, the carbon should last six to nine months. Prefilters are generally changed more frequently, and HEPA filters last for several years.

Buying an Air Filter

Truly effective portable air filters rarely are sold in stores. Some manufacturers of quality portable air filters that I have known and recommended for many years include **Aireox Research Corporation, E. L. Foust Company,** and **AllerMed Corporation.** Units can be purchased directly from the manufacturers, or from independent dealers such as **Allergy Resources, American Environmental Health Foundation, The Living Source, Nigra Enterprises,** and **Nontoxic Environments.**

For a built-in whole-house filter, check the Yellow Pages for a Heating, Ventilation, and Air Conditioning (HVAC) dealer.

AUTOMOBILE EXHAUST

While we don't usually think of automobile exhaust as an indoor air pollutant, it is present in many homes. If you park in an attached garage (or live in an apartment building with an attached garage) and warm up your engine before pulling out, exhaust fumes can enter the house through cracks around the edges of the door between the house and garage, through heater fresh-air-intake vents (yes, some are incorrectly installed in the garage), or through open windows. If you live on a busy street, automobile exhaust is just part of the stew of air pollutants you constantly breathe, whether indoors or out.

Gasoline and diesel engine exhausts are complex mixtures that contain hundreds of chemicals and are both mutagenic and carcinogenic. A prime component of auto exhaust is **carbon monoxide** (see Combustion By-products for health effects). A study conducted by the University of California at Davis and released in 1990 by the American Lung Association said that air pollution from motor vehicles alone could be linked to between 50,000 and 120,000 premature deaths in the United States each year and is responsible for $40 billion to $50 billion in annual health-care costs.

AUTOMOBILES

> **DANGER:** Motor fuel. Harmful or fatal if swallowed. Vapors harmful. Long-term exposure to vapors has caused cancer in laboratory animals. May cause eye and skin irritation. Avoid prolonged breathing of vapors. Keep face away from nozzle and gas tank. Keep away from the eyes and skin. Never siphon by mouth. Failure to use caution may cause serious injury or illness.
>
> **WARNING:** Chemicals known to cause cancer, birth defects, or other reproductive harm are found in gasoline, crude oil, and many other petroleum products and their vapors or result from their use. Read and follow label directions and use care when handling or using petroleum products.

Although pollution from automobiles generally is not considered *indoor* pollution, the related toxic problems certainly are worth mentioning.

In addition to the immediate dangers posted on gasoline pumps, Dr. Samuel Epstein, professor of occupational and environmental medicine at the University of Illinois Medical Center and a leading cancer researcher, has reported that leukemia and cancer can result from inhaling **benzene** fumes while refueling your car. Consumers are routinely exposed to 1 ppm (part[s] per million) benzene at full-service gas pumps, and 3 ppm at self-service pumps, which exceed the 1 ppm standard above which the Occupational Safety and Health Administration (OSHA) requires that workers be warned and protected.

Also, the interiors of most cars are made of **polyvinyl chloride** plastic and other **synthetic** materials. You know that "new car smell"? It's the odor of **vinyl chloride** fumes, which are carcinogenic.

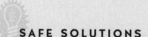

SAFE SOLUTIONS

When riding in a car, you can't remove the source of the contaminants, but you can do things to reduce the buildup of pollution levels within the car.

The most effective method is to buy an auto air filter. You'll need one that has a good amount of activated carbon and a particulate filter to remove irritating particles and toxic gases. There are some negative-ion generators sold as auto air cleaners (check the **Real Goods** catalog) that will remove particles but not gases. You can get a unit that will remove both for under $200 (see Air Filters).

Another thing to do that I've found to be very helpful is to use a sunroof for ventilation. If your car doesn't already have one, they can be installed for about $200. While this won't "clean" the air, it provides good ventilation and lets pollutants escape, while allowing fewer outdoor pollutants in than if you opened the window.

At the gas station, you might want to pay the extra few dollars to have the attendant pump your gas. Or, turn your head away from the tank as you are pumping the gas, so that at least you are not breathing the fumes directly. I try to hold my breath when I'm pumping, so that I don't inhale the fumes as much.

Remember, too, that if you drive a car that gets good gas mileage—my Geo Metro gets fifty-plus miles to the gallon—your trips to the gas pump will be less frequent and you'll be helping the environment as well.

SAFE SOLUTIONS

Check to see if automobile exhaust is entering your home, either from the garage or from the street. Remedial measures could include such simple things as weatherstripping around the door leading from the garage to the house, redirecting air-intake vents in your heating system, or installing a whole-house air-filtration system. If street pollution is really bad, you may want to consider moving.

SECONDHAND TOBACCO SMOKE

> **SURGEON GENERAL'S WARNING:** Smoking causes lung cancer, heart disease, emphysema, and may complicate pregnancy.
>
> **SURGEON GENERAL'S WARNING:** Quitting smoking now greatly reduces serious risks to your health.
>
> **SURGEON GENERAL'S WARNING:** Smoking by pregnant women may result in fetal injury, premature birth, and low birth weight.
>
> **SURGEON GENERAL'S WARNING:** Cigarette smoke contains carbon monoxide.

Tobacco smoke contains some of the most toxic air pollutants known, including **benzene, carbon monoxide, formaldehyde, ammonia, hydrogen cyanide,** and more than four thousand other chemicals, forty-three of which have been proven to cause cancer. Even if *you* don't smoke but are around people who do on a regular basis, you can have similar health risks.

It's now common knowledge that cigarette smoke poses a hazard not only to smokers, but to nonsmokers as well. Only 4 percent of the total smoke produced by a cigarette is actually inhaled by the smoker. The other 96 percent becomes sidestream waste, containing more than twice the concentration of pollutants the smoker inhaled. Passive smoking kills about 53,000 nonsmoking Americans every year. Researchers from the University of California Medical Center in San Francisco reported that nonsmoking spouses of cigarette smokers are 30 percent more likely to die of heart disease than other nonsmokers. Children of smoking parents have an increased incidence of upper respiratory infections, bronchitis, asthma, pneumonia, and a significant decrease in respiratory function.

Possible symptoms for the nonsmoker who inhales secondhand smoke include burning eyes, nasal congestion and drainage, sore throat, cough, headache, and nausea. Secondhand smoke is a significant health hazard for infants, children, pregnant women and their yet-to-be-born children, people with cardiovascular disease, asthmatics, and others with impaired respiratory function, heart disease, lung disease, or allergies.

Prolonged exposure to sidestream smoke can increase the risk of disease, including lung cancer, respiratory infection, angina, decreased blood oxygen levels, decreased exercise tolerance, decreased respiratory function, bronchoconstriction, and bronchospasm, in healthy people who do not smoke.

In 1992, an EPA panel reported designated secondhand smoke as a group A carcinogen.

SAFE SOLUTIONS

I've focused this section on secondhand smoke rather than aiming it toward smokers, because I'm assuming anyone who smokes knows the health risks by now. And tobacco smoke is considered to be an indoor air pollutant that must be addressed for everyone's good health.

If you smoke, stop. At the very least, be considerate of nonsmokers and do not smoke in their immediate presence. A simple "Do you mind if I smoke?" will let you know if you should step outside.

I do not allow anyone to smoke in my home. I have friends who smoke, and they all know and respect this rule. I have a friend who steps outside to smoke even when I am at *her* house. She goes out on the patio and talks to me through the window, or she opens the French doors and blows her smoke outside.

If you live with a smoker, do everything you can to encourage them to quit, or ask them to smoke outside. Or you could designate a "smoking room." In Victorian times, men retired to a separate room and put on their "smoking jackets" before enjoying their tobacco, so as not to disturb the delicate constitutions of the women they lived with. Now that's good manners!

COMBUSTION BY-PRODUCTS—
GAS APPLIANCES, KEROSENE HEATERS, FIREPLACES,
AND WOODSTOVES

> **WARNING:** Natural gas, like many petroleum-based substances such as gasoline, naturally contains benzene, a chemical known to cause cancer. The benzene in natural gas is destroyed when gas is burned in appliances. A warning odorant is added to natural gas so that leaks of unburned gas can be quickly detected. If gas is detected, contact your local utility company promptly.
>
> **WARNING:** Soot and formaldehyde, which may be produced when natural gas is burned, are also chemicals known to cause cancer. Properly operating appliances reduce the formation of soot.

The primary danger in using gas, kerosene, or wood to produce heat for cooking or warmth is the possibility of **carbon monoxide** poisoning. According to U.S. Consumer Product Safety Commission Product Safety Fact Sheet #13, "Each year hundreds of people die from carbon monoxide poisoning. Thousands of others suffer dizziness, nausea, and convulsions. You can't see, taste, or smell carbon monoxide. But it kills."

Carbon monoxide is produced when fuels do not burn completely. All fuel-burning appliances need air for the fuel to burn efficiently. When a generous supply of fresh air is available and the fuel is burning properly, there is little danger of poisoning. But when there is inadequate ventilation or the appliance is not operating properly, carbon monoxide is produced and can gradually overcome an unsuspecting bystander.

Carbon monoxide starves the body and brain of oxygen. Early symptoms of carbon monoxide poisoning are much like flu symptoms and include sleepiness, headache, dizziness, flushed skin, disorientation, abnormal reflexes, blurred vision, irritability, and an inability to concentrate. As poisoning progresses, the victim experiences nausea and vomiting, shortness of breath, convulsions, unconsciousness, and finally, death.

Most cases of carbon monoxide poisoning in the home involve gas appliances, such as kitchen ranges, space heaters, wall heaters, central heating systems, and clothes dryers. Other potential emitters are kerosene space heaters and wood- or coal-burning stoves and fireplaces.

These appliances also can emit other combustion by-product pollutants, including **formaldehyde, nitrogen dioxide, sulfur dioxide, carbon dioxide, hydrogen cyanide, nitric oxide,** and vapors from various **organic chemicals.** Even at the low levels produced from average use of these appliances, possible symptoms from exposure to these by-products include eye, nose, and throat irritation; headaches; dizziness; fatigue; decreased hearing; slight impairment of vision or brain functioning; personality changes; seizures; psychosis; heart palpitations; loss of appetite; nausea and vomiting; bronchitis; asthma attacks; and breathing problems. People with emphysema, asthma, angina, or chemical sensitivities should be particularly cautious. Because the effects of exposure to combustion by-products can be very subtle, it is somewhat difficult to connect symptoms with exposure.

The Consumer Product Safety Commission is concerned about long-term exposure to low levels of carbon monoxide among heart patients, the ability of nitrogen dioxide and other combustion products to cause an increase in respiratory disease in children, and the potential of formaldehyde as a human carcinogen.

SAFE SOLUTIONS

The most effective way for you to avoid combustion by-products is to use all-electric appliances—ranges, heaters, water heaters, and clothes dryers. Indoor air-pollution studies show that all-electric homes have significantly lower concentrations of combustion by-products than do homes with gas appliances. Because electric appliances are more expensive to run than gas appliances, be sure to inform your local utility company that you have an all-electric home and qualify for a special lower rate.

Most electric ranges are perfectly acceptable, with the exception of those that have self-cleaning ovens (they produce carcinogenic **polynuclear aromatics** that are on the EPA list of priority pollutants), and some new models, which have a distinct odor that can take a year or more to disappear. Buying a used, reconditioned range solves this problem, and is less expensive too. Also acceptable, but less efficient, are ceramic cooktops with electric heating elements hidden beneath a smooth ceramic slab.

If the wiring in your home is not adequate for an electric range, you can use a variety of small electric appliances, such as toaster ovens, coffee makers, convection ovens, crockpots, frying pans, woks, hot plates, or rice cookers, which can be operated on the standard 110-volt wiring. These can be purchased at most hardware and department stores. Choose appliances with a minimum of plastic parts and without no-stick finishes. If you have a health problem that makes you particularly sensitive to combustion by-product pollutants, it is well worth having the rewiring done for an electric range, or using small appliances despite their inconvenience.

The easiest way to convert from gas heat is to use electric space heaters. There are two basic types. Radiant, or quartz, heaters produce heat with exposed quartz tubes in a metal frame. They are inexpensive to buy, energy efficient, and produce fast "spot" heating, but they have two big disadvantages. First, they get very hot, so you have to keep them away from children, pets, curtains, shag rugs, or anything else that could get burned or catch fire. Second, since they are designed primarily for spot heating, sitting next to one could give you hot feet but leave your hands frozen. Convection heaters use a tube filled with water or oil, enclosed in a metal case, to warm the air slowly in an entire room. These are more expensive to buy and operate than radiant heaters and take longer to produce heat, but have the distinct safety advantage of remaining significantly cooler to touch.

In the past few years, new "ceramic" heaters have come on the market, which are small, boxy electric heaters that warm a room quickly.

Other acceptable heating methods are central forced-air electric, solar, and steam heat.

If you are sensitive to chemicals or have respiratory or heart problems, I cannot emphasize enough the importance of trying to replace your gas appliances and kerosene heaters. In my consulting practice I have seen many clients do everything I recommend except remove the gas from their homes, and their health problems remain. But almost as soon as they turn off the gas appliances, they start feeling better. It's amazing.

You can protect yourself somewhat from being poisoned by combustion by-products and still use gas appliances by taking the following precautions:

- Dilute pollutants with ventilation—open windows, flues, fans, and vents. Gases from combustion by-products concentrate initially in the area around the appliance and then spread to other areas of your home as the air circulates, so catch them at the source. During cooking, for example, a hood fan can remove up to 70 percent of pollutants produced.

- Check frequently to make sure your gas appliances are functioning properly. Clean clogged stove burners and blocked flues, fix cracks and leaks in pipes, and keep up on any maintenance suggested by the manufacturer. A poorly adjusted gas stove can give off 30 times the carbon monoxide of a well-adjusted stove.

- Make sure you are using your appliances according to instructions.

- If possible, put your gas appliances in a space outside of the living area, venting the fumes to the outside and placing a tight seal between the appliances and the living space to prevent gases from spreading throughout your home.

- Use a new-model gas stove with low-heat-input gas pilot light and nongas ignition system, which produces significantly fewer pollutants than an older stove with pilot light.

- Do not use a gas range or oven for heating a room.

In addition to the combustion by-products produced by gas, burning wood in woodstoves and fireplaces also produces other toxic by-products such as carcinogenic **benzo(a)pyrene.** It is easier to tell if these pollutants are present in your living space because they are extremely irritating to eyes, nose, throat, and lungs. Don't worry, I'm the last person who will tell you not to use your fireplace. Living in a forest by the ocean, my fireplace is burning almost constantly, all year round. However, because little research has been done on the effects of wood combustion by-products on indoor air pollution, take these precautions if you burn wood as your primary source of heat:

- Make sure woodstoves and fireplaces are installed and fitted properly and that the flue is open. Be certain that your fireplace was constructed to be used as a fireplace and is not there just for decoration. Have it inspected to make sure it has all necessary linings and clearances.

- Always keep the damper opened properly while the fuel is burning.

- Have your chimney inspected for creosote buildup when the weather starts getting cold, or periodically throughout the year if you use your fireplace often. Creosote buildup can cause flue fires and also may block the chimney, preventing escape of toxic fumes.

- Leave a window open a crack to allow pollutants to escape.

- Fix cracks or leaks in the stovepipe, and keep a regular maintenance schedule to insure that the chimney and stovepipe are clean and unblocked.

- Guard against negative air pressure indoors, and watch for downdrafts, which will push pollutants into your living space instead of carrying them up the flue.

A new product on the market is the single station carbon monoxide detector. Sold at most hardware stores (and by mail through *The Safety Zone*), they are designed to detect elevated levels of carbon monoxide and sound an alarm to alert you of a potential poisoning risk. If you have the potential to suffer from this hazard, it's probably a good idea to get an alarm.

ASBESTOS

Asbestos is a mineral fiber found in rocks, which has been shown to cause cancer of the lung. Not everyone who is exposed to asbestos develops cancer, but there is no level of asbestos exposure known to be safe.

The danger of asbestos comes from exposure to tiny fibers that are inhaled and become lodged in lung tissue. These fibers are so small that you cannot see them, and they pass right through the filters of vacuum cleaners.

Not all products containing asbestos pose a health risk. The risk exists only when the fibers are released.

SAFE SOLUTIONS

In most cases, the best thing you can do is to leave the material containing asbestos just the way it is.

Here are some common household products that may contain asbestos:

VINYL FLOOR TILES AND
VINYL SHEET FLOORING

There is some controversy as to whether or not asbestos fibers are released from asbestos-vinyl flooring materials during normal use. *Consumer Reports* magazine says no, but a team of French scientists found that heavily trafficked floors released significant amounts of fibers. Fibers can be released also if the tiles are sanded or seriously damaged, if the backing on the sheet flooring is dry-scraped or sanded, if the tiles are severely worn or cut to fit into place, if you use an upright carpet-sweeper–type vacuum cleaner on the flooring, or if you sweep the flooring with a stiff broom.

PATCHING COMPOUNDS AND
TEXTURED PAINTS

The Consumer Product Safety Commission banned the use of asbestos in patching compounds in 1977. According to the CPSC, asbestos is no longer added to textured paints. Older homes, however, may contain either of these materials, and sanding or scraping will release asbestos fibers. If walls seem in good condition, leave them alone.

CEILINGS

Some large buildings and private homes built or remodeled between 1945 and 1978 may contain a crumbly, asbestos-containing material that has been either sprayed or troweled onto the ceiling or walls. If walls and ceilings are undamaged, leave them alone.

STOVE AND FURNACE INSULATION

Asbestos-containing cement sheets and insulation may have been installed around wood-burning stoves or oil, coal, or wood furnaces. If the insulation on or around your stove or furnace is in good condition, it is best to leave it alone. If the insulation is in poor condition or pieces are breaking off, have it repaired or removed. The CPSC emphasizes that children should not play in an area containing insulation dust.

PIPE INSULATION

Hot-water and steam pipes in homes built or repaired between 1920 and 1972 may be covered with an asbestos-containing material, or pipes may be wrapped in an asbestos "blanket" or asbestos paper tape. Asbestos insulation also has been used on furnace ducts. If you have damaged insulation around pipes or ducts, leave the insulation in place and repair the protective covering.

WALL AND CEILING INSULATION

Homes constructed between 1930 and 1950 may contain insulation made with asbestos. Because this insulation is "sandwiched" behind plaster walls, you will not be exposed unless walls are torn down for remodeling. In this case, a contractor experienced with asbestos insulation should be used.

Not every brand of the types of materials just mentioned will contain asbestos, but some do. If you suspect there is a problem, try to determine from the label, from the installer, or from the manufacturer whether or not the material contains asbestos. Some plumbers and contractors who have experience working with as-

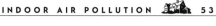

bestos products may be able to identify the products for you, or you can have them sent out for laboratory analysis.

If you suspect you have an asbestos problem that needs fixing, *do not attempt to do the work yourself.* Handling asbestos is a very delicate procedure that needs to be done with utmost care and proper protective devices. Call a qualified asbestos-removal contractor (get recommendations from your local EPA office) for a professional evaluation and estimate.

RADON

 One of the more dangerous contaminants you may find in the air in your home is **radon.** Some scientists believe that exposure to radon is the highest radiation danger the American public faces. It is known to cause lung cancer in high concentrations, but its health effects at lower levels of exposure are unsubstantiated and controversial. Even so, the Environmental Protection Agency has estimated that exposure to radon may be the second leading cause of lung cancer, after cigarette smoking.

Radon is a natural radioactive gas that results from the decay of **radioactive materials** that may be present in rocks, soil, minerals, water, or natural gas. Soil and building materials containing radioactive substances are thought to be the major sources of radon in the home. The main risk is not from radon itself, but from radon's progeny, which directly or by attaching to airborne particles may be inhaled into the lungs. Two of the progeny emit **alpha particles** that have the potential to inflict ten to twenty times the damage to biological tissue than similar doses of radiation from X rays.

Although the health effects of low-level exposure to radon are unclear, studies have shown that indoor concentrations of radon generally are much higher than outdoor concentrations and are especially high in tightly sealed energy-efficient homes. Because it takes 1,602 years for only half of the radon atoms to disintegrate, radon concentrations tend to become higher as time goes by, rather than disappear on their own.

The range of indoor concentrations found in homes is very broad, since concentrations of radon are affected by the amount and rate of radon being produced by the particular conditions in your home, the volume of space in which it accumulates, and the rate of air exchange. Problems with radon in homes tend to be regional, as radioactive materials from which it is generated occur in particular regions, either naturally occurring, or from having been dumped. You may have dangerously high levels of radon in your home, or none at all. It is difficult to determine the risk, since its presence cannot be detected either by your senses or by immediate symptoms. Radon is an invisible, latent, potential killer whose victims may die many years later, without ever making the connection that radon was responsible.

SAFE SOLUTIONS

First, you should do your best to determine whether or not you even have radon in your home. The homes more likely to contain radon are those built in uranium or phosphate mining areas, constructed with radioactive building materials, or that have radioactive materials brought to the home by water or natural gas.

The only way to know for sure if you have radon in your home is to get it tested. You can do this test yourself by ordering a radon test kit from *Air Check, Allergy Resources, Nontoxic Environments, Radon Solutions, or Radon Testing Corporation of America,* or you can hire a professional inspector.

But before you rush to buy a test kit, contact your local EPA office to obtain a map showing areas with potentially high radon levels. Regardless of where you live, if large portions of your home are made of stone, brick, or concrete, it should be tested.

If your radon test is positive, you will need to take some action. Small concentrations can be handled with good ventilation; for higher levels, you will need professional help.

Radon gas is generally produced under the house or in the basement and then seeps into the living space through porous materials and cracks.

Ventilation will reduce your exposure to radon. Simply opening the window will help, and will also reduce levels of other indoor pollutants. Block any entries through which radon can filter into your home.

Again, there is no clear evidence that radon in the home is

particularly harmful; however, because it is suspect, it would be worth determining if radon is in your home, taking precautions for protection, and keeping up on the latest research in this field.

PLASTICS

We use plastics in virtually every area of our lives. Plastics are a large, extremely diverse group of moldable synthetic materials made from petroleum or coal. They can be found as hard or soft solid forms, liquids that dry to solid coatings and finishes, adhesives, rigid or flexible foams, sheets, films, fibers, and filaments.

We are exposed to plastics in many different ways. There may be plastic vapors in the air we breathe, the plastic in clothing may rub against our skin, plastic may be absorbed into our food from packaging and storage containers, and plastic may be in the water we drink from plastic pipes or storage bottles.

It is important to get to know different kinds of plastics and how to recognize them, because some plastics can be harmful to our health, while others are not. When they were first introduced, we had no reason even to question their safety. But over the years, we have been finding more and more evidence that they are not as safe as we once thought. Some types of plastics are carcinogenic, others are endocrine disruptors, and still others can cause skin rashes—perhaps a minor complaint, but still a sign from our bodies that something is wrong.

Exposure to plastics has been linked to many kinds of interesting effects. One prominent health researcher has observed several cases in which a polyester-covered polyurethane foam mattress was a contributing factor in sexual impotence! Both polyester and polyurethane foam are plastics, and with an additional dose of polyester and urea-formaldehyde plastic resin in the bedsheets, it's not surprising that one's body might have difficulty responding.

There are basically two types of plastics: thermoplastics and thermosets. The difference between the two lies in their chemical structure. Both are made from chains of basic molecules, but the thermoplastic chains remain detached and separable, while the molecules in the thermoset plastics are tightly bonded in weblike structures. This distinction is very important, because it plays a key role in the relative safety of each kind of plastic.

THERMOPLASTICS

Thermoplastics become soft when heated, and harden when cooled, no matter how often the process is repeated. Think of this plastic as being like butter—it melts when heated, but becomes solid again when cooled. When butter is put into a mold and cooled, you have a stick of butter, otherwise, it just hardens in any shape it happens to flow into.

Most thermoplastics are easy to recognize because they are soft, bendable, and have a certain amount of flexibility because of their loose chemical structure. While this is an advantage for performance, it is a disadvantage for our health because these soft plastics tend to emit vapors of, or "outgas," plastic molecules, especially when they are heated. Have you ever noticed the smell of the interior of your car on a hot day, or when new synthetic carpets are installed, or when you open a plastic food container? These are all plastics vaporizing. You may notice after you have owned a plastic item for a while that it doesn't smell quite as much, but these plastics do continue to outgas for the life of the product. As long as a thermoplastic is in existence, it outgasses.

Each type of thermoplastic has different health effects. Some of the dangers are well documented, others are known and are only beginning to be suspected. Let's take a look at some of the more common thermoplastics you are likely to encounter on a daily basis, their health effects, and some examples of products made from these plastics.

Vinyl plastics, including **vinyl chloride** and **polyvinyl chloride (PVC),** are the most dangerous plastics. Products made from polyvinyl chloride/vinyl chloride include adhesives, artificial grass, baby pants, containers for toiletries, cosmetics, household chemicals, credit cards, crib bumpers, floor tiles, food packaging, garden hoses, handbags, inflatable toys such as beach balls and swimming pools, magnetic recording tape, pacifiers and teethers, paper finishes, phonograph records, playpen covers, raincoats and galoshes, shoes, shower curtains, squeeze toys, toys, umbrellas, upholstery (furniture and auto), wall coverings, and water pipes.

PVC releases vinyl chloride, which can cause cancer, birth defects, genetic changes, indigestion, chronic bronchitis, ulcers, skin diseases, deafness, vision failure, and liver dysfunction. Some PVCs contain added **plasticizers,** which makes the plastic even more unstable. Because plasticizers are not bound to the plastic chemically, they can be easily removed by water, oil, or heat. NASA banned the use of PVC in space capsules because the plasticizer outgassed and condensed in optical equipment. **DEHP,** a substance that appears to be a cancer-causing agent, is a plasticizer frequently added to PVC.

Perhaps the most dramatic experience I have ever had of the vaporizing of plastic was when I opened a metal tin of European cookies. I had checked the label carefully for artificial additives and preservatives, but inside was a polyvinyl chloride tray to hold the delicate cookies in place during shipping (these trays are also used for chocolates). The odor was horrible, and what was worse, the cookies were inedible—they were all tainted by the plastic.

Acrylic plastics are made from **acrylonitrile,** a suspected human carcinogen. Products made from acrylic plastics include acrylic fibers (clothing, blankets, carpets), adhesives, contact lenses, dentures, floor waxes, food preparation equipment, Lucite, nonwoven fabrics (carpet backing, disposable diapers, felt, filters, sanitary napkins, shoe liners), paints, paper coatings, Plexiglas, and wood finishes. Acrylonitrile has also been known to cause breathing difficulties, vomiting, diarrhea, nausea, weakness, headache, and fatigue.

Polyethylene is a suspected human carcinogen. Products made from polyethylene include carpet fibers, chewing gum, coffee stirrers, drinking glasses, electrical-outlet safety covers, food containers and wrappers, heat-sealed plastic packaging, kitchenware, paper coatings, plastic bags, plastic pails and garbage cans, squeeze bottles, swizzle sticks, and toys.

The most popular **fluorocarbon** plastic is **tetrafluoroethylene,** better known as Teflon. Tetrafluoroethylene can be irritating to eyes, nose, and throat, and can cause breathing difficulties. Teflon is used as a nonstick coating on clothes irons, cookware, ironing-board covers, plumbing, and tools.

Two common plastics are made from the **styrene monomer: polystyrene** (Styrofoam) and **ABS (acrylonitrile/butadiene/styrene)** plastic. Vapors released by the styrene monomer can be irritating to your eyes, nose, and throat, and they can also cause dizziness and unconsciousness. Products made with styrene plastics include air conditioners, automobile dashboards, building insulation panels, cleaning brushes, clocks, coasters, electronic products, floor polishes, flotation devices, ice buckets, insulation on soft-drink bottles, kitchen and bathroom wall tile, lighting fixtures, luggage tags, model cars and airplanes, paints, poker chips, serving trays, sewing-machine bobbins, silverware, throwaway hot-drink cups, toys, telephones, and typewriter carrying cases.

Polyester fiber and films can cause eye and respiratory-tract irritation and acute skin rashes. Products made from polyester include bedding, clothing, disposable diapers, food packaging, magnetic recording tapes, nonwoven disposable filters, sanitary napkins, tampons, and upholstery.

Nylon is a **polyamide** plastic. It is generally considered safe, but skin rashes and other types of dermatitis are common reactions to contact with nylon. Products that are made with nylon filaments and fibers include artificial grass, automotive upholstery, bristles on toothbrushes, hairbrushes, paintbrushes, clothing, fishing lines, hosiery, mascara, pen tips, rugs and carpets, surgical sutures, and tennis rackets.

THERMOSETS

Thermosets begin as soft plastics, but their shape is set by heat and cannot be altered once it is made. A thermoset acts in a way similar to cake mix—it starts out as a liquid, but once you bake it and it becomes solid, it stays solid, regardless of temperature. When you heat a thermoset plastic to very high temperatures (higher than you would encounter in normal, everyday use), it still doesn't melt; like a cake, it just disintegrates.

Because the plastic molecules in thermoset plastics are so tightly bonded, it is difficult for them to vaporize. For this reason, most thermoset plastics are very hard and relatively nontoxic in comparison to thermoplastics. There are, however, two thermoset plastics that pose significant hazards.

Urea-formaldehyde plastic resins, found in particleboard, plywood, building insulation, wet-strength paper (tissues, toilet paper, paper towels), and fabric finishes, are known to release high levels of formaldehyde, especially when new. The outgassing of formaldehyde decreases as the product ages, but even when some products are several years old, exposure is still great enough to cause health problems. Formaldehyde is a suspected human carcinogen and has been shown to cause birth defects and genetic changes in bacteriological studies. Symptoms from inhaling formaldehyde vapors could include cough, swelling of the throat, watery eyes, breathing problems, headaches, rashes, tiredness, excessive thirst, nausea, nosebleeds, insomnia, disorientation, and asthma attacks.

Polyurethane foam, used to make cushions, mattresses, and pillows, is the other thermoset plastic that can be dangerous. Exposure to polyurethane foam can cause bronchitis, coughing, and skin and eye problems. Polyurethane foam also releases **toluene diisocyanate,** which can produce severe lung problems.

Even greater than the everyday dangers posed is the danger of plastics in the event of a fire. Flames from burning plastics spread quickly, have extremely high temperatures, and produce large amounts of dense smoke. Ironically, plastics treated to be flame-retardant will produce more smoke when forced to burn than untreated materials. Many plastics produce toxic gases when they are burned; polyvinyl chloride turns into **hydrochloric acid,** burning polyurethane foam and polyester release toxic unreacted toluene diisocyanate. Since about 80 percent of fire victims are harmed not by flame but by smoke inhalation, the toxicity of the smoke plays a big factor in the harm that could result from a fire in your home. Natural materials such as wood and cotton fibers also produce toxic combustion by-products, but at a much slower rate than synthetic materials, allowing more time for a person to escape before deadly gases accumulate to lethal levels.

SAFE SOLUTIONS

Despite the long list of potentially dangerous plastics, some plastics seem to be relatively safe.

Cellulosic plastics are made primarily from cellulose fibers from wood or cotton, and have no adverse health effects that I am aware of. Examples of products made from cellulosic plastics include acetate fibers, automobile steering wheels, bodies and caps of pens and pencils, eyeglass frames, toothbrush handles, typewriter keys, and shoe heels.

Melamine formaldehyde plastics, such as Melmac dishware and Formica countertops, also seem to be relatively inert.

Phenolic plastic resins, more commonly called Bakelite, may release a small amount of formaldehyde when new, but this quickly dissipates. Handles of pots and pans and clothes irons are generally made from Bakelite.

Don't worry about replacing *every* plastic product in your home, a virtually impossible task. My television, VCR, laptop computer, and telephone are all made largely from plastic, because currently there are no alternatives available.

For the most part, you can live without plastic. Plastics have been popular only since World War II. Before that, everything was made from natural materials. There are many, many items still made from natural materials: wool diaper covers, wooden boxes, straw baskets, cotton shower curtains, glass jars, paper bags, leather shoes, wooden toys, glass dishes, and wood and glass clocks, to name just a few. So keep your eyes open, and when you have a choice, look for a natural material.

You might want to start your plastic cleanup by just looking around and taking inventory of all the plastics in your home. See what is easy to replace, and what can wait. Maybe start just by using a wicker basket for a trash basket next to your desk instead of a plastic one (it's more decorative, too). One by one, you'll find replacements.

LEAD

While adults can generally tolerate the low levels of **lead** that may be present in our homes, top officials in our federal government are now calling lead poisoning the nation's primary environmental threat to children. According to the EPA, one out of nine children under age six has enough lead in his blood for it to be a health problem. United States Public Health Service estimates place the figure as high as one in six.

Lead is a naturally occurring metallic element whose toxicity is well established. It is a cumulative poison, so while one small exposure may not seem harmful, repeated exposures can build up over time. Because lead is an element, it never decomposes into another substance that might be more easily tolerated, and it never leaves your body. Damage from consistent lead exposure is usually irreversible.

Early symptoms of lead poisoning include abdominal pains, loss of appetite, constipation, muscle pains and weakness, irritability, a metallic taste in the mouth, excessive thirst, nausea and vomiting, headache, insomnia, depression, and lethargy. Repeated low-level exposure has been found to produce anemia, stomach ailments, and permanent neuropsychological defects and behavior disorders in children, including noticeable learning difficulties, poor scores on IQ and development tests, and short attention spans. In very high doses, lead can cause brain damage, nervous system disorders, and death, although such heavy poisoning is unlikely from exposure around your home. There is no safe level for lead. James Mason, head of the U.S. Public Health Service, has stated that "the more we learn, the more toxic we find it to be."

PAINT

The household lead exposure people generally think of first is caused by lead-based paints. Manufacturers removed much of the lead from paint in the 1950s, and the federal government banned lead in paint altogether in 1978. While this means we don't have to worry about lead in a *new* can of paint, there is still great concern about the lead that is already on the walls in millions of homes across America. Seventy-five percent of all private housing built before 1980 has some lead paint, according to a 1990 study by the U.S. Department of Housing and Urban Development (HUD). Since lead was a standard ingredient in paint at that time, lead-painted walls may be found in houses in all older neighborhoods, whether well-to-do or poor.

Many children get lead poisoning not from eating paint chips, but rather from breathing fine paint dust stirred up by the opening and closing of windows with lead-painted window frames, or from the removal or disturbance of old paint during renovations. It can be found on the exterior and interior of houses—on walls, window and door trims, railings, baseboards, and radiators. One child seems to have gotten lead poisoning from playing in her sandbox after her father had sanded lead paint off the exterior of their home. HUD reported that 20 million lead-painted houses have too much lead dust or chippings—about 20 percent of the entire housing in America. Homes in the Northeast, Midwest, and Western states have more lead than the South.

It takes very little lead to cause lead poisoning. The Centers for Disease Control has set ten micrograms per deciliter as the level above which some sort of action should be taken. A child can reach lead/blood levels of three times that amount by ingesting lead equivalent to one granule of sugar a day, which could easily happen if a child touches a windowsill and sucks his thumb on a regular basis.

TAP WATER

Tap water is another source of lead—the EPA estimates that lead in water causes 10 to 20 percent of overall childhood lead exposure. If your water comes from a well, travels through old lead-soldered pipes (in your house or municipal water system), or is known to be very corrosive, you may have cause for concern.

DISHWARE

The glaze on ceramic and pottery dishware can also cause significant lead exposure. Lead is used to create bright colors and mask deficiencies in the pottery. It has been known to be a problem, especially in imported pieces. The federal government prohibits the sale of dinnerware that releases lead in amounts greater than 2,000 parts per billion (ppb), which prevents direct cases of lead poisoning. However, in 1986, the state of California passed legislation requiring written warnings on any dishware that releases lead in amounts greater than 224 ppb, based on the potential long-term health risk to young children and developing fetuses. In 1991, ten of America's most renowned dinnerware manufacturers were sued by the state and the Environmental Defense Fund for failing to alert consumers to high lead levels in some of their products.

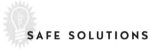

SAFE SOLUTIONS

If you are pregnant, try not to drink, eat, or breathe lead during pregnancy, as developing fetuses are the most vulnerable. Most important, do not start to strip paint or wallpaper to prepare the new nursery now if there is any chance that old layers of lead paint may lurk below.

Children are most likely to get lead poisoning between the ages of six months and six years, when lead dust from carpeting, toys, or the floor can most easily get in their mouths and lungs. Your doctor can order a blood-lead test for your child if you suspect your child has been contaminated.

If you live in a house or apartment built before 1980, inspect your building carefully for signs of paint chips or dust. Look at windowsills, baseboards, and especially doorframes, where friction can grind up paint layers. To remove dust, damp-mop or wipe with a solution of trisodium phosphate (TSP), which can be purchased at paint or hardware stores. (It will not be available in states where phosphates have been banned.) As with asbestos, it is better to leave lead paint in place if intact rather than create a hazard by disturbing it. But if you find you have a major problem that requires removal, hire a qualified contractor (contact your local HUD office for referrals). Complete removal might cost thousands of dollars, but you can significantly reduce the hazard by replacing doors, window frames, or contaminated carpeting, or by putting up wallpaper or paneling.

To remove lead from drinking water, you will need a reverse osmosis system or distiller. Inexpensive carbon filters will not remove lead (see Water Filters in chapter 5).

Before you buy ceramic or pottery dinnerware, ask about the lead used in glazes. Lead releases can vary from style to style from a single manufacturer, so be specific. When in doubt, don't buy it. Often local potters are well aware of the problem of lead in glaze and make a point to use lead-free glazes.

Do-it-yourself test kits can be used to determine the lead content of paint, water, or pottery. You can order **Lead Check** swabs by mail from *Air Check, Allergy Resources, Lead Check,* and *Nontoxic Environments.*

FORMALDEHYDE

> **WARNING** This product is manufactured with a urea-formaldehyde resin and will release small quantities of formaldehyde. Formaldehyde levels in indoor air can cause temporary eye and respiratory irritation and may aggravate respiratory conditions or allergies. Ventilation will reduce indoor formaldehyde levels.

Formaldehyde is a common chemical found in numerous household products, including adhesives, cosmetics, deodorants, detergents, fertilizers, paints, plastics, and textiles. It is a suspected human carcinogen, having been found to cause cancer in laboratory animals. The National Academy of Sciences estimates that 10 to 20 percent of the general population may be susceptible to irritation from exposure to formaldehyde at extremely low concentrations including cough, swelling and irritation of the throat, watery eyes, headaches, rashes, excessive thirst, nausea, nosebleeds, disorientation, and other symptoms.

PARTICLEBOARD

A major source of formaldehyde pollution in many homes is particleboard. Particleboard is made by pressing small wood shavings together with **urea-formaldehyde** resin. It is easy to recognize because you can see the pressed-together shavings on all sides. It is used extensively in the construction of inexpensive home furnishings, kitchen and bathroom cabinets, and in new-home construction (particularly as subflooring and in doors). While particleboard itself is simple to recognize, it is often hidden behind a thin wood veneer, so check carefully. Good places to look for exposed particleboard are inside cabinets, at the ends of shelves, in corners, and in drilled holes. Most wood items that are described as "veneered" or having a "genuine oak veneer" are generally filled with particleboard.

All products made with particleboard will release small quantities of formaldehyde. Formaldehyde emissions are greater when the product is new, and decrease with time, but it takes many years for the formaldehyde to evaporate entirely. Surprisingly, warning labels are not required on products made with particleboard, though they are on sheets of particleboard purchased at lumberyards.

INSULATION

Another common product made with urea-formaldehyde resin is urea-formaldehyde foam insulation (UFFI). The Consumer Product Safety Commission banned the use of UFFI in residences and schools in 1982, after receiving numerous complaints that exposure to this insulation caused respiratory problems, dizziness, nausea, and eye and throat irritations ranging from short-term discomfort to serious adverse health effects and hospitalization. Despite the fact that this ban was later overturned by the U.S. Court of Appeals, the CPSC continues to warn consumers that evidence indicates that substantial risk is associated with use of this product.

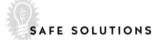

SAFE SOLUTIONS

Instead of particleboard, choose wood items made from solid wood whenever possible. Even plywood, although also made with a formaldehyde resin, is preferable to particleboard.

If you are insulating your home, choose any other insulation rather than UFFI. In general, fiberglass batts are the least toxic. There is some concern that fiberglass fibers may pose the same hazard as asbestos fibers, but I know of no evidence that suggests that fiberglass within walls might be released into your living space. If you want to check your indoor air for formaldehyde fumes that may already be present in your home, you can order a home test kit from *Air Check, Allergy Resources,* or *Nontoxic Environments.*

Some of the formaldehyde fumes from particleboard or UFFI can be sealed in; any kind of finish will help to some degree, although a sealant designed to be a vapor barrier, such as **AFM Hard Seal** (order by mail from *Allergy Relief Shop, Allergy Resources, American Environmental Health Foundation, The Living Source,* or *Nontoxic Environments*), will be more effective. They can reduce formaldehyde emissions up to 95 percent, but tend to break down after several years and require reapplication.

The most effective barrier for formaldehyde fumes is aluminum foil. Heavy-duty foil and foil-back paper (sold as foil vapor barrier at building-supply stores) are more durable than standard cooking foil. These will, of course, give a rather space-age look to your furniture and your walls, but they work quite well inside cabinets, where they are less visible and most needed to prevent fumes from building up inside the closed space. Use foil tape (available at hardware stores) to seal the edges and keep fumes from escaping.

If you do nothing else, at least open the window! As particleboard and UFFI continue to give off formaldehyde fumes, they can eventually reach very high concentrations in unventilated spaces. Try to leave a window open (even just a crack will help) in all rooms containing particleboard and throughout the house if your home is insulated with UFFI.

An appropriate air filter will also significantly lessen formaldehyde fumes, but don't expect a little air cleaner from your local department store to do the job. You'll need a heavy-duty machine with a lot of activated carbon or other adsorptive material especially formulated for formaldehyde removal, as described in Air Filters in chapter 2.

ELECTROMAGNETIC FIELDS

In the past few years there has been great concern about the possible health effects of the artificial electromagnetic fields that are created around us by electrical wires and appliances.

Electromagnetic fields (EMFs) are electrical and magnetic fields that exist naturally—generated by the sun, the moon, and the planets, and also by our bodies—or are man-made by electrical power generating stations. The activity of every living cell in our bodies is regulated by the flow of electromagnetic fields. Our metabolism is geared to the natural background levels of radiation and electromagnetic energies from the cosmos—the earth's electromagnetic field pulses at the rate of 7.83 hertz, and our body's own bioelectrical system pulses at about the same rate.

When electricity was first installed in American homes around 100 years ago, we encased ourselves in invisible cages of electromagnetic energy pulsing at 60 hertz. At its introduction, electricity was thought to be perfectly safe. Now researchers are not so certain. While the scientific community is not yet completely convinced that exposure to EMFs from the electrical wiring and appliances in our homes (or from nearby power lines) poses any health threat, accumulating scientific evidence has led many to believe there is cause for concern.

Laboratory studies on animal cells have clearly shown that EMFs from a 60-hertz alternating current emit radiation that can interact with individual cells and organs to produce biological changes. Verified epidemiological studies found that children who live near ordinary neighborhood electrical distribution lines were twice as likely to develop cancer as those who do not. Results of such studies are encouraging a major worldwide research effort.

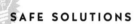

SAFE SOLUTIONS

Man-made electromagnetic fields from many environmental sources surround us constantly, and it is impossible to eliminate them entirely from our lives, even if we went to live on a mountaintop. You can, however, greatly reduce your exposure to man-made electromagnetic fields in your home, which often pose a greater risk than exposures from outdoors.

Let's start with the easy things first. Use battery-powered appliances and electronics whenever possible, as batteries produce a weaker electromagnetic field and rechargeable batteries can be recharged easily with solar energy instead of electricity (the *Real Goods* catalog has rechargeable batteries and a solar recharger).

Because EMFs get weaker with distance, you can protect yourself by keeping your distance from (or removing entirely) the more powerful emitters of electromagnetic fields in your home.

Dimmer switches	remove
Electric blankets	remove (or preheat bed, then unplug)
Photoelectric timer switches	remove
Microwave ovens	remove
Radiant heat installed in walls	don't use

Fluorescent lights	6 feet
Refrigerators and freezers	4 feet
Televisions and computers	3½ feet
Electric heaters	3 feet
Dial-faced electric clocks	3 feet
Blow dryer for hair	1 foot

Unplug appliances and electronics when not in use (as long as they are connected the wires are "hot" so that you can turn on the machine). At night, you may want to shut off all the circuits in your house (except for the circuit that powers the refrigerator), as the wires in your walls are "hot" all the time as well. If you do shut off your power, keep a flashlight and battery-powered clock next to your bed.

Take special care to make your bedroom as electromagnetically safe as possible, as this is the room where you probably spend most of your time while at home and that needs to be most conducive to getting good sleep so your body can rejuvenate itself.

If you can take on the more complex and expensive task of retrofitting your home, you might want to consider installing shielded wire. Simply twisting wires around each other (1 twist every 2½ inches) will reduce magnetic fields by about 80 percent. And install items that minimize the use of electricity, such as windows and skylights instead of artificial lighting, and climate-responsive heating and cooling rather than electric heating and air-conditioning.

Alternative energy sources (such as solar or wind) produce lower voltages of electricity and therefore more compatible electromagnetic fields.

The only way to really know how much EMFs you are being exposed to is to use a gauss meter to take readings. You can buy a gauss meter for about $150 from **American Environmental Health Foundation, Nontoxic Environments, Real Goods, TRA Instruments,** and **Teslatronics.**

A few years back, the staff of *Green Alternatives* magazine (unfortunately, they are no longer publishing) went on a field trip with a gauss meter and came back with a surprising report.

What did we learn in our Field Trip? That electromagnetic fields are unpredictable. In a lot of places where we expected to be absolutely cooked, such as the Bard computer lab or under the high-tension wires, the readings were moderate. Familiar objects, such as our computers and some of our cars, are dynamos of electromagnetic energy. And in a few places, such as the restaurant where we had lunch, there are wild, powerful fields for which there is no obvious explanation.

Above all else, we found that looks are deceiving. A person gets a more intense exposure to EMFs while working at a computer than from living next door to an electrical substation. Something that looks scary and industrial is not necessarily a threat. Friendly-looking household gadgets are not necessarily benign.

Mark Twain is said to have stated, "A little knowledge is a dangerous thing." The little knowledge we have about EMFs causes some to live in fear or move out of their homes, while others adhere to the "Well, I'm not dead yet" philosophy. Our Field Day with the gaussmeters at least gave us, and you, an idea of where EMFs are likely to be strongest. We just can't say for sure whether or not to worry.

The **S.A.F.E. Home & Office Company** catalog specializes in EMFs. They carry not only gauss meters, but also shielding materials, low-radiation computer monitors, low-EMF telephones, shielded clock radios, and reports on EMF research. They also do consultations, so all your questions can be answered.

John Banta, creator of the "Current Switch" video, also offers consultations and a variety of books on EMFs and EMF protection products through his **Electro-Pollution Supply**.

SMOKE DETECTORS

All battery-powered (ionization-type) smoke detectors contain radioactive materials and may be potential hazards. The radioactive materials are confined in metal containers designed to keep exposure to radioactive materials to a minimum, but since these alarms have been in use for only a short period of time, the real hazards are unknown. Any exposure to radioactive materials is suspected of creating potential adverse health effects.

SAFE SOLUTIONS

There are two types of smoke alarms on the market: ionization-type, which detects both visible and invisible signs of fire, and photoelectric detectors, which respond only to visible signs of combustion.

Interestingly enough, *Consumer Reports* magazine found that the photoelectric-type detectors overall are much more sensitive and effective than the ionization type! In this case, the product that is the best buy is also the best for your health. Photoelectric detectors are difficult to find in stores, but they can be ordered from **Real Goods, Karen's Nontoxic Products,** and **Natural Lifestyle.**

If you already have battery-powered smoke alarms and would like to switch, return your old smoke alarms to the manufacturer for proper disposal. The radioactive materials used in smoke alarms last for thousands of years, and similar materials produced in nuclear reactors must be buried deep underground.

Chapter 3

HOUSEHOLD CLEANING AND LAUNDRY PRODUCTS

ONE OF THE EASIER WAYS to create a nontoxic home is to replace all the heavy-duty chemicals we use to maintain our homes—ammonia, oven cleaners, furniture polish, scouring powder, disinfectant, glass cleaner—with simple, inexpensive, and natural materials you probably already have in your kitchen. These replacements are odorless or have subtle natural fragrances and work every bit as well as the chemicals you are accustomed to using. They also have the added benefit of being much less expensive than commercial cleaning preparations. You don't have to pay for advertising or packaging, or buy a different product for each cleaning need.

Labeling

Cleaning products are among the more hazardous products you will find in your home—so much so that they are the only household products regulated by the Consumer Product Safety Commission under the 1960 Federal Hazardous Substances Labeling Act. This means that cleaning products that can hurt you must carry various warnings on their labels. If a cleaning product contains a chemical that is hazardous, it must by law specify the hazard. Look at your cleaning-product labels and see if you find any of these words:

- **Toxic/Highly Toxic:** poisonous if you happen to drink it, if you breathe the fumes, or if it is absorbed through your skin
- **Extremely Flammable/Flammable/Combustible:** can catch fire if exposed to a flame or an electric spark
- **Corrosive:** will eat away your skin or cause inflammation of mucous membranes
- **Strong Sensitizer:** may provoke an allergic reaction

Hazardous cleaning products also must prominently display the degree of toxicity with one of the following signal words:

- **Danger** (or **Poison,** with skull and crossbones): could kill an adult if only a tiny pinch is ingested
- **Warning:** could kill an adult if about a teaspoon is ingested
- **Caution:** will not kill until an amount from 2 tablespoons to 2 cups is ingested

At one time these signal words accurately indicated the dose required to cause a toxic effect, but because of poor labeling practices, these words now suggest only a general degree of danger.

The label must also state "the common or usual name or the chemical name . . . of the hazardous substance or of each component which contributes substantially to its hazard." Other labeling requirements include a statement telling users how to avoid the hazard (and, if necessary, safe-use instructions), name and location of the manufacturer or distributor, instructions for handling and storage of packages that require special care, and a warning to keep out of the reach of children.

Manufacturers are required to keep records of all adverse

health effects associated with the substance they produce. There is no federal law requiring premarket safety testing by the manufacturer, however, and the hazards of some products have sometimes not been revealed until after complaints were received by the Consumer Product Safety Commission.

The real safety or danger of cleaning products is difficult to assess because manufacturers are not required to list exact ingredients on the label. You can't look at a label and be sure, for instance, that a certain furniture polish doesn't contain nitrobenzene (a substance commonly used in furniture polish that could be fatal if swallowed), or that a mold and mildew cleaner is free from pentachlorophenol (another commonly used deadly substance); however, these ingredients should be listed on an MSDS. Some product ingredients, though, are protected by trade secrets, and even the government and poison-control centers cannot find them out.

The best information we can get from poison-control centers is a general list of the chemicals commonly used in specific categories of products. Which brand-name products do or do not actually contain these substances is anybody's guess, unless the manufacturer voluntarily reveals the product's ingredients.

Perhaps the most disturbing fact about cleaning products is that the chemicals they contain can have devastating effects over time—and these warnings aren't mentioned on the label. That's how we are generally exposed to cleaning products—over time, daily, for years, even decades. We get so accustomed to using these products that we forget they may be dangerous. Yet the Hazardous Substances Act focuses on only the *immediate* effects the product can have *if not used according to instructions.*

Most cleaning products can be harmful during actual use, even when you follow the directions on the label exactly, although mention of this danger isn't required by law. Toxic fumes from these products may produce slight reactions such as headaches, fatigue, burning eyes, runny nose, and skin rashes. However, even if you do not have an obvious reaction while using the product after day-in/day-out exposure, year after year, your body may suddenly respond with cancer, heart disease, lung problems, or damage to the liver or immune system. Some substances in cleaning products may also cause birth defects and genetic changes.

Cleaning-product manufacturers are also not required to warn against product use by those who are at high risk because of specific medical conditions. For example, the labels on cleaning products in aerosol containers do not disclose that the aerosol mist can aggravate an existing lung condition, such as asthma. Asthma sufferers might have less trouble breathing if aerosol sprays and other volatile chemicals were not used in the home. The American Lung Association warns against the use of aerosol sprays, yet product labels do not reflect these specific health concerns.

If this is not enough, a study done by the New York Poison Control Center found that 85 percent of the product warning labels studied were inadequate. Some labels list incorrect first-aid information and others warn against dangers that don't even exist! A worker at my local poison-control center told me a story of a child who had swallowed some silica gel, a relatively harmless crystalline substance. Because this product was incorrectly labeled as a poison by the manufacturer, the mother tried to induce vomiting by putting her finger down the child's throat (she should never have done this without calling a poison-control center or doctor). The crystals came up and lacerated the child's esophagus, causing more harm than if they had just stayed in her stomach. Had the container not been mislabeled, the child would not have been harmed.

SAFE SOLUTIONS

Nontoxic cleaning requires very few specialized ingredients. I do all my cleaning with a squirt bottle of fifty-fifty vinegar and water, liquid soap, and baking soda. It couldn't be simpler.

You might need a few more items, though, to accomplish your specific cleaning needs. Here are some natural substances you might wish to have on hand to use as needed:

- *Baking soda:* available in bulk at natural-food stores
- *Salt:* any brand
- *Distilled white vinegar:* any brand
- *Lemon juice:* organically grown or home-grown lemons, if possible
- *Liquid soap:* available at natural-food stores

- *Borax:* a naturally occurring mineral that has no toxic fumes and is safe for the environment, but does carry a warning label that says, "Irritating to eyes and skin; harmful if swallowed; keep out of reach of children." It can be purchased in the cleaning-products department of every supermarket.

- *Scouring powder:* See Scouring Powders, p. 102.

- *Trisodium phosphate* (TSP) and *sodium hexametaphosphate:* naturally occurring minerals that are nontoxic to humans but may have environmental effects because they are phosphates. TSP can be purchased at any hardware, variety, or paint store. While the label does warn that it is for external use only, it is a skin irritant and should be kept out of the reach of children. I have found it to be relatively mild for the heavy-duty cleaning power it offers, and absolutely odorless. Order sodium hexametaphosphate by mail from **Allergy Resources** or **The Living Source.**

Although I do all my cleaning with homemade formulas, you may want to buy commercial products. Your local natural-food store will have many nontoxic cleaners to choose from, and you may even find some at your supermarket. If you need to order cleaning products by mail, these catalogs carry a good selection: **Allergy Resources, American Environmental Health Foundation, Cal Ben Soap Company, Granny's Old-Fashioned Products, Janice Corporation, Karen's Nontoxic Products, The Living Source, Logona USA, The Natural Choice, Nontoxic Environments, Real Goods** (they have some hard-to-find items such as heavy-duty soap with pumice, and nontoxic graffiti remover), and **Seventh Generation,** and **Soapworks.**

Frequently I am asked about cleaning products sold through multilevel marketing companies. In the past I haven't recommended them because I had difficulty obtaining ingredients lists (even when asked) and I suspected that they contained some ingredients of minor toxicity that were, nonetheless, on my list of things to avoid. Over the years, however, I've gone from being an absolute purist (brought on originally, I'm sure, by my own personal need for the least toxic products available) to having the attitude that it's better to make a less-toxic choice than continue to use a more-toxic product. And some of the newer companies have been willing to reveal their ingredients or at least answer questions about them.

Geo has a group of six products that clean everything from the easiest windows to the toughest grease and grime. They are made from natural-based colloidal concentrates and environmentally safe colors. I have a letter from the president of Geo, which states, "None of our products contain any petro chemicals or petro distillates."

Natural World offers a full line of cleaning products made primarily from natural-based ingredients. Their ingredients are readily available in distributors' literature.

While I have not had the opportunity to review all the ingredients of all the multilevel products, I have reviewed and rejected some on the basis of incomplete information. So ask for those ingredients lists, and make sure you know what is in the products you are buying, regardless of who you are buying them from.

Now, let's take a closer look at the dangers of some common cleaning products and how we can tackle these same cleaning chores with natural substances.

DRAIN CLEANERS

POISON: ☠ Call poison center, emergency room, or physician at once. Causes severe eye and skin damage; may cause blindness. Harmful or fatal if swallowed.

The primary component of drain cleaners is **lye**, an extremely corrosive material that can eat right through skin. Even a drop spilled on your skin or a dry crystal that falls on wet skin can cause damage. When ingested, lye quickly burns through internal tissues, damaging the esophagus, stomach, and the entire intestinal tract. The internal damage may be irreparable for those who survive lye poisoning.

Lye itself poses no danger from inhalation, but in liquid drain cleaners, lye is mixed with volatile liquid chemicals such as **ammonia** and **petroleum distillates,** which can release harmful vapors.

If you change only one cleaning product in your home, this is it. Drain cleaners get my vote for the most dangerous unnecessary product in the house.

SAFE SOLUTIONS

For all their dangers, lye-based drain cleaners are really not very effective. How many times have you tried to clear a drain with lye, only to have the clog just sit there, leaving you with a sinkful of corrosive, lye-contaminated water and wondering what to do next? Why endanger your family with a product that doesn't even work?

My favorite drain-opener is the handy-dandy plunger. Unlike lye-activated products, this old-fashioned standby works nearly every time. You can buy one that lasts for years at any hardware store, and they're very inexpensive. True, at times it takes more than a few plunges, but usually the clog will break down eventually.

If this doesn't work, lye won't work either, so call a plumber. He or she will use a long, flexible metal snake to push the clog away.

It's important, of course, to practice a little preventive plumbing. Use a drain strainer to trap food particles and hair, and remember not to pour grease down the drain. (Dump it in the garbage or into a "grease can" instead.)

There's also a nifty product called the **WorldWise Easy-Clear Sink Trap,** which replaces the curved part of your pipe under the sink and opens at the curve so you can pull the clog out. And if the clog is further down the pipe, you can use **Drain King,** a device that creates water pressure with water from your garden hose to push the clog through.

In addition, there are new enzyme products designed to remove soap, hair, grease, and other organic materials that coat the entire length of the pipe and cause slow drains. Most hardware stores now sell such products.

Regular use of one of these nontoxic methods will keep drains open or clear sluggish drains before they become full-fledged clogs:

- Pour 1 handful baking soda and ½ cup white vinegar down the drainpipe and cover tightly for 1 minute. The chemical reaction between the 2 substances will form a fizzy pressure in the drain and dislodge any obstructive matter. Rinse with hot water.
- Pour ½ cup salt and ½ cup baking soda or 2 tablespoons trisodium phosphate down the drain, followed by lots of hot water.

As a last resort, try pouring ¼ cup of 3-percent hydrogen peroxide down the drain. Wait a few minutes, then plunge. Repeat a second time if needed. This can open clogged drains that have defied other methods.

NOTE: Hydrogen peroxide bottles have labels that warn to keep out of eyes and out of the reach of children to avoid accidental ingestion. Used correctly, however, it is a safe and effective alternative to lye-based drain cleaners.

OVEN CLEANERS

> **DANGER:** Contact will cause burns. Avoid contact with skin, eyes, mucous membranes, and clothing. Do not take internally. Wear rubber gloves while using. Contains lye. If taken internally or sprayed in eyes, call a physician. Keep out of reach of children. Irritant to mucous membranes. Avoid inhaling vapors. Contents under pressure. Recommended for use only on porcelain, enamel, iron, stainless steel, ceramic, and glass surfaces. Do not get on exterior oven surfaces such as aluminum and chrome trim, baked enamel, copper tone, or painted areas, or on linoleum or plastics. For gas ovens, avoid spraying on pilot light. Keep spray off electrical connections such as door-operated light switch, heating element, etc.

Although oven cleaners contain several toxic ingredients, the greater dangers come from **lye** and **ammonia.** Like all-purpose cleaners, oven cleaners in **aerosol spray** containers are especially hazardous, because the spray sends tiny droplets of lye and ammonia into the air, where they can easily be inhaled or land in your eyes or on your skin.

Be especially wary of oven cleaners that advertise "no fumes." I have tried several brands, and all still smelled very strongly of ammonia.

SAFE SOLUTIONS

If you are like me, you probably hate to clean your oven. It is possible to never have to clean your oven if you are very careful about not allowing things to spill. If your casserole seems like it might spill over during baking, put a cookie sheet or sheet of aluminum foil on the lower rack. On those rare occasions when something does end up on the bottom of the oven instead of on your plate, wipe it up as soon as the oven is cooled, to prevent it from baking on even more.

Still, accidents do happen. I know of no commercial nontoxic oven cleaners, but I'll give you a tip from a friend of mine who runs her own nontoxic cleaning service and refuses to use chemicals. Here's how Gina cleans ovens.

Mix together in a spray bottle 2 tablespoons liquid soap (not detergent), 2 teaspoons borax, and warm water to fill the bottle. Make sure the salts are completely dissolved to avoid clogging the squirting mechanism. Spray it on, holding the bottle very close to the oven surface so the solution doesn't get into the air (and into your eyes and lungs). Even though these are natural ingredients, this solution is designed to cut heavy-duty oven grime, so wear gloves and glasses or goggles, if you have them. Leave the solution on for 20 minutes, then scrub with steel wool and a nonchlorine scouring powder. Rub impossible, baked-on black spots with pumice, available in a stick at hardware stores.

If you have an extremely dirty oven layered with years of baked-on grease, you may have to use a chemical oven cleaner *once* to get it clean before you can begin your nontoxic maintenance. For this *one* application, choose a nonaerosol product and follow these precautions from the Consumer Product Safety Commission for safer use of oven cleaners.

- Read the directions before each use, and follow them.
- Wear protective gloves and goggles.
- Open windows in the kitchen, and be sure that children and other members of the family are out of the room.
- If you use an oven cleaner that requires boiling water, place the can in the oven before adding boiling water, so that you will not be overcome by ammonia fumes.
- If the fumes begin to affect you, close the oven door, leave the room, and get fresh air.

FURNITURE AND FLOOR POLISHES

> **DANGER:** Harmful or fatal if swallowed. Keep out of reach of children.

Regarding furniture and floor polishes, both accidental ingestion and inhalation of fumes during normal use (especially if an aerosol spray is used) are harmful. In addition, some of the more toxic ingredients can be easily absorbed through the skin. The primary danger is from exposure during use, but once it's on the furniture, polish can give off residual fumes.

Phenol, suspected of causing cancer in humans, is used in many furniture and floor polishes. Allowing phenol to touch your skin can cause it to swell, peel, burn, or break out in hives and pimples. A small amount of phenol, taken internally, can cause circulatory collapse, convulsions, cold sweats, coma, and death. Keep this chemical away from your body!

Another chemical frequently used in furniture and floor polishes is **nitrobenzene,** which is extremely toxic and easily absorbed by the skin. An accidental spill on the skin can cause skin discoloration, shallow breathing, vomiting, and death. Repeated exposure can cause cancer, genetic changes, birth defects, and damage to heart, liver, kidney, and central nervous system.

Because furniture and floor polishes are labeled "Harmful or fatal if swallowed," I would think these products could contain enough of these toxic chemicals to kill. Do you really want this stuff around your kids? Remember, younger children can't read warning labels. What could happen when one day they decide to surprise you by polishing the furniture?

Furniture and floor polishes might also contain harmful **acrylonitrile, ammonia, detergents, artificial fragrances, naphtha,** and **petroleum distillates,** and may be dispensed as **aerosol sprays.**

SAFE SOLUTIONS

It's easy to make your own furniture polish. The active ingredient in most polishes is plain mineral oil, which you can purchase at a drugstore and apply sparingly with a soft cloth. Mineral oil is an odorless petrochemical product that is relatively safe to use; its only real danger comes from repeated, regular ingestion. You'll be using the same active ingredient without all the extra solvents and perfumes. If you like lemon-scented polish, you can add 1 teaspoon of lemon oil to 2 cups mineral oil.

The idea behind furniture polish is to get an oil absorbed into the wood, but it doesn't matter what kind of oil you use. It could be any oil, even one right in your kitchen cabinet. I just use plain mayonnaise. Just open the bottle, put a little on a soft cloth, and rub it in. Your furniture will smell like a sandwich for a few minutes, but the odor disappears quickly and the mayonnaise leaves a soft, nonsticky finish.

You can also mix your own "salad dressing" polishes.

- 1 teaspoon olive oil, mixed with the juice of 1 lemon, 1 teaspoon brandy or whiskey, and 1 teaspoon water (make fresh each time)
- 3 parts olive oil mixed with 1 part white vinegar
- 2 parts olive or vegetable oil mixed with 1 part lemon juice
- For oak: Boil 1 quart beer with 1 tablespoon sugar and 2 tablespoons beeswax. Cool, wipe onto wood, and allow to dry. Polish when dry with a chamois cloth

Don't worry about the odors any of these natural polishes might leave. The food smells quickly dissipate, and they don't become rancid.

SILVER POLISHES AND OTHER METAL CLEANERS

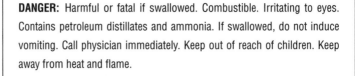

DANGER: Harmful or fatal if swallowed. Combustible. Irritating to eyes. Contains petroleum distillates and ammonia. If swallowed, do not induce vomiting. Call physician immediately. Keep out of reach of children. Keep away from heat and flame.

The main chemicals of concern in metal cleaners are **ammonia,** which can burn the skin and produce irritating vapors, and unknown **petroleum distillates.** "Petroleum distillates" is not the name of a particular chemical, but rather of a whole group of chemicals of varying toxicity that are made by distilling petroleum. We have no way of knowing which petroleum distillate may be used in this product; all we are told is that it is fatal if swallowed. Since the manufacturer is required to warn on the label only of the dangers of accidental ingestion, we do not know if the vapors of this product might also be harmful, or if it can be absorbed through the skin.

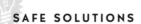

SAFE SOLUTIONS

It is so easy to remove tarnish from silver without chemicals, I can't imagine why anyone would want to use smelly polish! Instead of rubbing for hours, you can *magnetize* tarnish away. I've been recommending this method since my very first book, and recently saw a Magic Silver Cleaning Kit being advertised on late-night TV for only $19.95 (consisting of a sheet of aluminum and "magic crystals").

Here's how you can perform this trick at home for only pennies. The basic ingredients needed are aluminum (either in the form of a pot, pan, or aluminum foil) and some kind of salt (table salt, rock salt, or baking soda work fine). In the salty water, the aluminum will act as a magnet and attract the tarnish away from the silver. After submerging the pieces of silver for a few minutes in water containing both the aluminum and salt, you can literally wipe them dry and the tarnish will be gone (badly tarnished silver may need to go through the process several times). There are many ways this can be done. Here are a few methods you can try to see which is most convenient for you.

- For very large items, such as trays or candelabra, run very hot water into your kitchen sink and add a sheet of aluminum foil and a handful of salt. Let sit for 2 or 3 minutes, then rinse and dry.

- For silverware, put a sheet of aluminum foil in the bottom of a pan, then add 2 or 3 inches of water, 1 teaspoon salt, and I teaspoon baking soda. Bring to a boil, then add silver pieces, making sure water totally covers the silver. Boil another 2 or 3 minutes. Remove from pan, rinse, and dry.

- For small items, such as jewelry, fill a glass jar half full with thin strips of aluminum foil. Add 1 tablespoon salt and cold water to fill the jar. Keep covered. To use, simply drop small items into the jar for a few minutes, then remove, rinse, and dry.

Washington Toxics Coalition reports that this mixture gives off toxic **hydrogen sulfide.** However, I have used this method for years and never noticed any odor or experienced ill effects.

Vermont Country Store sells cotton "silvercloth," which is embedded with silver particles and somehow acts like magic to prevent tarnish. I remember my grandmother taking the silver out of zippered bags of silvercloth, then returning them to their bags after our Sunday dinner. Often these old ways are still the best.

To clean brass and copper, use lemon juice. Rub it on with a soft cloth, rinse with water, and dry. If this doesn't work, try applying one of the following mixtures using lemon juice:

- Make a paste of lemon juice and salt.
- Sprinkle a slice of lemon with baking soda.

- Make a paste of lemon juice and cream of tartar. Apply and leave on for 5 minutes before you rinse with warm water and dry.

If you don't have a lemon around the house, other kitchen staples clean brass and copper equally well: hot white vinegar mixed with salt; hot buttermilk; hot sour milk; tomato juice; and Worcestershire sauce.

Brass will look brighter and need polishing less often if rubbed with a bit of olive oil after each cleaning.

Clean chrome by wiping it with a soft cloth dipped in apple cider vinegar, or by rubbing with a lemon peel. Rinse with water and dry with a soft cloth.

There are a few nontoxic metal polishes on the market; Washington Toxics Coalition recommends **Twinkle.** Check labels of polishes at your local supermarket and hardware store. If the polish is toxic, it is required by law to contain a warning label. Those without warnings are probably relatively safe.

AMMONIA AND OTHER ALL-PURPOSE CLEANERS

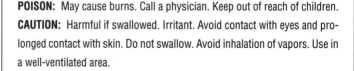

> **POISON:** May cause burns. Call a physician. Keep out of reach of children.
> **CAUTION:** Harmful if swallowed. Irritant. Avoid contact with eyes and prolonged contact with skin. Do not swallow. Avoid inhalation of vapors. Use in a well-ventilated area.

Ammonia is great for attacking household grease and grime, but it also attacks the skin—rashes, redness, and chemical burns during exposure are common. Because it is a very volatile chemical, its fumes are extremely irritating to eyes and lungs. Ammonia fumes can be especially harmful to anyone with respiratory problems. Children with colds or bronchitis and those with asthma will have greater difficulty breathing with ammonia in the air. Ammonia also can cause severe eye damage if it is accidentally splashed in your eye or if you absentmindedly rub your eyes with ammonia on your hands.

If products come in **aerosol spray** cans, the risk is increased, as the spray makes it much more likely that actual droplets of ammonia will end up on your skin and in your eyes and lungs.

SAFE SOLUTIONS

Create your own all-purpose cleaning solutions by mixing various natural substances together in proportions and combinations that reflect the type of cleaning job. Start by mixing one teaspoon of any one or more of the following into one quart warm or hot water in a spray bottle or bucket: TSP (use for heavy-duty cleaning), liquid soap, or borax. Add a squeeze of lemon juice or a splash of vinegar to cut grease.

If you want to buy a less toxic commercial preparation, your natural-food store should have a selection of soap-based all-purpose cleaners that do not contain ammonia.

BASIN, TUB, AND TILE CLEANERS

> **WARNING:** Causes eye and skin irritation. Vapors may irritate. Use only in a well-ventilated area. Do not get in eyes or on clothing. Avoid prolonged breathing of vapors. Not recommended for use by persons with chronic heart conditions or chronic respiratory problems such as asthma, emphysema, or obstructive lung disease. Harmful if swallowed. For prolonged use, wear gloves. Keep out of reach of children.
>
> **CHEMICAL HAZARD:** Contains bleach. Do not mix with other household chemicals such as ammonia, toilet bowl cleaners, rust removers, vinegar, or acid. To do so will release hazardous gases.

Bathroom cleaners are made from the same ingredients as other all-purpose cleaners—**ammonia, detergents, artificial fragrances,** and **aerosol propellants**—and have similar dangers. Note that they should only be used in well-ventilated areas. How many bathrooms are well ventilated or even have windows? And how many people do the logical thing and take the spray bottle of tile cleaner into the shower with them, further confining ventilation behind a shower curtain or glass door?

SAFE SOLUTIONS

A sprinkle of baking soda works great to bring sparkle and shine to bathroom surfaces (follow with a hot water rinse if you're concerned about killing germs). Or use a nonchlorinated scouring powder such as one of the **Bon Ami** products. To remove mold or mildew from the bathroom, see below.

MOLD AND MILDEW CLEANERS

> **DANGER:** Eye irritant. Keep out of reach of children. Use only in well-ventilated area.

Mold and mildew cleaners may contain **phenol, kerosene,** or **pentachlorophenol,** all of which may be harmful through skin absorption or inhalation, or fatal if swallowed. These products also may contain **formaldehyde,** suspected of causing cancer in humans and a strong irritant to eyes, throat, skin, and lungs.

The labels warn that mold and mildew cleaners are a dangerous eye irritant, yet they are another product usually packaged in either pump or **aerosol spray** containers, sending the harmful mist into the air.

SAFE SOLUTIONS

Prevent mold growth by creating an environment in which it cannot live. Mold grows in dark, damp places, so keep rooms dry and light. During wet winters, you may have to keep the heat on if you live in a shaded area, next to a creek, or in any especially moist location.

You can make your own mold and mildew cleaner by mixing borax and water, or vinegar and water, in a spray bottle. Spray it on and the mold wipes right off. Borax also inhibits mold growth, so you might try washing down the walls in your bathroom with a borax solution and just leaving it on, or sprinkling borax in damp cabinets under the sink.

If you have a major mold problem, the best solution is to use heat. Put a portable electric heater in the room (any inexpensive quartz heater from the hardware store will work), turn it up to the highest setting, close the door, and let it bake all day. The mold will dry up into a powder that brushes right off. Please use caution and common sense when employing this method. Check on the heater periodically, and do not leave the heater on overnight or while you are away from your home. For concentrated areas, use a hand-held hair dryer to dry up the mold in just a few minutes.

Allowing air to circulate also will help keep things dry. Hang clothes so there is space between them, and if you don't launder clothing damp with perspiration, at least allow it to dry before putting it back in the closet. Always hang wet towels after bathing to allow space for wetness to evaporate before throwing them in the hamper. If you have the space in your bathroom, get into the habit of hanging up your wet towel after bathing, then replacing it with a fresh one right before your next bath or shower. Check the walls behind the furniture to see if mold is growing there, and rearrange furniture, if necessary, to allow plenty of air flow. Small fans can increase air flow, if needed.

DISINFECTANTS

CAUTION: Keep out of reach of children. Keep away from heat, sparks, and open flame. Keep out of eyes. Avoid contact with food.

Disinfectants contain a number of volatile chemicals that are dangerous to inhale. The ingredient most frequently found in disinfectants is **cresol,** a chemical easily absorbed through the skin and through the mucous membranes of the respiratory tract. Cresol can cause damage to the liver, kidneys, lungs, pancreas, and spleen, and also can affect the central nervous system, resulting in such common symptoms as depression, irritability, and hyperactivity. Experts warn that there is danger of poisoning by both ingestion and inhalation. Disinfectants pose a hazard even in their closed containers, since vapors can leak out and build up to high levels in closed rooms. Disinfectants also may contain other toxic germ killers: **phenol, ethanol, formaldehyde, ammonia,** and **chlorine.**

Ironically, most of us use a disinfectant when there is an illness in the family, just when the sick person is most vulnerable to toxic effects. Some people are so concerned about cleanliness that they overdisinfect and are constantly surrounded by that "fresh, clean smell"—actually dangerous fumes.

SAFE SOLUTIONS

You may not even need to use a disinfectant. Like the television commercials say, disinfectants will "kill germs on contact." They can *reduce* the *number* of germs but will not kill *all* germs present, only some of them. Germs are very friendly with one another and will quickly multiply soon after disinfecting.

If you want to eliminate disease-causing bacteria and viruses, you must sterilize items by immersing them in boiling water. To reduce germs on large surfaces (such as walls or floors), try using a solution of one-half cup borax dissolved in one gallon hot water.

Regular cleaning with plain soap and water will keep germs under control. Even just a rinse of hot water will kill some bacteria. And keep things dry—bacteria, mildew, and mold cannot live without dampness.

If, for some reason, you need a liquid disinfectant, the safest I know of is an aqueous solution of benzalkonium chloride 1:750 (available at drugstores under the brand name Zephirin). It is usually used for medical purposes, but it can be substituted for any liquid disinfectant and produces far fewer fumes.

RUG, CARPET, AND UPHOLSTERY SHAMPOOS

> **CAUTION:** Do not take internally. In case of eye contact, flush thoroughly with water. Keep out of reach of children.

The active ingredient likely to be found in most rug, carpet, and upholstery shampoos is **perchloroethylene,** a solvent commonly used as a spot remover. It is a known human carcinogen, and its immediate effects can be light-headedness, dizziness, sleepiness, nausea, tremors, loss of appetite, and feelings of disorientation. Long-term exposure may result in damage to the liver or central nervous system.

Rug, carpet, and upholstery cleaners may also contain **naphthalene,** which, according to *The Condensed Chemical Dictionary,* is "toxic by inhalation." Headaches, confusion, nausea and vomiting, excessive sweating, and urinary irritation can all result from exposure. Naphthalene is also suspected of causing cancer in humans. **Ethanol, ammonia,** and **detergents** are other common ingredients in these products.

Rug, carpet, and upholstery shampoos frequently leave residues after use. While I have heard no reports of the possible health effects from exposure to these residues, I don't think I would want my baby to be crawling around on a carpet cleaned with such dangerous substances.

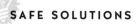 SAFE SOLUTIONS

The safest carpet cleaners on the market are those with a baking-soda base, but these are really only scented baking soda in fancy packages. Regular unscented baking soda works just as well, is less expensive, and doesn't contain **artificial fragrance,** which contributes to indoor air pollution.

To deodorize your carpets with baking soda, sprinkle it liberally over the entire carpet (make sure the carpet is dry first). By "liberally," I mean it should look as if it had snowed on the carpet. You will need several pounds for a nine-by-twelve-foot room. Wait fifteen minutes or longer, then vacuum. You can even leave it on overnight. I tried this once with an old wool oriental area rug that had been sitting in my great-aunt's attic. It had that usual musty, moldy smell, and after two applications of the baking soda, the odor was entirely gone.

Wipe up spills immediately, before they become stains. Plain water will generally work, but if you need a stronger spot remover, try a solution of ¼ cup borax dissolved in 2 cups cold water, or undiluted vinegar or lemon juice. Carbonated water works well, too.

Here are some tips for removing specific stains.

- *Blood:* Gently sponge the stain with cold water, and dry with a towel. Repeat until stain is gone.
- *Grease:* Cover the stain with baking soda, rubbing lightly into the rug. Leave on for an hour, then brush off. Repeat as needed.
- *Grease and oil:* Cover spots with cornstarch. Wait an hour, then vacuum.
- *Ink:* Put cream of tartar on the stain and squeeze a few drops of lemon juice on top. Rub into the stain for a minute, brush off the powder with a clean brush, and sponge immediately with warm water. Repeat if needed. If the ink is still wet, immediately put a mound of table salt on the wet spot. Let it sit for a few moments, then brush up. Continue to reapply and remove until all moisture is absorbed and the stain is bleached out.
- *Soot:* Cover the stain thickly with salt, then sweep it up carefully.
- *Urine:* Rinse with warm water, then apply a solution of 3 tablespoons white vinegar and 1 teaspoon liquid soap. Leave on for 15 minutes, then rinse and rub dry.

SPOT REMOVERS

> **CAUTION:** Eye irritant. Vapor harmful. Keep out of reach of children.

The most commonly used solvent in spot removers is **perchloroethylene,** the same solvent used in dry cleaning. Your major risk from perchloroethylene comes from exposure when actually using the product. Perchloroethylene fumes are carcinogenic, highly toxic, and can cause light-headedness, dizziness, sleepiness, nausea, loss of appetite, and disorientation. Exposure to large amounts of perchloroethylene fumes can be fatal.

SAFE SOLUTIONS

Spots are easiest to remove the minute they occur, so get in the habit of attacking spots when they happen, before they become stains.

One day many years ago, my literary agent invited me to join her for dessert at a luncheon she was having in a fancy restaurant with an important editor from a major publishing house. I ordered an ice cream creation that was swimming in a pool of bittersweet chocolate sauce. I took one bite and the entire scoop of ice cream landed on the skirt of my red cotton corduroy dress. My agent immediately ordered a bottle of club soda and doused my dress thoroughly. It didn't all come out, but when I washed it later in plain soap and water, the chocolate stain disappeared.

You can make your own good, all-purpose spot remover by dissolving ¼ cup borax in 2 cups cold water. Sponge it on and let it sit until it dries, or soak the fabric before washing in soap and cold water. This works well for blood, chocolate, coffee, mildew, mud, and urine.

Try this for fruit juice or tea stains: Stretch the fabric over a basin and pour boiling water over the stain.

Glycerin works well to soften some spots—grass or milk, for example. It is a by-product of soap manufacture and is available at most drugstores. Glycerin soap will also work. Try rubbing grass or milk stains with glycerin and rinsing with warm water.

Undiluted vinegar or lemon juice may also work to remove some spots.

These alternatives to using chemical spot removers are worth trying, especially since chemical spot removers are so dangerous to use.

DRY CLEANING

Many garments, made from both natural and synthetic fibers, are labeled "Dry clean only."

Dry cleaning isn't really "dry"; instead of detergent and water, items are "washed" with detergent and a solvent that removes spots and stains without being absorbed by the fiber. Dry-cleaned fabrics don't shrink or stretch, dyes don't fade or run, delicate fabrics don't tear or waterspot, and wools don't mat.

Perchloroethylene (perc) is the most popular dry-cleaning solvent in use today. Inhaling fumes from this solvent can cause cancer, liver damage, depression of the central nervous system, light-headedness, dizziness, sleepiness, nausea, loss of appetite, and disorientation.

Other toxic chemicals that also may be used in the dry-cleaning process are **benzene, chlorine, formaldehyde, naphthalene, trichloroethylene,** and **xylene**.

SAFE SOLUTIONS

Do dry-cleaned items pose a hazard? Yes and no. Inhaling perchloroethylene fumes is dangerous, but perchloroethylene is a very volatile substance that evaporates thoroughly, leaving no residue. Dry-cleaned items do go through a drying process, but many times the items are still damp when covered with their protective plastic. Studies done by the Environmental Protection Agency listed fumes from slightly damp dry-cleaned items as a common indoor air pollutant. The solution is simple: As soon as you bring home dry-cleaned items, remove the plastic covering (tie it in a knot and dispose of it in a place where babies won't find it and accidentally suffocate while playing with it) and hang the item in a well-ventilated area (preferably outdoors) to encourage evaporation of the solvent. This could take up to a week, and the warmer it is, the faster the solvent will dry. If you have an extra room in your home, you might want to set up a space where items that have just been dry-cleaned can be hung near a small space heater. Close the door to keep fumes out of the rest of the house, and then open windows in the extra room to ventilate the solvent fumes to the outside.

You might decide that you don't want to dry-clean everything marked "Dry clean only," and that's okay, too. These labels frequently are sewn into items that don't really need dry cleaning; manufacturers just recommend dry cleaning out of fear that the consumer will complain the garment is inferior after they wash it incorrectly. Even professional dry cleaners agree that you can wash almost anything without harm—if you know how to do it.

Wash cotton garments by just throwing them into the washing machine with natural soap, borax, baking soda, and/or sodium hexametaphosphate (see Chlorine Bleach). Wash whites in hot water and colors in warm water to prevent colors from fading. About a tablespoon of white vinegar per tub of laundry also will help keep colors colorfast. Using borax in the wash will help retard the formation of mildew. Dry cottons in medium heat to prevent shrinking, and remove them from the dryer as soon as they are dry to minimize wrinkles.

Linen also can be tossed in the washing machine. Pretend it's a colored cotton and follow the same instructions. Remove from the dryer and press while it's still damp.

Washing silk fabrics in the washer or by hand generally is discouraged, but when I used to wear silk shirts I always washed them by hand and they all turned out fine. Wash each item separately by swishing it around in a basin of very cold water with a bit of mild soap. Do not rub. Rinse with cold water and gently remove excess water by rolling the fabric in a towel. Let silk garments drip dry in the shower stall, and then press them with a warm (not hot), dry iron. If the label says "Washable Silk," the garment can go in the washer *and* dryer (though I've never tried this myself).

Hand wash wool in cool or lukewarm water (to prevent shrinkage) with mild soap or a few tablespoons of vinegar. Sweaters and knits should be reshaped on a towel to their original size while still damp. Roll up the sweater in the towel to absorb excess moisture, then dry by hanging it over the back of a wooden chair or over a towel bar.

Instead of taking your down jacket or sleeping bag to the dry cleaner, you can wash it in your bathtub with warm water and mild soap or baking soda. Dry it in a tumble dryer at a cool temperature.

A "dry-cleaning" product of sorts is Sweater Fresh (available by mail from **Natural Lifestyle**). Just spray garments, toss them in the dryer, and tumble for a few minutes. Garments come out clean and fresh without washing, soaking, or dry cleaning. Works on cotton, wool, rayon, and silk, and can be used on blankets and pillows.

The future of professional garment care seems to be a move away from toxic dry cleaning to nontoxic "wet cleaning." Indeed, the industry may be forced to make this change for economic reasons. It seems that perc can migrate right through the walls of dry-cleaning establishments and contaminate the products of the stores next door. Consequently, supermarkets are starting to refuse dry cleaners as neighbors, so if cleaning establishments want to stay where the customers are, they are going to have to change their ways.

Wet cleaning combines hand washing, spot cleaning, steaming, and high-tech washing machines (using only special detergents and water) and clothes dryers. These machines are much more sophisticated than your home washing machine They use computer microprocessed agitation so that fabrics don't become tangled and lose shape, and microsensors measure moisture content so garments can be removed from the dryers before they shrink. To find a wet cleaner in your area, contact **Aqua Clean Systems**.

CHLORINE BLEACH

> **CAUTION:** Keep out of reach of children. May be harmful if swallowed or may cause severe eye irritation. Never mix chlorine bleach with cleaning products containing ammonia, or with vinegar. *The resulting chloramine fumes are deadly.* It also should not be used on silk, wool, mohair, leather, spandex, or on any natural fiber that is not colorfast, as it can damage or discolor the fabric and cause colors to run.

While the greatest danger of chlorine bleach is accidental ingestion, the fumes inhaled during use also pose a hazard. Product labels warn only against drinking liquid bleach, but toxicology books report that chlorine is "toxic as a [skin] irritant and by inhalation." Even though the amount of fumes released is well within recognized safety limits, many people report adverse reactions to chlorine fumes at these low levels and even to chlorine residues left in fabrics after laundering.

SAFE SOLUTIONS

I use sodium hexametaphosphate instead of bleach. This pure mineral powder makes "your whites whiter" and "your brights brighter" by dissolving the mineral deposits and soap scum that make fabrics look dull and dingy.

To give you some idea of how well this works, before I was married I asked a former boyfriend to not bleach his clothes with chlorine bleach because the residue left on his clothes made me sneeze every time I got near him. So he followed my washing instructions, but began to complain after a few months that his shirts weren't "white" enough (dull, dingy, soap-scum buildup). As a businessman, he needed "bright-white" shirts to wear with his three-piece suits. I was experimenting with sodium hexametaphosphate at the time and gave him some. He loved it! It solved the problem with one washing, and he still uses it (even though he's now married to someone else).

To use sodium hexametaphosphate, add ¼ to 1 cup per 5 gallons of water, depending on water hardness, in your regular wash to prevent dulling film from forming. To determine the proper amount you should use, start with ⅛ cup sodium hexametaphosphate in a washerload of water and keep adding until the water feels slippery between your fingers. After adding the sodium hexametaphosphate, add half the amount of soap you normally would use.

To remove years of accumulated detergent film from laundry, run the items through a whole wash cycle using twice as much sodium hexametaphosphate as you would normally use, and no soap or detergent.

As a second choice, buy a powdered nonchlorine bleach, available in the laundry section of any supermarket or natural-food store. This product contains sodium perborate or borax as a bleaching agent instead of chlorine. This is a big improvement over chlorine bleach, but it still contains some ingredients, such as **artificial fragrance,** that you may want to avoid if you are allergic.

LAUNDRY DETERGENTS

> **DANGER:** In case of eye contact, get prompt medical attention. Keep out of reach of children.
> **WARNING:** Harmful if swallowed, irritating to eyes and skin. Keep out of reach of children.
> **CAUTION:** May be harmful if swallowed.

Manufacturers don't agree on how harmful laundry detergents might be, and some detergents with similar formulas have no warning at all on the label.

It can't be said too often that detergents cause more household poisonings than any other household product, most often when children accidentally ingest colorful powders packaged in easy-to-open boxes.

A lesser hazard comes from the residues left on clothing and bedsheets, which can cause severe skin rashes, or from "springtime fresh" fragrances that linger long after articles are laundered. There have also been reports of flu and asthma symptoms associated with breathing air that contains detergent dust.

SAFE SOLUTIONS

Detergents were developed especially to clean synthetic fibers and are unnecessary on natural fibers such as cotton, linen, silk, and wool. These can be washed using laundry products made with natural soap.

There is a big difference between detergent and soap. Detergents are formulated from **petrochemicals** and may contain **bleaches, synthetic whiteners,** and **artificial fragrances.** Some detergents have been banned because of the environmental hazards they create. Soap, on the other hand, is made from natural minerals and fats and has been used with no ill effects for hundreds of years.

Natural soap flakes are available at many supermarkets and natural-food stores, or you can grate bar soap to use in the laundry. You can also order soap-based laundry compounds from **Cal Ben Soap Company** and **Soapworks**.

One problem with soap that our grandmothers encountered was that it can leave a residual scum on fabrics. However, this can be remedied by washing garments with sodium hexametaphosphate (see page 95).

You don't always need to use soap to get clothes clean. Often, the purpose of laundering is not so much to dispel dirt as to freshen clothing and remove perspiration and odors. For this you can use about a cup of plain baking soda, white vinegar, or borax (available in the cleaning-products section of your supermarket), or a tablespoon of trisodium phosphate (sold at hardware stores) per washerload of clothes. All these natural substances are excellent for removing smells, and they don't add any odors of their own.

Another solution is a new product that may revolutionize the way we do laundry. It's just a simple disk that you drop into your washing machine with your clothes. Metallic elements, including silver and copper, in the activated ceramics release electrons, which in turn produce ionized oxygen. This form of oxygen breaks up dirt and organic compounds, turning plain water into a natural cleanser. I have never used it myself, but I have seen piles of testimonials that say it really does work (everybody is skeptical at first). It costs about $49 for three disks, which last for 500 laundry loads or more. I haven't seen it in stores, but you can order it from **The Living Source, The Natural Choice, Nontoxic Environments, Real Goods,** and probably many other mail-order catalogs. I wouldn't be surprised to find them advertised on television one day soon.

FABRIC SOFTENERS

> **CAUTION:** Keep out of reach of children.

Fabric softeners leave a residue on fabrics to control static cling. They never really wash out, so you are constantly exposed whenever you are in contact with a fabric. Residues can be very irritating to skin, and can cause allergic reactions such as stuffy nose and watery eyes.

Fabric softeners also are usually very strongly scented. People with allergies to perfume should be particularly careful about using these products.

SAFE SOLUTIONS

Fabric softener is one of those products that didn't even exist before synthetic fibers became popular. They were developed solely to reduce static cling that builds up on synthetic fabrics. If you wear natural fibers, you don't need to use fabric softeners at all, because there is no problem with static cling. Go through your closet, separate your natural fibers from synthetics, and at least refrain from using fabric softener in your natural-fiber laundry. If you have lots of natural/synthetic blends, try laundering them without fabric softener and see if you really need to use it.

If you find you do need a fabric softener, the safest and most convenient type is the unscented sheet variety that goes into the dryer, rather than liquid added to the wash (which might be accidentally swallowed) or an aerosol spray that is applied to dry cloths (which could end up in your eyes or lungs).

Baking soda added during the rinse cycle also acts as a fabric softener.

SPRAY STARCH

> **CAUTION:** Contents under pressure. Keep out of reach of children.

Spray starch is not generally considered to be an especially toxic product, and the label warning reflects this, pointing out only the dangers of the aerosol can.

Spray starch may contain such toxic chemicals as **formaldehyde, phenol,** and **pentachlorophenol,** but probably the biggest danger in using a spray starch comes from the mechanics of the spray. The **aerosol spray** is used to distribute the harmful chemicals mixed with a fine cornstarch powder, which could end up in eyes and lungs. Not that cornstarch is harmful, but it is a particle and could act as a carrier for the other, more harmful substances.

SAFE SOLUTIONS

You can make starch by dissolving one tablespoon of cornstarch in one pint of cold water. That's all the commercial spray starches are—just a little cornstarch mixed with chemicals. Pour the mixture into a spray bottle and squirt to apply (shake before using).

I don't even use starch. Most of my clothes are cotton, and I like the softness of the unstarched fabric against my skin. I have found that if I want my cotton shirts to look "crisp," I can take freshly laundered items to a dry-cleaning establishment, where I can request "press only—no starch" for a nominal fee. The high heat of their pressing machines adds a certain "hold" to the fabric that I can never achieve with my iron at home (and besides, I don't have to iron them myself).

DISHWASHER DETERGENTS

> **CAUTION:** Injurious to eyes. Harmful if swallowed. Avoid contact with eyes, mucous membranes, and prolonged skin contact. Keep out of reach of children.

As with many other cleaning products, the primary danger of dishwasher detergent is accidental ingestion and, to a lesser degree, exposure during use. Most dishwasher detergents contain **chlorine** in a dry form that is activated when it comes into contact with water in the dishwasher, releasing chlorine fumes into the air, which leak out of the dishwasher and into the kitchen. While low levels of chlorine are considered safe for the most part, many people report such symptoms as headache, fatigue, burning eyes, and difficulty breathing when exposed to even the small amount of chlorine released during normal dishwashing.

Also, a very thin film of detergent can remain on the washed dishes. Run a load of dishes through your dishwasher and compare them to dishes washed by hand. You may be able to see, smell, feel, or even taste the difference. If there is a residue, you are ingesting dishwasher detergent in small amounts every time you eat or drink. The long-term health effects are unknown.

SAFE SOLUTIONS

Using sodium hexametaphosphate in your dishwasher works well. The same substance that can be used as a bleach substitute, this mild mineral powder dissolves grease and doesn't leave water spots on the glasses. Its one disadvantage is that it won't remove dried-on food, but for regular washing, it works just as well as any commercial chlorinated brand.

Or, mix two tablespoons of baking soda with two tablespoons of borax (or premix baking soda and borax fifty-fifty, and use four tablespoons in your dishwasher).

You could also try some of the few brands of dishwasher detergent that do not give off strong chlorine fumes, such as those you can order from *Cal Ben Soap Company* and *Soapworks* (also look in the cleaning-products section of your local natural-foods store). These still should be stored safely and used with caution, as they may contain other harmful ingredients.

Never use dishwashing liquid as a substitute in a dishwasher, as the bubbles can clog the drain and inhibit the action of the water spray.

GLASS CLEANERS

Most glass cleaners are nothing more than **ammonia** mixed with water and a little **blue dye.** It is interesting that ammonia bottles are labeled "Poison," yet glass cleaners have no warning labels at all! Glass cleaners containing ammonia can release highly irritating fumes and can cause eye damage if accidentally sprayed into the eye.

Glass cleaners in **aerosol spray** containers are even more dangerous, because the aerosol spray distributes tiny droplets of ammonia into the air, where it can be easily inhaled or float into your eyes.

SAFE SOLUTIONS

Interestingly enough, *Consumer Reports* found that plain water is more effective than half the commercial glass cleaners on the market!

I am going to recommend only one glass cleaner. Because it works so well, I don't know why you would want to try anything else: fifty-fifty water and vinegar in a pump spray bottle (or you can apply it with a sponge from a bucket). I wipe it off with an old cotton terrycloth towel, but any rag (or even crumpled newspaper) will do. This works so well that you can now buy it in the supermarket mixed with a little **green dye,** but I prefer to make it myself.

You might run into one problem with this, and it will only happen the first time you use it. Some chemical glass cleaners contain a wax that can build up on the glass and cause it to streak terribly when you use vinegar and water. If you have been using this type of glass cleaner, you might have years of buildup that will have to be removed before you can use the natural cleaner. Use a little rubbing alcohol to get it off, and then you can clean your windows chemical-free!

Here are some additional window-cleaning tips.

- Never wash windows when the sun is shining directly on them; the cleaning solution will dry too fast and streak.

- When washing, use side-to-side strokes on one side, and up-and-down strokes on the other, so you can tell which side might need some extra polishing.

- *For foggy windows:* Wash windows with plain soap rubbed directly onto a soft, damp cloth. Rinse and dry. The soap will leave a transparent film that will make the water molecules bead up instead of sticking to the glass as a mist.

SCOURING POWDERS

Almost all scouring powders contain **chlorine** bleach, which acts as a whitener and stain remover. The powdered chlorine produces chlorine fumes when it comes in contact with water, which can be highly irritating to eyes, nose, throat, and lungs. Some people also experience headaches, fatigue, and difficulty breathing.

One warning that should be on the scouring-powder can (but isn't) is the same one you'll find on a chlorine-bleach bottle: *Never mix chlorine with ammonia; the resulting chloramine fumes can be deadly.* Ammonia is hidden in many cleaning products, so you may not always know that you're mixing them. You could, for instance, use an all-purpose cleaner with ammonia in your toilet bowl, then sprinkle in some scouring powder. The combination is of course less of a hazard than if you poured chlorine bleach into the toilet bowl with the ammonia; but even the level of chloramine fumes produced by ammonia and scouring powder could be dangerous, depending on your (or your child's) individual ability to tolerate these fumes.

Detergents and **talc** are also used in scouring powders. The danger of talc is that it may be contaminated with carcinogenic **asbestos,** and when you sprinkle scouring powder in your sink, a small amount always goes into the air and possibly into your lungs. There is *no* safe level for asbestos exposure.

SAFE SOLUTIONS

Dry baking soda, borax, or table salt sprinkled on a wet sponge acts as an effective abrasive for scouring.

Bon Ami Cleaning Powder and **Bon Ami Cleaning Cake** (available in many hardware stores) are made from nothing more than soap and ground feldspar. **Bon Ami Polishing Cleanser** (available in every supermarket) contains added nontoxic detergents and nonchlorine bleach.

AIR FRESHENERS AND ODOR REMOVERS

Most air fresheners don't "freshen" the air at all—they cover up the offensive odor with a more pleasant one, or interfere with your ability to smell by releasing a nerve-deadening agent or coating your nasal passages with an undetectable oil film.

While little (if any) scientific research has been done on the health effects of air fresheners, they are made from a number of chemicals known to be toxic in amounts larger than is found in an air freshener: **naphthalene, phenol, cresol, ethanol, xylene, and formaldehyde.** Many people with allergies and respiratory problems are bothered by the smell of air fresheners; the possible effects of long-term, low-level exposure to these chemicals is unknown.

SAFE SOLUTIONS

Air freshener is one of those products that is highly advertised but probably completely unnecessary.

You can rid your home of undesirable odors simply by opening a window or turning on a fan. This will also help reduce any toxic fumes that are building up indoors.

Track down odors in your home and find out what's causing

them. For mold smells, keep the area dry and light and, if necessary, use a small bag of silica gel (you can buy it at a camera store) to absorb excess moisture from the air. Silica gel changes color when it is saturated; you can reactivate it by drying it out in the oven. Just a note about silica gel: Many packets are labeled "Do not eat" and show a skull and crossbones. According to my local poison-control center, however, this is a "gross mislabeling . . . silica gel is inert and is no more dangerous to swallow than sand."

To reduce food smells, empty the garbage frequently and clean the can when needed. Sprinkle ½ cup borax in the bottom of the garbage can to inhibit the growth of odor-producing mold and bacteria.

If you have some heavy-duty odors to remove and don't want to get an air filter, try zeolite. Zeolites are a complex group of naturally occurring minerals, most of which are derived from the alteration of volcanic ash. They have a complex lattice structure made of hydrated aluminosilicate, which is arranged in a honeycomblike framework. These channels provide enormous internal surface areas within the zeolite crystals, which are lined with negatively charged ions and have a natural electrostatic attraction to positively charged pollutants.

The most common naturally occurring zeolite is the mineral clinoptilolite (chemical composition Na_2K_2,Ca).

It has been very successful in removing sulfur dioxide, hydrogen sulfide, formaldehyde, and ammonia, as well as many other intense and complex odors such as those found in locker rooms, nursing homes, beauty parlors, nail shops, and new cars, or from cigarette smoke, smoke damage, skunk odors, and mold and mildew. Zeolites also can pick up toxics such as cadmium, cobalt, copper, mercury, lead, and zinc, as well as radioactive materials.

The amount of zeolite you might need to solve an odor or gas problem depends on the amount of the pollutant present. One advantage to zeolite is that because heat causes the rock to release pollutant molecules, you can put your zeolite out in sun to renew it. Theoretically, it can be reused indefinitely, but it hasn't been in use long enough to determine what it's real lifespan might be. And, it's easy to tell when the zeolite needs a sunning—it will begin to smell.

You can order zeolite by mail from *Allergy Resources,* *Marge Smith,* and *Van Cleave & Associates.*

If you use air fresheners to scent the air, try natural fragrances, which are even more pleasant. Why not use the real thing—fresh flowers or pine boughs—to provide a delicate scent? Or you can make sachets of fragrant herbs and flowers. Go to the herb section of your natural-food store and sniff the different jars. I like the smell of ground cloves in my kitchen in the wintertime, and peppermint in the bathroom—just put them in a small basket or jar, or in a small sachet bag. You can also toss dried herbs into a pot of water simmering on the stove. The heat will release the fragrant essential oils. Beware of premixed, packaged potpourris—buy only those with natural scents. You can make your whole house smell wonderful, and it costs a lot less, too.

DISHWASHING LIQUIDS

Dishwashing liquid is just a liquid **detergent** with some **dye** and **artificial fragrance.** Some labels warn, "Do not use with chlorine bleach," indicating that they probably also contain **ammonia,** which, when mixed with chlorine, can produce harmful, if not fatal, fumes. There are no general warning labels, but it is still a detergent, and according to the Center for Science in the Public Interest, detergents are responsible for more household poisonings than any other household product. Their fruity smells are particularly attractive to children. Here's another case of a product we use daily and usually consider totally benign, which should actually be placed well out of the reach of children.

I am also concerned about the coloring used in liquid detergents. I have been unable to find any information that indicates these dyes are regulated for safety in any way. Dishwashing detergent is not a food, drug, or cosmetic, so these colors are not regulated by the FDA. The Consumer Product Safety Commission regulates cleaning products, but they are concerned only with the "hazardous ingredients." Some artificial dyes used in food products are allowed even though they are known to cause cancer; it makes me wonder about the safety of soaking your hands in these colors three times a day.

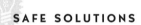

SAFE SOLUTIONS

Use a plain liquid soap, such as **Dr. Bronner's Pure Castile Soap,** available at most natural-food stores. Or you can rub your sponge with bar soap, although I have found that with this method you have to be very careful not to drop the dishes—they get very slippery!

If you like lemon-scented dishwashing liquid, use a few slices of fresh lemon in the dishwater. This will also act to help cut grease.

If you live in a hard-water area and you end up with water spots on your glasses, add a few teaspoons of sodium hexametaphosphate (order from a chemical supply house) to your dishwater and use only about half the amount of soap you would normally use. Your dishes will dry spotless!

Chapter 4

Home and Garden Pest Control

THE BEST WAY TO control pests is by natural means. Natural pest-control methods are even more effective than chemical pesticides because many pests are beginning to develop immunities to the chemicals. Some of our worst pests are now resistant to practically all our chemical weapons. So we come back to Mother Nature and common sense as our best defense.

Home and garden pesticides contain chemicals specially formulated to kill. Fly sprays, flea bombs, ant and roach killers, and rat and mouse poisons are used in or around 91 percent of all American households. In many ways our gardens are microcosms of agricultural methods; the same pesticides and fertilizers used by agribusiness are on our local nursery shelves, in smaller bottles with more appealing labels. According to the National Academy of Sciences, "suburban gardens and lawns receive heavier pesticide applications than most other land areas in the United States," including agricultural areas.

When we use pesticides and fertilizers in our gardens, we contaminate the land in our own yards, pollute our own water, and create invisible clouds of poison in our own air. A 1987 study under the auspices of the National Cancer Institute found that children who lived in households where outdoor pesticides were regularly used were six to nine times more likely to develop some forms of childhood leukemia; the figure increased four times when indoor pesticides were regularly used. In addition, our children or pets can accidentally ingest stored pesticides, with possibly fatal results.

Pesticides are the number-two cause of household poisonings in the United States. About 2.5 million children and adults are affected each year by such common household items as fly spray, ant and roach bait, and insect repellents, both from accidental ingestion of liquids in storage and inhalation of sprays during normal use. According to poison-control center reports on pesticide exposures, 70 percent of the incidents involve children less than five years of age, and more than half of those who die from pesticide-related incidents are children.

Of approximately 1,400 different active pesticide ingredients used in more than 35,000 formulations, more than 100 are known to cause cancer, birth defects, and mutagenic changes, although authorities believe there could be more, since most pesticides have not been adequately tested for these effects.

Pesticides are stored in the fatty tissue in the body, and can accumulate over time to dangerously high levels. When you exercise and burn fat or go on a weight reduction diet, pesticides are released into the bloodstream.

Immediate health effects from inhaling some common household pesticides during use include nausea, coughing, breathing difficulties, depression, eye irritation, dizziness, weakness, blurred vision, muscle twitching, and convulsions. Long-term exposure from repeated use and lingering residues can also damage the liver, kidneys, and lungs, and can cause paralysis, sterility, suppression of immune function, brain hemorrhages, decreased fertility and sexual function, heart problems, and coma.

Not only is a pesticide hazardous during the actual application, but residues can stay in an area for a very long time. Pesticides can remain active in the air for days or weeks; some can even last up to twenty years! When several types of pesticides are used, residues can intermingle, and when they combine, these become even more toxic. It's frightening to consider what toxic compound could be created from the pesticides in your food mixed with the pesticide residues in the air, mixed with pesticides in your tap water, mixed with your pet's flea collar, etc. Fortunately, we can choose not to use these potentially very harmful products.

Labeling

All pesticides, whether for home and garden or commercial use, are regulated by the Federal Insecticide, Fungicide, and Rodenticide Act (FIFRA). Although it was originally passed in 1947 to protect farmers from ineffective and dangerous pesticides, amendments in 1972 shifted the emphasis from safeguarding the pesticide user to public health and environmental protection. This act allows federal control of all pesticide applications and regulates both intrastate and interstate marketing and use of pesticides.

FIFRA is intended to insure that the use of a pesticide will not cause "any unreasonable risk to man or the environment, taking into account the economic, social, and environment costs and benefits of the use of any pesticide." Unfortunately, economic and social benefits have taken precedence over environmental and health costs in the past. Because there are safe, workable, and cost-effective alternatives available that make it unnecessary in most cases to use toxic pesticides at all, zero pesticides should be our goal, or at least minimal use of nontoxic pest controls.

Since October 1977, the EPA has required laboratory safety tests at the manufacturers' expense before any new pesticide is allowed on the market. Included must be tests for acute-exposure effects, the lethal dose in animals, and for cancer, genetic mutations, birth defects, and infertility under chronic exposure.

Pesticides that were in use before 1977, however, have not undergone such testing and still continue to be used. A further complication is that many of the safety tests on which earlier registrations were based were sloppy or fraudulent. In the early 1980s, Industrial BioTest, the nation's leading pesticide-testing laboratory at the time, was found to have faked many of its test results. So we can't even be sure of the safety of the pesticides that supposedly have been tested. In 1987, Consumers Union examined the EPA's records of fifty common household pesticides to see if the agency had enough data to determine their safety. In 72 percent of the cases, the EPA lacked this crucial information.

FIFRA requires that all pesticides be registered. It classifies pesticides for household or restricted use, gives the EPA power to ban harmful pesticides, and requires informative and accurate labeling.

Like hazardous cleaning products, pesticide labels must indicate the degree of toxicity by use of one of the following signal words:

- **Danger** (or **Poison,** with skull and crossbones): could kill an adult if only a tiny pinch is ingested

- **Warning:** could kill an adult if about a teaspoon is ingested

- **Caution:** will not kill until an amount from 1 ounce to 1 pint is ingested

But, as with cleaning products, the accuracy of these signal words cannot be relied on.

In addition, labels require precautionary statements and information on proper treatment in case of poisoning, what types of exposure require medical attention, what ways the pesticides might be poisonous to humans and domestic animals (though if it says nothing, don't assume it is completely safe), protective clothing or ventilation requirements, and environmental cautions such as if the pesticide will harm birds, fish, or wildlife (often precautions are given such as "Do not use near lakes or streams").

Also, the common or chemical name of the active ingredients must be listed, with the percentages of active ingredients and inert ingredients. Since October 1988, all EPA List One (toxic) inert ingredients must be labeled with the statement "This product contains the toxic inert ———." Inerts on List One are "of toxicological concern" because they cause cancer, have neurotoxic or other chronic effects, cause adverse reproductive effects, or have a particular toxic effect to the environment. If the name of the inert ingredient does not appear on the label, it might be a "potentially toxic inert with high priority for testing," an inert "of unknown toxicity," or an inert "of minimal concern." While the law does offer some protection, lack of cautionary labeling does not guarantee no toxic inerts are present.

Every pesticide on the market must be registered with the EPA (this registration number must be on the front panel of the label written as "EPA Registration No. ——"). A code for the factory that makes the pesticide (called the "establishment number") must also be on every container. Usually it can be found under the registration number.

Other requirements include the brand name, the common scientific name for the pesticide, the type of formulation (liquid, wettable powders, emulsifiable concentrations, dusts, etc.), child hazard warning ("Keep out of reach of children"), net contents, directions for use, a reminder that it is a violation of federal law to use a pesticide product in any manner inconsistent with its labeling, and name and address of the manufacturer.

The EPA was unable to furnish me with a list of pesticides used in household products, or examples of pesticides that fit into their signal-word categories. But here is a list of pesticides' relative toxicities from the book *Bugbusters: Getting Rid of Household Pests Without Dangerous Chemicals,* by Bernice Lifton (New York: McGraw-Hill Paperbacks, 1985), based on a list compiled by the University of California at Berkeley.

- *Most Dangerous:* aldicarb, carbofuran, demeton, disulfoton, fensulfothion, fonophos, methamidophos, mevinphos, parathion, phorate, schradan, TEPP

- *Dangerous:* aldrin, bufencarb, carbophenothion, chlorpyrifos, DDVP, dichlorvos, dicrotophos, dieldrin, dinitrocresol, dioxathion, DNOC, endrin, EPN, methyl parathion, mexacarbate, monocrotophos, nicotine, paraquat, pentachlorophenol, phosalone, phosphamidon, propoxur

- *Less Dangerous:* akton, azinphos-methyl, binapacryl, BHC, chlordane, chlordimeform, caumaphos, crotoxyphos, crufomate, diazinon, dicapthon, dichloroethyl ether, dimethoate, dinobuton, endosulfan, ethion, fenthion, heptachlor, lead arsenate, lindane, metam sodium, naled, oxydemeton methyl, phosmet, toxaphene, trichlorfon

- *Least Dangerous:* Captan, carbaryl, 2, 4-D, daminozide, DDT, dicofol, diquat, Malathion, maneb, naph-

thaleneacetic acid, oxythioquinox, perthane, pro-
pargite, quinomethionate, ronnel, rotenone, TDE,
temephos, tetrachlorvinphos, tetradifon

I found a general-purpose household pesticide spray on a
local supermarket shelf containing DDVP as its active ingredient.
It was labeled "Caution" by the EPA, but DDVP is listed as "Dangerous" on the University of California list (see above). It is ultimately not worth your effort to pick your way through this
semantic jungle to find out how dangerous a product is since effective, nonchemical alternatives are available.

SAFE SOLUTIONS

The keys to success in any natural pest control program for controlling pests in your home is to prevent pests from entering your
home in the first place and to make it impossible for them to live
there. If bugs are driving you nuts, it's probably because you are
putting out the welcome mat by providing them with perfect living conditions. If you don't take these two steps, the best you can
do is get rid of the pests temporarily, for they will return again and
again. But once you have pest-proofed your home, you will be
permanently protected from almost all unwelcome visitors.

The first thing to do is figure out how pests are getting into
your home, and do something to keep them out. For example, if
you have ants, follow the line of ants around to see where they're
coming in, then seal up the hole with white glue. They're sure to
find another entry point, but after a few days of keeping a sharp
lookout and wielding a swift glue bottle, you'll fill all your holes
and eliminate the ant problem for good. Also, you might need
screens on your windows to block flying insects.

Second, make your home an unpleasant place for pests to be:

- *Take away their food supply by keeping living areas
  clean.* Be especially careful to sweep up food
  crumbs, wipe up spills when they happen, wash
  dishes immediately, and deposit leftover food in its
  proper place. Store food in tightly closed, impenetrable metal or glass containers. Empty garbage
  cans frequently, and if necessary, accumulate

garbage in a plastic bag with a twist tie to eliminate the enticing odors of decaying food. Dispose of disposable diapers using good hygiene, as they, like food waste, attract pests.

- *Dry up their water supply.* Repair leaky faucets, pipes, and clogged drains. Insects have to drink somewhere—don't let poor plumbing turn your home into the "neighborhood bug bar."
- *Get rid of any clutter that they can hide in.* Clean out your attic, basement, and closets. Remove piles of old clothing, newspapers and magazines, and boxes. Check out-of-the-way places especially well (under stairwells, for instance), where unused items often get tossed.

You can eliminate the pests already living in your home with homemade potions of natural ingredients you probably already have right in your kitchen. Or you can use mechanical methods to control them, such as zapping them with extreme temperatures, using fragrances that are offending (to them, not to you!), or trapping them. These methods are more effective than chemicals, easier, and safer for children and pets.

In the garden, use "organic" methods. Organic gardening is based on an understanding of how nature creates healthy plants. The ultimate goal is to have a healthy living plant/soil ecosystem that does not need added pesticides of any kind, artificial or natural.

Organic gardening takes more awareness, study, and planning than gardening with artificial fertilizers and toxic pesticides and even to begin to describe its many methods is beyond the scope of this book. It's a skill to hone over a lifetime—there is much to learn. But I've found organic gardening to be a very rewarding pastime, and there are plenty of resources of information, tools, and supplies. Order these catalogs and dig in: **Bountiful Gardens, Real Goods, Gardener's Supply, Gardens Alive!, Harmony Farm Supply, The Natural Gardening Company,** and **Peaceful Valley Farm Supply. Acres, U.S.A.** and **agAccess** specialize in books on all aspects of organic gardening and agriculture.

LAWN CARE

Though no warnings are posted to alert us to their danger, some of the more toxic pesticides available are used routinely for lawn care. Pesticides commonly used on lawns are the insecticides **chlorpyrifos** and **Diazinon** (common name **Dursban** and others), the herbicides **2, 4-D** and **Banvel,** and the fungicides **benomyl** and **Daconil.** The adverse health effects associated with these pesticides are numerous.

More than four million American households pay up to two hundred dollars a year to have their lawns maintained with these hazardous chemicals.

The $1.5 billion lawn-care industry has grown dramatically in the last few years, thanks to the tanker spray truck. By premixing pesticides and fertilizer in large quantities and applying them from a nozzle, lawn-care companies can treat dozens of lawns each day during the entire season. This means that more pesticides and fertilizers than ever before are being applied on a regular basis within immediate neighborhoods. The chemicals evaporate into the air during and even after application, contaminating land and local water supplies.

Because lawn-chemical spraying is not just a personal hazard but a community hazard as well, many communities are adopting right-to-know ordinances that require the company that sprays to notify residents before spraying will take place and after spraying has occurred. Because of such ordinances, the industry is beginning to post signs voluntarily, but don't count on it.

Considering the health and environmental effects of lawn-care chemicals, it's ironic that chemical lawn care is not good even for the health of the lawn. While you may see improvements for the first two to four years, the lawn later begins to disintegrate.

On top of the pesticides, the act of mowing the lawn with a power mower also produces air pollution. In only a half-hour, a gas-powered lawn mower emits more exhaust than an automobile driven 187 miles! According to the EPA, 20 percent of our nation's air pollution is caused by power equipment used to tend lawns and gardens.

SAFE SOLUTIONS

Share these tips on natural lawn care with your neighbors to stop pesticide spraying in your neighborhood altogether:

- *Let your grass grow.* Close and frequent mowing weakens grass plants. Grass that is 2½ to 3 inches tall shades weed seedlings (preventing their growth) and holds moisture in the soil. Mow when the grass is dry and in the evening or cooler time of day, and keep your mower blade sharp. Leave nitrogen-rich grass clippings behind to degrade into soil-building compost. Rake up any large clumps to use for compost or mulch.

- *Fertilize naturally.* Grass clippings, compost, and manure return needed bacteria and enzymes, along with nutrients, to the soil. Include clover or other nitrogen-fixing plants in your lawn to make it self-fertilizing.

- *Cut dandelions* at the root, several inches below the ground, and reseed bare spots. Despite the advertising to the contrary, most won't grow back. Or just learn to live with them. They look bad only twice a year, and a quick mowing will solve that.

- *Dethatch* in late spring or early summer, then reseed.

- *Dry out fungus,* dethatch, add soil bacteria, and reseed. Fungus grows only in wet, thatchy, overfertilized lawns.

- *Aerate* twice a year (compacted soil promotes weeds). Add a soil loosener like compost or gypsum, then reseed.

- *Reseed* bare spots and thinning lawns to prevent weed growth.

- *Water* in the evening, deeply and infrequently. Allow the grass to dry thoroughly between waterings.

- *Choose the right species.* An 80:20 mix of fescue and rye grows well in most areas, although it is best to choose a grass native to your area. Pick varieties that resist drought and disease; need little mowing, fertilizer, or water; and are suited to available light and traffic.

- *Use your lawn space to grow a wildflower meadow,* an organic edible garden, or anything else you'd like.

Your local nursery may carry natural lawn-care products; also, ask if they know of a lawn-care company that uses natural methods. Or order lawn-care products by mail from **Gardens Alive!** and **Gardener's Supply.** You can purchase an old-fashioned manual-push reel lawnmower from **Gardener's Supply** and **Real Goods** (they also have gas-free solar-powered mowers).

GARDEN PESTICIDES

HAZARDS TO HUMANS AND DOMESTIC ANIMALS

CAUTION: Harmful if swallowed, inhaled, or absorbed through skin. Causes moderate eye injury. Avoid breathing spray mist. Avoid contact with eyes, skin, or clothing. Wash thoroughly with soap and water after handling. Wear a long-sleeved shirt and long-legged pants when spraying. Spray with the wind to your back. Do not spray on windy days. If clothing becomes wet from spray during use, remove clothing after spraying, wash affected body areas thoroughly with soap and water, and launder clothing before wearing again.

Do not use on household pets or humans. Do not allow children or pets to go onto a treated area until the treated area has dried. Do not contaminate fishponds. Food utensils such as spoons and measuring cups must not be used for food purpose after use in measuring pesticides. Keep out of reach of children. [A toll-free medical information number also must be provided.]

ENVIRONMENTAL HAZARDS: This pesticide is highly toxic to birds, fish, and other wildlife. Birds, especially waterfowl, feeding or drinking on treated area may be killed . . . [this warning label went on for several pages in a little booklet attached to the bottle].

We spend a lot of time and money, and create a lot of toxic dangers, trying to eradicate what we think of as garden pests, but actually many pests are beneficial. Insects seem to be Nature's way of picking up the garbage. Attracted by odors and electromagnetic signals put out by nutrient-deficient, weakened, and diseased plants, they remove them from the food chain. Fully healthy plants give signals that generally are unappealing to these creatures.

SAFE SOLUTIONS

Virtually all healthy plants can produce their own natural pesticides, which usually make up about 5 to 10 percent of a plant's dry weight. These include inhibitors to block the protein-digesting enzymes of the attacking pest; enzymes that can dissolve part of the outer skin of insects; and powerful antibiotics than can kill viruses, bacteria, fungi, and nematodes.

Fifty years ago, soil scientist William Albrecht did a classic experiment in which he grew two plants in different pots next to each other. The soil in the pots was identical except that some of the minerals had been removed in one. As the two plants grew, they were wrapped around each other. The plant in the deficient soil developed fungus and insect problems, while the plant in the fully mineralized soil grew healthily, with no insect problems or disease—even with the weakened and diseased plant wrapped around it.

Weeds, too, appear to be Nature's way of correcting deficiencies. They help to create conditions that return missing elements back to the soil. If you know how to read what weeds are telling you about the health of the soil, you can work with Nature and correct the imbalance a lot faster than it will take the weeds. Just getting rid of the weeds will not solve the fundamental problem of deficient soil and food.

So the first thing to do to control all the helpful things we consider to be pests is to create healthy soil by using organic gardening methods.

Also, you can use natural and harmonious ways to handle unwanted insects, animals, and plants. These include traps, companion plants that deter harmful insects, beneficial insects and organisms, and natural botanical pesticides and repellents.

Natural botanical pesticides are less toxic than their synthetically derived counterparts, but they do need to be used with care and as a last resort. Here's a rundown on the health and environmental effects of the more popular botanical pesticides.

- *Nicotine* is extracted from the tobacco plant. It is a violent poison that injures the human nervous system and is also toxic to other mammals, birds, and fish.

- *Rotenone* is moderately toxic to humans and many animals, and highly toxic to fish and other aquatic life.

- *Pyrethrins* are extracted from the seeds of a type of chrysanthemum. They are relatively nontoxic to humans, but slightly toxic to fish and other wildlife.

- *Sabadilla* (red devil dust) comes from the seeds of the South American lily. Generally it is toxic only on contact, but is harmful to bees.

If you do use natural pesticides, use them sparingly. Because they are marketed as being nontoxic, safe, and organic, there is a danger that we will assume they are not harmful at all and end up using them in even greater quantities than artificial pesticides.

Natural pesticides have become so popular that they are now available in most nurseries and garden centers, right next to the toxic pesticides. Ask your local nursery for advice on controlling pests in your garden, or order natural pest controls by mail from **Real Goods** or any of the organic-gardening catalogs listed at the beginning of this chapter.

RAT AND MOUSE KILLERS

> **DANGER—POISON:** Keep out of reach of children. This bottle contains a deadly poison—arsenic. Poisonous if swallowed. Do not get in eyes or on skin or clothing. Wash thoroughly after handling.

Rat and mouse killers are the most harmful pesticides available for home use. They can contain **arsenic, strychnine,** or **phosphorus,** all of which kill quickly if ingested.

SAFE SOLUTIONS

Though some experts say cats will reduce the number of rats and mice in the area only by about 20 percent, I've found that my two cats keep the rat and mouse populations in my house well under control, and we live out in the countryside. It wouldn't hurt also to look for and fill holes and cracks in your building structure that mice can crawl through. Seal up the holes with white glue—it's less toxic than caulk.

Professionals recommend the old-fashioned mousetrap. The preferred bait is not cheese, but peanut butter sprinkled with a bit of cornmeal or oatmeal. Use plenty of traps—for an average home, twelve is probably plenty. It's better to use more traps for a short period of time than to use one trap and expect each rodent eventually to pass by. Rats and mice are very clever and have a way of avoiding traps, especially if they're always in the same place. So keep your bait fresh, use enough traps, and change their locations every few days for maximum effectiveness. You might try placing your traps in open paper bags. If your rodents can still find the traps, it will make your disposal job much easier.

Another way to kill mice is by sprinkling an attractive poison around the area. Instead of using a chemical, make a mixture of one part plaster of Paris and one part flour with a little sugar and cocoa powder added to make it taste good. They eat it, and they're gone. Note: Do not use this method if you have children or pets.

If you have a major problem with rodents, call a professional pest-control company for detailed advice on how to "rodent-proof" your home. They can give you good advice on how you can block pests from coming into your home, but don't let them sell you on the whole poison routine. Just say you want to try whatever can be done without chemicals first.

HOUSEHOLD INSECTICIDES

> **CAUTION:** Keep out of reach of children. Use only when area to be treated is vacated by humans and pets. Not to be taken internally by humans or animals. Hazardous if swallowed or absorbed through skin. Do not get on skin, in eyes, or on clothing. Avoid breathing of vapors or spray mist. Do not smoke while using. Should not be used in homes of the seriously ill or those on medication. Should not be used in homes of pollen-sensitive people or asthmatics. Do not use in any rooms where infants, the sick, or aged are or will be present for any extended period of confinement. Do not use in kitchen areas or areas where food is prepared or served. Do not apply directly to food. In the home, all food-processing surfaces and utensils should be covered during treatment or thoroughly washed before use. Remove pets, and cover fish aquariums and delicate plants before spraying.

According to the EPA, no insecticides that are sold for general home use have warning labels stronger than "Caution." Any products that pose greater danger are available only for application by licensed pest-control operators.

Most insecticides kill all types of flying and crawling insects—ants, fleas, cockroaches, mosquitoes, flies, and silverfish. One of the more commonly used pesticides in home sprays is pyrethrin, which is the crushed, dried flowers of *Chrysanthemum cinerariifolium*. It's harmless for humans or pets to swallow, but kills bugs on contact. The problem with commercial pyrethrin formulations is not the pyrethrin, but the fact that it is mixed with other pesticides, frequently dispensed in **aerosol sprays,** and diluted with "inert ingredients" of unknown type or toxicity.

SAFE SOLUTIONS

You can order pure pyrethrin powder by mail, or if you have a patch of garden, you can grow your own *Chrysanthemum cinerari-*

ifolium and gather the blossoms when two or three outer rows of petals have opened. Dry blossoms either in the sun or in an oven set at the lowest temperature. Grind dry flowers into a powder using a coffee mill, blender, or mortar and pestle. Place 10 grams of powder in a light-proof bottle and add 4 ounces alcohol. Shake the mixture occasionally, and let it stand for 24 hours at room temperature. Pour the finished mixture through coffee-maker filters and use as is, spraying through a small spray bottle, for roaches, flies, fleas, beetles, lice, and other insects.

A truly ingenious new alternative is **Insect Aside.** It is a hand-held bug vacuum. Just suction up the bugs, and they are held in a disposable cartridge lined with nontoxic sticky gel until you are ready to throw them away.

ANTS

Wipe up ants with a wet sponge when you see them. They rely on one another for direction. Without a trail, others get lost.

To keep ants out, sprinkle powdered red chili pepper, paprika, dried peppermint, or borax where ants are coming in. Or use the botanical approach: Plant mint around the outside of the house. Ants won't come inside, because they don't like the smell.

COCKROACHES AND SILVERFISH

Cockroaches are especially fond of vegetables, meat, starches, grease, sweets, paper, soap, cardboard, bookbindings, ink, shoe polish, and dirty clothes. And they're not fussy about their places of residence, either. They might be living in your telephone, electric clock, radio, or even your refrigerator. So how do you get rid of them?

While they aren't particularly appealing to live with, it might be comforting to remember that cockroaches really aren't a pest. The World Health Organization does not include cockroaches on its list of insects that are hazardous to health (fleas, bedbugs, lice, mites, scorpions, and some spiders are included), and there are no reported instances in the scientific literature of roaches transmitting human disease.

For limited infestations, use cockroach traps—either buy the commercial "motels" with the adhesive strip, or make your own (see instructions below). Use several in each room where you've seen roaches. When the traps start working, leave a few cockroaches inside to attract others. Clean traps by immersing them completely in a bucket of hot, sudsy water; then make sure to wash your hands thoroughly.

Here's how to make your own nontoxic roach traps.

- Rub grease on the inside of the neck of a quart mason jar. Set the jar upright and put a piece of banana inside for bait. Place a tongue depressor against the side of the jar, and the cockroaches will "walk the plank" to their deaths.

- Wrap masking tape around the outside of an empty jam jar. Fill the jar half-full with a mixture of beer, a few slices of banana, and a few drops of anise extract, or use boiled raisins, pet kibble, or pieces of apple, potato, or banana peel as bait. Finally, smear a band of petroleum jelly around the inside rim so the cockroaches can't climb out.

- Soak a rag in beer and place it in a shallow dish overnight in an infested area. In the morning, you can easily dispose of the drunken roaches.

You also could put cucumber rinds or bay leaves in the infested area, or spread around any of the following mixtures. Repeat weekly for several weeks to kill newly hatched roaches.

- Equal parts flour or powdered oatmeal mixed with plaster of Paris
- Equal parts baking soda and powdered sugar
- 2 tablespoons trisodium phosphate (TSP), ¾ cup borax, ½ cup granulated sugar, and 1 cup flour
- 2 tablespoons flour, 1 tablespoon cocoa powder, and 4 tablespoons borax

If none of the above methods works (and you probably won't need to do this), as a last resort use boric acid, available in hardware and building-supply stores. Make sure to get *technical* boric acid and not *medicinal* boric acid. Medicinal boric acid is a white powder that can easily be confused with sugar or salt; a tablespoon accidentally eaten can kill a small child. Technical boric acid, used in industrial manufacturing, is just as dangerous but is tinted blue for easy identification. It also has the added benefit of being treated electrostatically, so it will cling to the cockroach—when other cockroaches rub against the roach, they'll pick it up. There are several brands of commercial roach killers made of 100 percent boric acid, but buying plain boric acid is cheaper. Sprinkle it around in out-of-the way corners and it will continue to kill roaches as long as it is there. Boric acid is preferable to chemical sprays because it is a nonvolatile powder, but it is still a poison, so don't use it around food or in cabinets where food is stored, or where children or pets may come in contact with it.

Everything that works for cockroaches also works for silverfish.

FLIES

During the day, you can encourage flies to leave by darkening the room and opening the door to the outside light. Because flies are attracted to light, they will quickly fly outdoors.

Repel flies by hanging clusters of cloves around the room, or by scratching the rind of an orange or lemon to allow the unappealing (to them) citrus oil to escape. You will hardly notice the pleasant aroma.

If a fly happens to come in anyway, keep a flyswatter on hand, or make your own flypaper. Simply boil equal parts sugar, corn syrup, and water together and place it on brown paper. The flies can't resist this sticky treat. If this seems like too much trouble, you can buy adhesive fly strips at most hardware stores.

FOOD-STORAGE PESTS (BEETLES, WEEVILS, MOTHS, AND MITES)

Food-storage pests enter the home through contaminated groceries. Inspect all packaged foods at the store before putting them in your cart. Look for loose package flaps and tiny holes in the packaging. Be particularly watchful with any grain products (including whole grains, flour, cereals, pasta, baking mixes), dried fruits, beans, powdered milk, and pet foods. Buy only small amounts of these products, which can be eaten in a short period of time.

Store foods in tightly closed containers in a cool, dry cabinet, or in the refrigerator. Packets of silica gel (available at camera stores) will absorb moisture and help keep cabinets dry. Check food supplies once a week in summer and once a month in winter, and throw away (in the outside garbage) any contaminated foods before the infestation spreads to other containers. If you buy foods in bulk, you might think about getting an extra refrigerator to put in the garage for storing extra supplies. Not only will the foods be protected from insects, but they will stay fresher, too.

Putting a bay leaf in each container will help to repel stray pests, but will not eradicate an infestation. If you want to try this, put the bay leaves in small cotton bags to prevent them from crumbling into the food. You wouldn't want to bake a cake with bay-flavored flour.

INSECT REPELLENTS

> **CAUTION:** Harmful if swallowed. Avoid contact with eyes and lips. Do not allow children to rub eyes if hands have been treated. Do not apply on or near: rayon, spandex, or other synthetics. May damage furniture finishes, plastics, leather, watch crystals, and painted or varnished surfaces including automobiles.

I don't know about you, but I don't think I'd want to rub something on my skin that could take the paint off my car!

The most commonly used pesticide in insect repellents is **DEET** (common name for **diethyl toluamide**). According to the British medical Journal *Lancet,* exposure to DEET has been reported to cause brain disorders, slurred speech, difficulty walking, tremors, and even death. *Consumer Reports* has documented at least a dozen cases of acute neurotoxicity in children who had been exposed to or accidentally swallowed DEET; some of the children died.

Obviously, while not everyone who uses a DEET-based insect repellent will suffer these effects, it makes you think twice, especially since up to 56 percent of DEET enters the bloodstream after it is applied to the surface of your skin, and it can remain in the body for up to two months.

SAFE SOLUTIONS

Most people use insect repellents to keep mosquitoes away. The main strategy for dealing with mosquitoes is to keep them from biting you and from buzzing in your ear when you are trying to sleep. So if you don't care if they're still flying around as long as they're not bothering you, dip a cotton ball in some vinegar and rub it on your exposed skin. The vinegar evaporates immediately, and, no, you won't smell like a pickle.

Two other natural repellents are oil of citronella and oil of peppermint, both available at most natural-food stores. These are very strong, however, and can result in a rash when applied directly to the skin, and bad irritation to eyes when rubbed in accidentally. Dilute these oils with vodka or vegetable oil (a few drops to one ounce of either) and then apply them, like perfume, at strategic points. Or, burn citronella candles or torches (available at most hardware stores).

Mosquitoes also hate the smell of garlic. The recommended method for using this repellent is to eat lots of garlicky food. The trick here is to get all your friends to eat a lot of garlic so none of you will notice one another's bad breath—or at least so none of you will care—and you'll all be protected from mosquito bites.

If you don't even want the mosquitoes in the same room with you, wait until they light upon a wall and then suction them up with the long attachment on your vacuum cleaner.

Basil planted outside your window will prevent mosquitoes from coming in, or you can keep a few basil plants inside. Not only will you keep mosquitoes away, but you'll have an endless fresh supply of this wonderful herb. Once you've tasted fresh basil, you'll never go back to using the dried leaves in the jar.

There are also a number of herbal insect repellents. Look for them at your natural-food store or order by mail from **Green Ban, Simmons Handcrafts,** or **Lakon Herbals** (their **Bygone Bugs** is made from organically grown herbal ingredients).

For a severe mosquito problem, pretend you live in an old movie and get some romantic-looking mosquito netting for your bed from **Real Goods.**

If necessary, and depending on circumstances, wear protective clothing. This could mean using big rubber bands to tighten pant cuffs around boots, a cotton turtleneck shirt, a hat with protective netting, a silk balaclava for your face, and cotton work gloves. This is, of course, overkill for most people, but even just putting on a loose fitting shirt on summer evenings will keep some insects off your skin. **Real Goods, Gardener's Supply,** and **Nontoxic Environments** all carry nylon protective headgear and suits.

MOTHBALLS

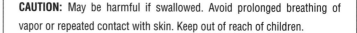

> **CAUTION:** May be harmful if swallowed. Avoid prolonged breathing of vapor or repeated contact with skin. Keep out of reach of children.

Mothballs are made from 100 percent **paradichlorobenzene,** a volatile chemical that can cause headache; swollen eyes; loss of appetite; nausea; severe irritation to your nose, throat, and lungs; depression; and injury to your liver and kidneys when you are exposed to it over a long period of time. It is harmful if swallowed, and because mothballs look so much like candy, they are very attractive to children. If a two-year-old child were to eat even one mothball accidentally, he or she could develop seizures in less than an hour.

I have always found the warning label on mothballs amusing. It clearly states, "Avoid prolonged breathing of vapor," yet by the very design of the mothballs, you must be constantly exposed to these fumes. The odor of mothballs hidden in a closet can permeate your entire home; certainly, mothballs in the bedroom closet can infiltrate the room and increase to very high levels if the room is not ventilated adequately. The vapors from mothballs also are absorbed by clothing and blankets, making your exposure very direct when you are around these items.

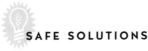

SAFE SOLUTIONS

Instead of buying paradichlorobenzene, look in natural-food stores and closet shops for herbal products that act as repellents. They might contain lavender or other herbs, or cedar oil, chips, or needles. Not only are these products safer and equally effective, their scent is far more pleasant than the musty smell of mothballs. Make sure the product is of natural origin, as you may find synthetic imitations. You can order natural moth repellents by mail from **Hummer Nature Works, Seventh Generation, Vermont Country Store,** and **Walnut Acres. Gardener's Supply** sells a disposable cardboard trap that lures clothes moths inside, where it ensnares them on a sticky surface.

You also can make your own herbal moth repellents. Make sachets of any of the following:

- dried lavender
- equal parts dried rosemary and mint
- dried tobacco
- whole peppercorns
- cedar chips or other wood soaked in real cedar oil

Your natural-food store should carry most of these items; pet stores will have cedar chips. It may be difficult to find cotton sachet bags; if so, try cotton baby socks, or sew your own.

The moths you see flying around are not the moths that eat your woolens. Two varieties of clothes moths cause damage. They are too small to notice and are not drawn to light like other varieties. It is the larvae of these moths that eat fabric, not the moth itself.

Your best protection is to store and maintain your woolens correctly to prevent larvae from hatching. Simply wearing all your clothes at regular intervals will cause any larvae to fall off. Or, you can occasionally air items in the sun, then brush them to crush larvae and remove dried-up pests. Washing will kill clothes moths in all stages of development, as will pressing with a steam iron, running through a hot dryer, or placing items in a warm (140°) oven for an hour. You could also place small items in the freezer for several days. When you buy new woolens, it is a good idea to put them through one of these treatments before storing them with your other items to kill any larvae that might be present at the time of purchase. This is especially important if you make a point of buying unmothproofed woolens.

Once you know your woolens are free from moths, store them properly. Place them in drawers or boxes containing natural repellents, or, if you are storing them over the summer, protect them in airtight containers, such as paper packages or cardboard boxes with all edges carefully sealed with paper tape. You will have secured your woolens against the munching of moth larvae, and your home will be free of dangerous fumes.

LICE SHAMPOOS

Every parent with a school-age child might someday have to deal with a child picking up head lice at school. Contrary to what we might think, head lice is a condition that cuts across all social and cultural boundaries—it can show up on anyone.

At one time the most common treatment for head lice was a shampoo that contained **lindane,** a very toxic chemical easily absorbed through the skin. One child's death was reported to have been the result of lindane poisoning after treatment for head lice, and lindane now is known to cause convulsions, seizures, and cancer in laboratory animals. When I checked my local drug-store shelves, none of the half-dozen shampoos available contained lindane. Nevertheless, keep an eye out for this very dangerous chemical.

The popular active ingredient nowadays is pyrethrin. As with general purpose pesticide sprays, the toxicity problem lies not with the pyrethrin, but with the added **petroleum distillates.** Because the petroleum distillates frequently are not identified, I would hesitate to put chemicals of unknown toxicity on my child's scalp, especially since the scalp area is very porous, and chemicals put on the hair are easily absorbed into the bloodstream.

SAFE SOLUTIONS

A very effective, and much less toxic, alternative is to use a combination of shampooing, soaking, and combing with a nit-removing comb especially designed to eliminate lice (available at your local pharmacy). Here is the procedure:

1. Wet hair thoroughly with warm water and apply a coconut-based shampoo. Coconut oil contains dodecyl alcohol, which is deadly to adult lice (any shampoo that lists sodium lauryl sulfate as an ingredient contains coconut oil. Or you can use a bar soap that has a coconut-oil base). Work the soap or shampoo into a thick lather, covering the entire head and all the hair.

2. Rinse with warm water and repeat the lathering process, this time leaving suds on hair. Tie a towel around the lathered hair and leave it on for 30 minutes.

3. Remove the towel and comb the soapy hair with a regular comb to remove tangles; then use the nit-removing comb on 1-inch sections of hair (following the instructions that come with the comb). If the hair dries during combing, dampen it with water. Depending on the length of hair, the combing can take 2 hours or more. Very curly or woolly hair can take even longer.

4. After removing lice, wash the hair a third time, rinse, and dry. Inspect the hair when dry for any lice you missed, and remove them.

This won't be fun, but *everyone* in the household must be treated when one member of the family has head lice. Lice don't care which head of hair they live in, and the infestation can last longer than necessary when family members spread lice back and forth. During the elimination process, everyone must comb his or her dry hair daily to check for lice. Also vacuum upholstered furniture daily, change pillowcases and bedsheets, and launder clothes. As an extra precaution, you might want to run pillows and blankets through your clothes dryer to kill lice.

Check after seven to ten days to see if any missed lice nits have hatched; if so, you have to go through the whole process again.

TERMITICIDES

The two questions regarding pesticides that I am most often asked have to do with termite treatments—how toxic are they, and what can be done for nonchemical treatment?

Termites play an essential role in nature by helping to clear the forest of dead trees. Since large areas of our homes are made from dead wood, it's not surprising that termites are responsible for structural damage in excess of $750 million each year in the United States alone.

Since World War II, the most popular method of termite control has been to spray potent, long-lasting pesticides—such as **chlordane, aldrin, dieldrin,** and **heptachlor**—directly onto or into the soil around a building's foundation, and in the crawl space or basement. Chlordane has been found in the soil of treated areas thirty years or more after treatment. After persistent health and environmental problems became associated with the use of these pesticides—poisoned fishponds, contaminated well water, seepage into the indoor air of treated homes—several states banned them. The EPA discovered that 90 percent of the homes *properly* treated with termiticides still had detectable residues in the air one year later. Under public pressure, the manufacture of these pesticides ceased in 1987, and since April 15, 1988, their sale has been prohibited.

The new popular termiticide is **chlorpyrifos** (commonly known as **Dursban, Lorsban,** or **Pyrinex**). Injected underground, it can continue to be effective for almost twenty years. Consumers Union found that chlorpyrifos has not been adequately tested to determine if it causes cancer, genetic mutations, or nerve damage. It is extremely toxic to fish, birds, and aquatic invertebrates.

SAFE SOLUTIONS

The best way by far to control termites is to make your home unattractive or inaccessible to them.

- Subterranean termites need food, warmth, and moisture in order to survive. Keep the area under your house cold and dry, and they'll look elsewhere for food.

- Do an annual inspection. It takes a well-established termite colony almost three months to eat a pound of wood, so catching them early can make it easier to control any problems that do arise.

- Use copper or galvanized-steel termite shields. Properly installed, these shields prevent termites from reaching the woodwork from the earth. Use them at basements, crawl spaces, or chimney foundations; on concrete piers with saddle and wood posts; and at entrances with wood steps or floors. Buy termite shields ready-made, or buy a roll of sheet metal at a building-supply store. Unroll the sheet metal over foundation walls, and bed edges down at a 45-degree angle. If this sounds too confusing, call a few contractors and see if you can find an experienced person locally to help you with this.

When building or remodeling, there are a few preventive measures you can take. Some of these tips also can be applied to already-existing structures.

- Design and construct foundation walls and supporting piers in a way that minimizes the possibility of future cracks or fissures through which termites can attack.

- Wood in contact with the ground should be heart tidewater red cypress or heart redwood or treated with a natural wood preservative (see **The Natural Choice** and **Sinan Company** catalogs).

- Provide good cross ventilation for unexcavated areas under the house.
- Screen all openings for ventilation under the house and in the attic with eighteen-mesh metal screening.
- Remove all wood scraps and stumps from the soil surrounding the house.
- Wooden floor joists should be at least 24 inches above the ground, and wooden construction on the exterior of the house should be at least 6 inches above the ground.

To get rid of termites without toxic chemicals, cut out and re-place infested wood, or call local pest-control companies to find out what kinds of nontoxic alternatives they offer. New methods range from freezing to electrocution.

AS A LAST RESORT

If you absolutely *must* use chemical pesticides and you feel there is no other alternative, follow these "Pesticide Safety Tips" rec-ommended by the Environmental Protection Agency:

- Always read the label before buying or using pesti-cides. Use pesticides only for the purpose(s) listed and in the manner directed.
- Do not apply more than the specified amount of the pesticide. Overdoses can harm you and the en-vironment.
- Keep pesticides away from food and dishes.
- Keep children and pets away from pesticides and sprayed areas.
- Do not smoke while spraying.
- Avoid inhalation of pesticides.

- If you mix pesticides, do it carefully to avoid splashing. (I wouldn't mix pesticides at all! Unless you are a chemist, how could you know what toxic horror you might be creating?)

- Avoid breaks or spills of pesticide containers.

- If you spill a pesticide on your skin or on your clothing, wash with soap and water and change your clothing immediately.

- Store pesticides under lock in the original containers with proper labels. Never transfer a pesticide to a container such as a soft-drink bottle, which would attract children.

- Dispose of empty containers safely. Wrap single containers of home-use products in several layers of newspaper, tie securely, and place in a covered trash can. Never burn boxes or sacks. Dispose of large quantities in special incinerators or special landfills. (Call your local EPA office to find out where.)

- Wash with soap and water after using pesticides, and launder your clothes before wearing them again.

- If someone swallows a pesticide, check the label for first-aid treatment. Call or go to the doctor or the hospital immediately and keep the pesticide label with you. (If my child swallowed a pesticide, I'd probably race to the emergency room, and not call first.)

Chapter 5

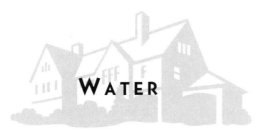

WATER

I T USED TO BE THAT we could take for granted turning on the tap and having clean water pour out. Not anymore. Today, the responsibility for clean water lies with us. Buying the proper equipment will be a major investment, but not any more than buying any other major appliance, and it is well worth every penny for its contribution to your family's health.

We are exposed to more water pollutants than just those we drink or use in cooking. According to a study done by the Massachusetts Department of Environmental Quality Engineering published in the *American Journal of Public Health,* 29 to 46 percent of water pollutant exposure (depending on the chemical and the concentration) occurs *through the skin* in children, and 50 to 70 percent in adults! For a normal adult, taking a fifteen-minute bath can be equal to drinking a quart of the same water; a fifty-pound child can absorb up to ten times as much contamination from swimming in a pool for an hour as drinking a quart of water. In addition, we breathe the fumes of certain pollutants released from running water. The EPA has now identified **chloroform** released from hot, running shower water as a major indoor *air pollutant*—so there's a hazard in breathing water in the form of steam, too.

The EPA has identified more than 700 pollutants that occur regularly in drinking water, both from municipal sources and from water taken directly from the earth through wells or springs. At least 22 are known to cause cancer; it is not known exactly how many pollutants are carcinogenic, since not all have been tested.

It has been estimated that the 700 known pollutants may represent as little as 10 percent of the actual number of contaminants that may be present in municipal drinking waters; testing procedures have not yet been invented to detect all the dangerous substances that could be present.

The most common water pollutants are the **trihalomethanes,** or **THM**s, the most common of which is chloroform. THMs are formed when **chlorine** used as a disinfectant combines with the natural organic matter in the water (dead leaves and humus in soil, silt, and mud). According to the EPA, THMs are present in virtually all chlorinated water supplies in the United States. Chloroform can cause liver and kidney damage and central nervous system depression, and is a suspected human carcinogen. In 1992, a Medical College of Wisconsin study that made front-page headlines found that people who regularly drink tap water containing high levels of chlorine by-products have a greater risk of developing bladder and rectal cancers than people who drink unchlorinated water.

The second most common water pollutant is **fluoride.** It is added to many water supplies as a public service, to reduce dental cavities in children. Much controversy has surrounded the use of fluoride, because in large amounts it can weaken the immune system and cause heart disease, genetic damage, birth defects, and cancer. The U.S. Public Health Service recommends an "optimum" intake of 1 mg of fluoride per day, but that level is frequently exceeded when you combine the fluoride found in tap water, the fluoride in toothpaste and mouthwashes, and the fluoridated water used in reconstituted fruit juices and other processed foods and beverages. There is some question even as to whether fluoride prevents cavities. Perhaps in the right amount it does, but this is a case where more is not necessarily better. Studies at the University of Arizona found that "the more fluoride a child drank, the more cavities appeared in the teeth," and that "scientists noticed an increase in cavities and missing and filled teeth in children participating in fluoridation programs."

Pipes used to transport water throughout the system and within your home also can contribute pollutants. **Cadmium, copper, iron, lead,** and **zinc** can leach into the water from metal pipes. Cadmium can cause kidney damage, anemia, heart problems, high blood pressure, birth defects, and cancer; lead can be responsible for headaches, nerve problems, mental retardation and learning disabilities in children, birth defects, and, possibly, cancer. Carcinogenic **asbestos** can be released from asbestos cement pipes. The plastics industry insists that **polyvinyl chloride (PVC)** pipes are safe, yet studies show that a variety of toxic and carcinogenic substances leach from these pipes into the water, among them **methyl ethyl ketone (MEK), dimethyl-formamide (DMF), cyclohexanone (CH), tetrahydrofuran (THF), carbon tetrachloride, tetrachloroethene, trichloroethane, di-(2-ethylhexyl) phthalate (DEHP),** and **dibutyl phthalate.** Water standing in PVC pipes for any length of time will also become contaminated with carcinogenic **vinyl chloride.**

This list of pollutants does not even begin to cover what else might be in your particular water supply. Water is sometimes referred to as a "universal solvent," because it picks up a bit of everything that it passes by. Both our surface waters and groundwaters are now contaminated from years of industrial dumping, and your water supply could contain anything from **nitrates** to **pesticides** to **industrial solvents.**

The EPA has jurisdiction only for the quality of water that comes from your tap—if you get your water from a source that services more than fifteen individual year-round hookups (if your source is the well in your backyard, you're not covered). All chemical additives—whether they are added for a specific purpose or they find their way into the water supply accidentally—fall under the EPA's jurisdiction. The quality of our public water is controlled by the National Interim Primary Drinking Water Regulations (Code of Federal Regulations Title 40, Part 141), developed by the EPA in accordance with the Safe Water Drinking Act, an amendment to the Public Health Service Act. By this law, the EPA monitors *eight* inorganic chemicals and *ten* organic chemicals, leaving an estimated *thirty thousand* possible hazardous pollutants without regulation.

I know these statistics sound incredible. It seems logical for us to expect that the EPA could do a better job of providing clean water in our taps. But we must remember that most municipal water treatment facilities were built in the early 1900s for the purpose of disinfecting water, rather than purifying it. Our water treatment facilities were designed to kill disease-causing bacteria and not to remove chemical contaminants.

But now researchers are finding that, for all the toxic chemicals that are added to our water, we are not even protected from bacteria. In 1993, a parasite called **cryptosporidium** contaminated the water supply in Milwaukee, sickening 400,000 people and causing 100 deaths. Because *cryptosporidium* was only recently recognized as a threat, there are no laws requiring utilities to check specifically for this parasite.

The federal government estimates that it would take billions of dollars and ten to fifteen years to upgrade our water treatment facilities. An EPA report estimates that about 30 million Americans each year are drinking from public water systems that violate one or more health standards.

BOTTLED WATER

Bottled water generally can be relied upon to be bacteriologically safe and free of chlorine.

Many consumers believe that bottled waters are of higher quality than tap water, although legally this need not be true. Many bottled waters are only processed tap water, and their quality varies widely depending on the quality of the local water and the type of filtration used. Buying "pure" water in a plastic bottle defeats the purpose, because the plastic quickly leaches into the water. Federal and state regulations for bottled water are confusing and changeable; and some bottled waters are even exempt from regulation!

I drank bottled water for several years, at great expense, until I found out that the fluoride levels in my favorite brand were five times higher than those in tap water! High pollutant levels are allowed in bottled water based on an industry-wide assumption that bottled waters are consumed as a beverage—a health-conscious alternative to an alcoholic beverage or soda pop—and not as the primary source of drinking water.

SAFE SOLUTIONS

There are many excellent brands of bottled water on the market today—too many to list here—that can be enjoyed as a refreshing beverage even if not as a regular source of drinking water.

Bottled water is defined by the Food and Drug Administration as simply "water that is sealed in bottles or other containers and intended for human consumption." Federal regulations require that bottled waters marketed across state lines meet federal standards for drinking water. Those bottled waters sold only within individual states need meet only state requirements, which can vary from federal standards.

The purity of bottled water is controlled under the federal Food, Drug, and Cosmetic Act (*mineral waters* and *soda waters* specifically are exempt and thus are not regulated at all). Legally accepted sources for bottled water are wells, springs, and public water right from the tap. No requirements specify that the source of the water or any treatment it has undergone be listed on the label, but if any information is given at all, it must be truthful and not misleading. Manufacturers have an excellent selling point in telling if the water has come from a well or a spring, so if the source of the water is not revealed, chances are the water is treated tap water.

Bottled waters are divided into two types: still (without bubbles) and sparkling (with bubbles). Even though there are no state or federal regulations for the labeling of bottled-water containers, the labels do use certain generalized descriptive terms.

- *Drinking water:* tap or well water processed in some way before bottling
- *Spring water:* water that emerges from the earth's surface under its own pressure, sometimes through a pipe. Water in bottles labeled "Spring water" must come from a spring; "Natural spring water,"

unlike plain spring water, may not be processed in any way before it goes into the bottle. Beware of companies with the word "spring" in the company name rather than in the name of the product, or companies referring to the product as "spring-fresh," "springlike," or "spring-pure." Do not mistakenly assume that this water is from a spring.

- *Mineral water:* water containing a legally specified level of minerals. "Natural mineral water" is sparkling or still water, usually from a spring, which contains only the naturally occurring minerals. Regular "mineral water" may have had minerals added or removed.

- *Sparkling water:* water that contains bubbles made by carbon dioxide gas. "Naturally sparkling" water contains the bubbles when it is underground; when the water is drawn from the spring, the natural carbon dioxide is removed separately and reinjected during bottling. Some still waters also are carbonated, with either natural or manufactured carbon dioxide.

Club sodas and seltzer water are *not* controlled by federal regulations. Both are merely filtered and carbonated tap water; club soda also contains added mineral salts. The quality of these waters will differ greatly, depending on the local water and the method of filtration used.

According to tests done by Consumers Union in 1980, none of the thirty-eight brands of bottled waters tested for pesticides had detectable levels of trihalomethanes or other pesticides. Amounts of other pollutants, such as nitrates, cadmium, iron, and lead, were well within federal limits, and none of the brands contained harmful quantities of bacteria. However, the tests did find a number of brands that had excessive levels of sodium and fluoride. Home-delivered bottled waters either come from a natural spring or are processed tap water distilled or purified using reverse osmosis. Most come in five-gallon plastic bottles nowadays, so you might not want to trust these, either, for your regular drinking water.

If you do want to drink bottled water, choose one bottled in glass directly from the natural source. The FDA suggests you select one that is controlled by federal regulations, preferably one that indicates its source. Most companies have a water-analysis report available for inspection, which they should send on your request.

Thus, if you know what to look for on the label, you can choose your water wisely.

WATER FILTERS

All water pollutants fall into five basic categories.

- *Microorganisms:* microscopic plants and animals more commonly known as bacteria, viruses, protozoans, algae, and cysts. Not all are harmful, but many cause water-quality problems more frequently than any other pollutant

- *Particulates:* all the minute bits of material that do not dissolve in water—metals (such as lead), rust, dirt, sand, and other sediments

- *Dissolved solids:* solid materials like fluoride, nitrates, sulfates, and salts, which decompose in water

- *Volatile chemicals:* all nonparticulate substances that can be vaporized—chlorine, chloramine, chloroform and other trihalomethanes, chlorinated hydrocarbons, pesticides (DDT, dieldrin, lindane, heptachlor), radon gas, benzene, carbon tetrachloride, trichloroethylene, xylene, toluene, and hundreds of others

- *Radioactive particles:* minute bits of radioactive materials

To find out what's in *your* water, start by calling city hall, your local water district office, or your local department of health services. Be prepared for them to give you the runaround. You might not get any information from them, or they may send you the results of tests done five years ago.

You may want to ask if your water is tested on a regular basis. The Safe Water Drinking Act requires that the water be tested periodically; the interval between tests depends on the number of customers served by your water system. A survey conducted by the Congressional General Accounting Office found, however, that more than half the water suppliers were not doing the required testing. Also, remember they are only testing for eight inorganic chemicals and ten organic chemicals—there may be many other contaminants in your water. Moreover, water quality changes constantly, and pollutants that may not have shown up on the last water analysis report may be present on the next one. Some people choose to have their water tested independently, although this can be expensive and is not always accurate.

Even without test results, you can learn a great deal about the condition of your water by asking the following questions:

1. Where does the water come from (a reservoir, groundwater)?

2. What type of pipe is used to transport the water? Does it add lead, asbestos, or vinyl chloride? (You also need to find out what type of pipe has been installed in your home.)

3. Is chlorine used to disinfect the water (or chloramine, or some other chemical)?

4. Is the water fluoridated?

5. Is there agriculture in the area that would result in excessive pesticide or nitrogen fertilizer runoff? Are there factories nearby producing industrial waste?

6. Where is the city dump in relation to municipal water supplies? Could hazardous materials from the dump be leaching into the water?

One limitation to the water-quality data that come from your local waterworks is that the reports will tell you the quality of the water as it leaves the treatment plant, *not as it comes out of your tap.* The levels of chlorine, metals, bacteria, and particulates may have changed by the time the water is pumped through the distribution system to your home. For many years, the EPA failed to detect excessive lead in some drinking-water supplies; it was ultimately found by independent laboratories testing samples submitted by homeowners.

SAFE SOLUTIONS

When I learned how unreliable bottled water can be, even though I was loyal to one brand, I decided it was time to purify my water supply myself.

Buying a water filter requires a little homework and careful consideration. There is no one filter right for every water supply and every family.

The first step is to find out which pollutants are in your water and need to be removed. Because each water-purification method removes different pollutants, you must determine which type of equipment is right for your water supply.

If your water supply is not regulated or if you would like to have your water independently tested, look in the Yellow Pages under "Laboratories—Analytical." Ask these laboratories what testing they do and get estimates from several, because prices and services can vary.

In response to consumer demand for home water-quality testing, there are now low-cost mail-order services specifically designed for homeowners. Contact **Allergy Resources, American Environmental Laboratories,** and **National Testing Laboratories** for information on their test kits.

It is important also to keep in mind that no water-purification device can make your water 100 percent pure 100 percent of the time. Using current technology, we can reduce pollutants to a level that significantly lessens their health effects. When we choose a device, we are choosing also our level of risk.

There are five factors to consider.

1. Which pollutants need to be removed from your water
2. How much it costs both to purchase the unit and to maintain it over time

3. Convenience

4. What type of device to buy

5. Effectiveness of pollutant removal

Compromises will need to be made in each of these areas. The units that are most effective are not the least expensive. Are you willing to turn a unit on and off, or do you want purified water to flow instantly from your tap? Do you want to remove just the pollutants found in your water supply, or do you want broad-spectrum removal to protect yourself from possible unknown contaminants?

The cost of a water-purification device also is a prime consideration for many people who want cleaner water. Units of varying effectiveness range in price from thirty-nine dollars to several thousand dollars. In general, it costs more to buy a more effective device, but not always. Almost any device is better than none at all, *if used properly.* Buy the best you can afford, but remember to take into consideration the overall cost of the unit over time, including replacement components, if any.

With convenience high on the priority list for choosing products these days, some people are willing to sacrifice water quality for having the water come right out of the tap or through an auxiliary faucet. Others are willing to turn devices on and off and collect drinking water in containers to have the purest water possible. If you aren't willing to keep up with the user participation and regular maintenance required for some devices, it's better to choose an automated device or one that requires less upkeep. Most units actually can pollute water if not properly maintained, so make sure you are willing to do what it takes to keep your unit operating optimally.

The type of water purification device you choose will depend on the final use of the water you are purifying.

For drinking water, you can simply use a point-of-use device that will purify water only at the specific tap at which it is used. Point-of-use devices that attach to shower heads and bathtub taps are also available. Or you can choose a point-of-entry device that will purify water where it enters your house, providing clean water from every tap. Generally speaking, point-of-use devices produce drinking water of higher purity, and some people choose to use a combination of both.

Evaluating the efficiency of a water-purification device can be difficult, primarily because much of the advertising for such devices is false and misleading. In many cases salespeople are unable to give accurate information on technical aspects of their devices, although I have consistently found that manufacturers and sellers of good-quality products are more than willing to reveal every detail about the devices they produce and represent. Beware of such sales tactics as refusing to give out information over the telephone, door-to-door salespeople wanting to sign you up for thousands of dollars' worth of equipment, phony "water officials" who call nights or weekends, and companies who will test your water for free, then try to sell you a unit.

A new wrinkle that has appeared for buyers and sellers of water-purification devices is that some states are now requiring state certification for filters sold that claim to improve health or the quality of tap water. It may seem safe to assume that any good filter sold by an honest dealer *would* be certified; however, because of the intricacies and enormous expense of some certification programs, some manufacturers are withdrawing their claims rather than certify their products. This will make it more difficult for consumers to compare products, but if you understand what each type of filtration can and cannot do, you will be able to make a wise choice.

What to Buy

While there are more than four hundred companies making water-filtration devices, there are only three basic methods of water purification used in devices designed to further decontaminate the already potable water that comes from your tap: activated carbon (in granular or block form), reverse osmosis, and distillation. Even though there are different brands and different designs available, each method can only remove certain pollutants and not others. However, any particular method will remove all types of similar pollutants.

If you know you have lead in your water, for example, buying a unit to remove lead will, in addition, automatically remove arsenic, asbestos, cadmium, dirt, and all other particulates. If you want to remove fluoride, all other dissolved solids will be removed also. A unit that removes chlorine and trihalomethanes will take care of any other volatile chemicals that may be in the water.

To remove *particulates* or *dissolved solids,* you should buy a *distiller* or *reverse osmosis* device.

To remove *volatile chemicals,* use an *activated carbon* device.

To remove *microorganisms,* water *distillers* work best.

COMPARISON OF POLLUTANTS REMOVED BY WATER-PURIFICATION METHODS

	ACTIVATED CARBON (GRANULAR)	ACTIVATED CARBON (BLOCK)	DISTILLATION	REVERSE OSMOSIS
Asbestos	Some	Yes	Yes	Yes
Bacteria and viruses	No	Yes*	Yes	Some
Chlorine	Yes	Yes	No	No
Fluoride	No	Some	Yes	Yes
Heavy metals	No	Yes	Yes	Yes
Minerals	No	No	Yes	Yes
Nitrates	No	No	Yes	Yes
Organic chemicals	Yes	Yes	Some	Some
Salts	No	No	Yes	Yes

*Pore size must be smaller than 1 micron to remove *cryptosporidium.*

For all-around protection you'll want to invest in either a reverse osmosis unit or a distillation unit that also includes an activated carbon filter. There are advantages and disadvantages to each, so I'll discuss them separately to help you decide which is best for you.

ACTIVATED CARBON

The least expensive water purification method is activated carbon. Even though it is relatively ineffective on particulates, dissolved solids, radioactive particles, and microorganisms, it is the best at removing volatile chemicals. If your water is chlorinated (as most municipal supplies are), you could benefit from using a carbon filter. So if you can't afford anything else, it is better to get an activated carbon filter than to do nothing—*if* it's the right type.

Activated carbon works by the process of *ad*sorption. Each little particle of carbon is like a honeycomb containing minute pores that attract and trap pollutant molecules. As water passes through and the micropores are filled, fewer and fewer pores remain available, until finally the carbon is fully saturated and begins to release the pollutants back into the water! The game you play with activated carbon is "change the filter in time," and it can be difficult to tell exactly when to change it.

For this reason, you *must* change the carbon regularly. How often you'll need to change the carbon depends on the size and amount of carbon in the unit and the volume of volatile chemicals in your water. All carbon units come with instructions to change the carbon after so many months or so many gallons, but a good way to gauge this for yourself is to purchase an inexpensive chlorine test kit (like you would use to test the chlorine in your swimming pool) and test your water periodically to find out exactly how long the carbon is effective with your water. Tests done by Rodale Product Testing Labs show that the effectiveness of contaminant removal declined sharply after about 75 percent of the rated life on all the filters tested. They suggest changing the carbon more often than recommended. Another way is to try to figure out how much water you use on a daily basis and compare that to the estimated life of the carbon cartridge. Mark the date on your calendar and change the carbon when that time has passed, even if you think it is unnecessary. It doesn't hurt to change the carbon too often. At the very least, change it once a year.

The amount of pollutants that can be adsorbed by a filter cartridge containing activated carbon depends simply on the amount of carbon in the cartridge. The more carbon, the more micropores available. The little carbon filters that you screw on to your faucet are practically worthless. They're just as good as any other carbon filter for about the first glass of water, but they become saturated very quickly and then cause more harm than good.

Another common problem with carbon filters is bacteria growth. Bacteria tend to grow inside carbon cartridges and can multiply to potentially hazardous levels. While there is no evidence that these bacteria are common causes of disease in users of water with carbon filters, there is no practical way to monitor the amount or type of bacteria that may be present in home filters. Some granular carbon units offer a "backwashing" function to control bacteria growth, which involves switching a lever or attaching a separate device to flush hot water through the carbon in the reverse direction. Although backwashing will remove some bacteria, it is not as effective or reliable as changing the carbon completely. "Bacteriostatic" filters have been embedded with silver to control bacteria growth. EPA studies, however, have found that in addition to being potentially harmful to health, the silver does not actually reduce the bacteria count.

Still, activated carbon filters can be effective when used properly. For maximum efficiency, look for a good selection of micropore sizes within the carbon, an adequate amount of carbon (EPA studies showed that units with small amounts of carbon were only marginally effective at removing trihalomethanes, whereas units with larger amounts removed trihalomethanes up to 98 percent), good contact time between the water and the carbon to allow the pollutant molecules to be adsorbed, and a smooth flow of water through the carbon. *Consumer Reports* found that the popular pour-through pitcher-type filters remove only about half the pollutants after just twenty gallons—a practically worthless investment. Carbon block units are generally preferred—the carbon lasts longer because there is more of it, and the compressed design inhibits bacteria growth. The least expensive brands come with a hard plastic housing for the cartridge. Though this does not seem to affect the water quality if the water comes in contact only briefly with the plastic while passing through, water sitting in the filter over a long period of time may absorb polymers from the plastic. Plastic units are fine for most people, but if you are extremely sensitive to plastic, you might want to get a stainless steel unit.

Carbon blocks come in two basic styles: over-the-counter units that sit on top of the counter with diverter tubes to and from the tap, and undersink models mounted to the pipes, which dispense filtered water through the main tap or through an additional tap especially mounted for that purpose.

There are many carbon block filters on the market. Compare them according to the price of the original unit and the price of the cartridges and their estimated life. I did a cost comparison once, and there was a difference of more than $200 between the least and most expensive units to filter the same amount of water.

There are two special types of granulated carbon filters you might want to consider—one is for the showerhead and the other filters water for the whole house. Because skin absorption of water pollutants and inhalation of volatile chemical fumes during showering has now been proven to be a problem, I strongly suggest that you do something to protect yourself from these other modes of exposure. A whole-house filter is attached to the incoming cold water line of your home, so all water is filtered, even in the toilet. You have clean water for bathing, teeth-brushing, and dishwashing; all taps dispense clean water.

A showerhead filter screws right into your showerhead and filters the water only at that point. I know many people who have these simple showerhead filters and I have heard some amazing stories. One friend used to have a horrible rash all over her body that required cortisone treatments. Soon after she began filtering her shower water, the rash went away completely and has not returned. If you have a skin problem, you really may want to try this. I have had one on my showerhead for years, and I love it.

A new development in carbon filters is the use of KDF to enhance the carbon. KDF is a high-purity copper/zinc alloy that is melted together and flaked to make a "golden sand." It has two properties. First it uses chemical oxidation reduction to neutralize harmful chemicals, including chlorine, hydrogen sulfide, and iron. These substances are actually chemically changed into harmless substances (chlorine to chloride, etc.), which are then mechanically filtered out. KDF also produces .04 volts of electricity and acts like little magnets to attract and permanently trap pollutants like heavy metals. Because the KDF removes many pollutants, the carbon in the unit is then free to take out other volatile chemicals that are not removed by the KDF. Together, KDF and carbon work much more efficiently than carbon alone.

REVERSE OSMOSIS

Reverse osmosis purifies water by forcing it through a membrane that allows water molecules through, but not pollutants. Plants purify water by a similar method—as the water passes through the natural cellulose, nutrients are removed and waste fluids disposed. Reverse osmosis is a very good method of removing particulates and dissolved solids, but will not remove most microorganisms, and barely touches volatile chemicals. For this reason, most reverse osmosis membranes are used in conjunction with a carbon filter. If particulates and dissolved solids are not a problem in your water supply, the added expense of a reverse osmosis membrane is unnecessary.

A reverse-osmosis unit is ideal for someone who values convenience over effectiveness. It will remove significant amounts of almost all pollutants to some degree, hides under the sink, and gives more than two gallons per day of somewhat purified water at the flip of a lever. Periodically you have to change the membrane and the special particulate prefilter, but otherwise there is no involvement with the process. If nothing else, it's better than drinking tap water.

These units do have certain drawbacks, however. The biggest disadvantage is that the quality of water diminishes with use, and filtration may be inconsistent, depending on water pressure.

If you choose a reverse-osmosis system, opt for one that has three separate canisters for the three filtration methods. Some inexpensive models wrap the membrane around a core of carbon and have all three filtration steps in one unit. The three-canister models are more efficient, and you have more control over maintenance. When you first use your reverse-osmosis unit, it is very important to process at least twenty gallons of water through the system before drinking water from the system. Some membranes are preserved with formaldehyde, which needs to be removed, and flushing water through will remove some plastic residues.

Important note: If your chlorinated municipal water flows through galvanized pipes, or if you don't have chlorinated water, you will have to take precautions to protect your reverse-osmosis membrane. "Spurs" build up inside galvanized pipes, which are perfect breeding grounds for bacteria. While these bacteria are harmless to drink, they feed on the reverse-osmosis membrane, making it useless. To remedy this problem, either add about a teaspoon of chlorine bleach to the prefilter every month (a time-consuming and toxic procedure) or purchase a point-of-use ultraviolet unit to kill bacteria (available from **Nigra Enterprises**).

DISTILLERS

For high-quality, consistently pure water, nothing beats a distiller. Distillation comes closest to duplicating nature's own hydrologic cycle for water purification. The heat of the sun causes water to evaporate from the earth's surface, leaving impurities behind; then it gets condensed, and pure water returns to the earth as rain, hail, sleet, or snow.

Water distillers work by boiling the water to turn it into steam, and then condensing it into "pure" water. Boiling the water destroys bacteria and other living materials, leaving them behind in the boiling tank, along with particulates and dissolved solids that are too heavy to rise with the water vapor.

Early distillers concentrated only on the removal of microorganisms and solid materials. Newer designs have special volatile gas vents or double-distilling processes that enhance volatile chemical removal. Most are also coupled with activated carbon postfilters to remove any chemicals that may remain after distillation.

One danger with stainless steel distillers is that they add aluminum to the water. In a laboratory test done by the Rodale Press Product Testing Department, all of the metal distillers tested produced water with at least traces of aluminum; some distillers increased the aluminum content of the water by up to 130 percent, bringing the aluminum levels to the maximum limits generally considered acceptable. Because aluminum exposure has been linked with nervous system diseases and brain disorders, the fact that stainless steel distillers add this particular metal to the water is cause for concern. You can avoid this problem by choosing a glass distiller.

The major disadvantage to distillers is that you have to "make" the water. It's not automatic; you usually have to turn on the power supply and hook up the hoses to the water source. I can tell you from experience, this is not a big deal. I have a **Rain Crystal** glass distiller mounted near my kitchen sink. It's as simple to turn on as turning on a light bulb, and my husband ran the input water hose directly to the cold water shut-off valve under the sink. Distillers are not inexpensive, but I consider the investment a small price to pay for consistently pure water, gallon after gallon, for the rest of my life.

Many department, discount, and hardware stores now offer drinking-water filters. You may find something that is appropriate for you there; however, bear in mind that these units probably were chosen by a buyer who had little knowledge of water purification and based the decision primarily on price, rather than on ability to purify water.

Many multilevel marketers of household products sell some kind of activated carbon filter, most of which contain carbon cartridges made by the same manufacturer. These are entirely adequate carbon filters and differ more in price than performance. You can probably find similar quality for less money, however.

If you'd like some help from a knowledgeable person while making your decision, look in the Yellow Pages of your telephone book under "Water Filtration and Purification Equipment." In addition to sources for filters you can install yourself, there will be listed companies that can install and maintain systems for you. Also, you can order water filters by mail from health- and environment-oriented catalogs such as **American Environmental Health Foundation** and **Nontoxic Environments,** or from an independent dealer such as **Nigra Enterprises.**

Some unusually good water purification units I have recommended over the years include an enhanced carbon unit called the **Seagull IV,** the **Rain Crystal** Pyrex glass water distiller, and a three-canister reverse osmosis/carbon system with a high rejection rate called the **Water Safe WS/RO5.** A KDF shower filter can be ordered from **Real Goods, Home Health, The Natural Choice,** and **Natural Lifestyle.**

Chapter **6**

DRUGS AND MEDICATIONS

> **WARNING:** Keep this and all medications out of reach of children. In case of accidental overdose, contact a physician or poison-control center immediately. As with any drug, if you are pregnant or nursing a baby, seek the advice of a physician before using this product.

MOST HOME MEDICINE CABINETS are filled with over-the-counter nonprescription drugs—painkillers, antacids, allergy medicines, cough syrups, laxatives, and sleeping pills. It's a multibillion-dollar industry offering more than 200,000 products.

An over-the-counter drug, as opposed to a prescription drug, is a drug product you can buy without a prescription and use when *you* think it is useful or necessary, without a doctor's guidance. Over-the-counter drugs are formulated only to relieve symptoms and not to cure the underlying disease. They just make you less miserable so you can continue your daily routine while your body works on curing itself with its natural healing powers.

The biggest danger in having any kind of drug or medication in your home is the risk of accidental poisoning from an overdose.

Children especially are attracted to the brightly colored pills and can quickly consume too many, with serious consequences.

Many drugs and medications have dangerous side effects. I'll be discussing the specific risks associated with some of the more common nonprescription drugs later in this chapter, but if I don't cover everything in *your* medicine cabinet, you can go to your local library and look up information on more than 2,500 popular pharmaceuticals in the *Physician's Desk Reference*. There you'll find other books written for the general public about the health effects of both nonprescription and prescription drugs. Your favorite bookstore also will carry books on the subject. You should do this extra research because often a product's side effects aren't listed on its label.

By using over-the-counter medications, we are, in effect, playing doctor with ourselves, and as our own self-care physicians, we want to prescribe the proper treatment. Yet how often do we take medications or give them to other members of our household without stopping first to find out *all* the facts—the proper dosage, possible side effects, and other health effects, or if in fact this is the right drug for the symptoms? Since 1962 the Food and Drug Administration has been reviewing the active ingredients found in over-the-counter drugs. In many cases they have found that, while some active ingredients may be "safe," *they are not effective at doing what the consumer believes the drug is supposed to do.* We may be taking medications we don't even need, because we are misdiagnosing our symptoms!

Symptoms are signals from the body that something is wrong and that the body is doing something about it. When you run a fever, your body is heating up to kill germs; when you cough, it is to clear your lungs; a headache may be a sign that you are under too much stress and should take more leisure time for yourself. It's not always a good idea to stifle your symptoms, and never a good idea to ignore them completely, as they are part of your natural healing process.

Over-the-counter medications are meant to provide temporary relief for occasional symptoms, and are not to be used on a regular basis. As the label says, "If symptoms persist, see your doctor." You may have a more serious illness that requires medical attention.

Labeling

Only active ingredients are required to be listed on the labels of drugs and medications, and they probably contain many additional ingredients you might want to watch out for: **alcohol, caffeine, artificial colors and flavors, sugar, saccharin, preservatives**—the list is endless and there is no way of knowing if any are in the product.

SAFE SOLUTIONS

To be more comfortable while your body is healing itself, there are some natural things you can do.

The oldest form of medicine, as well as the basis of modern pharmacology, is the use of herbs and plants. Herbs and medicinal plants can be taken in many forms, including tinctures (the most concentrated form, usually in an alcohol base), teas, pills, and pressed juices for internal use, and ointments and shampoos for external use.

Homeopathic remedies are another choice. Homeopathy is a medicinal system that stimulates our own innate healing and immune processes by using the energetic essences of plant, mineral, and animal substances captured by a water-based pharmaceutical process. One of the main principles of homeopathy is that like cures like, which means that a substance that creates a specific set of symptoms in a healthy person, when given in a large dose, will cure similar symptoms in a sick person, when given in a specially prepared minute dose. Almost every pharmacy in France carries homeopathic medicines, and in Germany 16,000 physicians use this medically recognized system. Your natural-food store will have a well-stocked department full of natural remedies. Also check out the **Home Health** and **Self Care** catalogs, and **Natural Health** magazine.

When you need extensive health care, consider also exploring alternative therapies, which can be used either alone or in conjunction with modern medical practices. Acupuncture, ayuvredic medicine, chiropractic, bodywork, and many other holistic modalities are worth looking into and are becoming accepted by medical doctors as "complementary medicine."

Now let's look at some specific complaints and their safe solutions.

ARTHRITIS, FEVER, AND ACHES

The most common reason people take nonprescription drugs is for pain relief. One evening spent watching television will verify this point, since your favorite shows will be interrupted every ten minutes by commercials for Bayer aspirin, Anacin-3, Extra-Strength Excedrin, Motrin, Advil, Tylenol, and Aleve. Most pain relievers also lower fevers and reduce the inflammatory distress of arthritis, and these drugs are frequently advertised to relieve all these symptoms.

Painkillers, or analgesics, work by blocking the transmission of pain impulses to the brain, and should not be taken for more than ten days in succession by adults, or for more than five consecutive days by children.

Most analgesics contain one of three active ingredients: aspirin, acetaminophen, or ibuprofen.

Aspirin is by far the most widely used painkiller. More than 20 billion doses are sold each year; that's about 100 aspirin tablets for every man, woman, and child in America. Aspirin has been widely used for years and is considered by the FDA to be "safe and effective" when taken in the recommended dosage—no more than 4,000 mg in a twenty-four-hour period. However, in some cases, aspirin can:

- interfere with blood-clotting, and regular use can cause iron-deficiency anemia;
- trigger or aggravate peptic ulcer and cause stomach upset, heartburn, or bleeding in the stomach;
- produce allergic reactions in an estimated 2 out of 1,000 people and in some asthma sufferers. Reactions can range from rashes, hives, and swelling to life-threatening asthma attacks;
- stimulate the brain and spinal cord, followed by central nervous system depression, which appears

as respiratory failure, circulatory collapse, coma, and death; and

- in high doses, interfere with liver function.

Early signs of aspirin toxicity include ringing in the ears, hearing loss, headache, dizziness, vomiting, rapid breathing, extreme irritability, and bizarre behavior. Pregnant women should check with their physicians before taking aspirin. Children under age eighteen with chicken pox or flu should not be given aspirin, as they may develop Reye's syndrome, an often fatal liver disorder.

The FDA also considers acetaminophen to be "safe and effective" when taken in the recommended dosage—no more than 4,000 mg in a twenty-four-hour period. Milligram for milligram, acetaminophen is as effective as aspirin for pain relief and fever reduction, but is not recommended for reducing the inflammatory effects of arthritis.

Acetaminophen (one popular brand name is Tylenol) is used by many people who are allergic to or who get upset stomachs from taking aspirin. For this reason, it appears to be safer than aspirin, but in some ways it's not. You can be allergic to acetaminophen, too, and overdoses can cause severe liver damage and even death.

Ibuprofen (such as the brand-name product Motrin) is a relative newcomer to the painkiller market, having been available for many years only as a prescription drug. Possible side effects include nausea, vomiting, stomach cramps or pain, constipation, diarrhea, heartburn, stiff neck, headache, fever, dizziness, depression, insomnia, blurred vision, or swelling of hands and legs. You should not take ibuprofen if you are allergic to aspirin or have a history of dizziness, bronchospasms, liver disease, hypertension or heart disease, nasal polyps, stomach ulcer, or intestinal bleeding. According to *Physician's Desk Reference*, "It is especially important not to use ibuprofen during the last three months of pregnancy unless specifically directed to do so by a doctor, because it may cause problems in the unborn child or complications during delivery."

SAFE SOLUTIONS

HEADACHES
Approximately nine out of ten headaches are the result of the body's reaction to apprehension, anxiety, depression, worry, and

other emotional states. FDA investigators found that over-the-counter pain relievers provide little if any relief for this type of headache. Other common types of headaches are migraine headaches and hypertensive headaches, caused by a sudden rise in blood pressure. Authorities say that these types of headaches should not be treated with over-the-counter analgesics either. The other types of headaches are caused by inflammation—of the sinuses, of membranes surrounding the brain, or even from developing brain tumors. For these conditions, medical care is recommended, not over-the-counter drugs. So when is it appropriate to take an analgesic for a headache? If it's caused by a fever or a hangover; otherwise the FDA says no.

Headaches can be caused also by a great variety of food allergies or by many substances you might have around the home. If headaches are a recurring problem for you, it might benefit you greatly to play detective and keep a diary of everything you eat, every exposure to a chemical, every activity, and every time you get a headache. This seems like a lot of trouble, I know, but it's very rewarding when you no longer have headaches because you've found the cause, instead of just covering up the effects.

For temporary relief from occasional headaches, regardless of the source, drink a cup of strong peppermint tea and take a short nap. Or try teas made from rosemary, catnip, or sage.

Massage can also help a great deal. Gently rub the area where the pain is, or relax your neck by letting your head droop forward as far as it will go, then turning your head slowly in the widest possible circle. Lying in a warm bath with a cold washcloth on your head will lessen pain by drawing blood away from your head. And, finally, I have a friend who swears that the best cure for his rare headaches is a steaming bowl of Chinese hot and sour soup, without MSG. It works every time.

FEVER

A fever generally is considered to be any body temperature higher than the average 98.6°F, although keep in mind that "normal" body temperature fluctuates within a one-degree range of 98.6°F. Any chronic or extreme symptoms and temperature higher than 102°F warrant immediate medical attention. But for those in-between fevers, there are a few things you can do.

First, decide if you really want to lower the fever. In many cases, fever can be beneficial, as it seems to increase the mobility of your white blood cells and enhance their ability to kill germs. One problem with taking aspirin to reduce fever is that it interferes with the body's natural defense cycle, so while you may reduce your fever, it might take longer for you to get well.

The simplest way to reduce fever is by placing a cold washcloth on the forehead. It has to be changed and rinsed regularly, as it quickly absorbs heat from the skin. For a serious fever, overall sponging of the body, taking a cool bath or shower, or wrapping the patient in a wet sheet for short periods of time will help.

Various herbal teas have been used to treat fever, including boneset, yarrow, vervain, and barberry berries. Your natural-food store may carry these herbs, or see if you can find an herb shop in your community. If it's too much trouble to go hunting for these herbs, open your spice cabinet and take out your cayenne pepper—yes, *hot* red pepper. Add small amounts to warm water, milk, or tea, or fill empty gelatin capsules and take a couple with a glass of water.

You can get dehydrated very quickly with a fever, so keep drinking liquids. Add as much lemon juice as you can to everything and take some extra vitamin C.

HEARTBURN, CONSTIPATION, DIARRHEA, AND NAUSEA

Between the television commercials for painkillers are the commercials for antacids—liquids, gels, tablets, capsules, powders—to relieve the heartburn, sour stomach, and acid indigestion caused by excess stomach acid. It seems there's something wrong with everybody's stomachs—if it's not heartburn, it's "irregularity." Diarrhea isn't quite so popular in the TV commercials, but it's all part of the same gastrointestinal problem. Nausea is sometimes related to gastrointestinal function, but can also be a sign of food poisoning, hormonal changes (during pregnancy or menstrual cycle), a food allergy, or motion sickness.

Antacids work by chemically neutralizing excess hydrochloric acid in the stomach. They are considered to be relatively safe, in comparison with other groups of drugs; however, they do contain ingredients that can be dangerous to some people, particularly if they are taken in large amounts over a long period of time.

Some antacids contain **aluminum compounds,** which can be risky for people with kidney problems or who are on kidney dialysis. The level of aluminum in your blood doubles when you take an aluminum-containing antacid. Heavy use may affect your body's metabolism in its ability to process certain essential minerals, which may lead to bone abnormalities.

Bicarbonate compounds are also widely used as antacids, including **sodium bicarbonate** (baking soda) and **potassium bicarbonate.** Because they are readily absorbed into the body, they can measurably increase the alkalinity of blood plasma and other body tissues. Sodium bicarbonate also increases the sodium level in the body, which may be risky for those with high blood pressure.

Most laxatives are not especially harmful, but the FDA believes that there is a widespread overuse of laxatives, due largely to misleading advertising. Laxatives should be used only in cases of infrequent, difficult, or uncomfortable bowel movements as an occasional, temporary measure, and not on a regular basis or for an extended period of time. Prolonged use of laxatives can seriously impair normal bowel function, and people can become dependent on laxatives. It is normal for bowel movements to occur in the range of three movements per day to three movements per week, and any sudden change in your normal pattern which lasts for more than a couple of weeks is cause for you to seek professional help, not treat yourself with a laxative.

The FDA also frowns on diarrhea remedies. Over-the-counter products are effective for only the mildest forms of diarrhea, which usually go away by themselves in a day or two. One of the more popular antidiarrheal drugs, **diphenoxylate hydrochloride,** may cause more harm than it does good. It is an addictive narcotic substance, and overdose could be fatal. To prevent overdose, the drug is formulated with other substances that can cause dry skin, flushed face, rapid heartbeat, and other unpleasant side effects.

SAFE SOLUTIONS

Most gastrointestinal difficulties can be related to the food you eat, so if your stomach and intestines are giving you trouble, they are probably just unhappy with what you're putting in them.

Do you eat a lot of processed foods? If so, you probably have a diet high in sugar and fat and low in dietary fiber, which helps the gastrointestinal tract work smoothly. Are you drinking enough water and other beverages? A diet that contains lots of fresh fruits, vegetables, and whole grains provides adequate amounts of fiber and fluids to keep your gastrointestinal tract well regulated.

HEARTBURN

If you occasionally have heartburn and need an antacid, don't reach for an over-the-counter drug. An interesting study in Great Britain showed that antacid tablets containing the usual aluminum hydroxide, magnesium, and sodium bicarbonate didn't work at all to reduce heartburn. What did work for about half the patients was a formula that contained alginic acid, a natural substance derived from seaweed. If you'd like to try this, get some sodium alginate tablets from your natural-food store, chew one or two tablets thoroughly (do not swallow them whole), and then drink a glass of milk.

Losing weight can also help heartburn, as can eating smaller meals, especially in the evening, and avoiding lying down for several hours after the meal. Alcoholic beverages; chocolate; coffee; tomatoes and tomato products; citrus fruits; and fried, fatty, or spicy foods all stimulate your stomach to produce excess acid. Cigarette smoking also greatly contributes to heartburn—if you smoke, there's a good chance that by giving up your cigarettes you'll also be giving up your heartburn.

Frequent heartburn may also be a symptom of hiatal hernia. A medical doctor will want to fix the problem with an expensive operation—try a chiropractor first, who should be able to put your stomach back into place with a quick adjustment of your abdominal muscles.

CONSTIPATION

For occasional constipation, try prunes, prune juice, or large doses of vitamin C. Your natural-food store probably carries some herbal laxatives that are very effective, in addition to psyllium husks—another natural substance, which is FDA-approved as a safe and effective laxative (drugstore laxatives often are just psyllium with sugar and flavorings).

DIARRHEA

Diarrhea, like fever, is one of the body's healing mechanisms—if you get it, it probably means that your body wants to expel whatever is in your gut. It may want to get rid of a toxic virus or bacteria, or cleanse your system of a mild case of food poisoning. Or, you might have an allergy to the food the body wants to eliminate. So it might not be in your best interest to inhibit diarrhea, but again, don't ignore chronic or severe symptoms. Let everything come out, and sip warm water to keep from getting dehydrated.

NAUSEA

To relieve nausea, try a cup of raspberry leaf or basil tea. During pregnancy, 10 to 20 mg per day of vitamin B_6 can help.

My favorite remedy for nausea is ginger ale. I had a medical doctor once who was very old and knew a lot of folk remedies. He told me to drink ginger ale—ginger ale specifically, and not other carbonated beverages (my mother always gave me 7-Up, thinking it was the bubbles that helped)—because the *ginger* helped the nausea. Instead of drinking commercial ginger ale, I make my own with fresh ginger and honey. Here's the recipe (I know it's a little complex and not what you want to do when you're sick, but you can make the syrup and keep it indefinitely in the refrigerator, if you can resist drinking it in the meantime as a refreshing beverage).

Nausea-Relief Ginger Ale

6 ounces fresh gingerroot (available at most supermarkets)
2 cups water   1¼ cups honey

1. Peel and finely chop the ginger (you should have about 1 cup).

2. In an enamel or stainless-steel saucepan, bring the ginger and water to a boil, then simmer for 5 minutes. Remove from heat and let stand for 24 hours, covered with a cloth (a kitchen towel works fine).

3. Strain through two layers of cheesecloth (buy at hardware store), and squeeze the pulp in the cloth to extract all possible juice.

4. Return juice to saucepan, add honey, and bring to a boil over moderate heat, stirring to dissolve the honey. Simmer for 5 minutes.

5. Cool, pour into a bottle, and refrigerate.

To USE: Mix a soupspoon of syrup in a glass of carbonated mineral water or club soda, more or less to taste.

ALLERGIC HAY FEVER

Each year millions of allergy sufferers take antihistamines to relieve their symptoms. During an allergic response, the body produces an irritating substance called histamine, which attaches itself to the secretory cells of the nose, eyes, and lungs. Antihistamines block the histamine receptor sites on these cells, preventing the condition that causes the symptoms.

In general, antihistamines are considered to be safe and effective. There are only two notable side effects: dry mouth and drowsiness. If you'd like to stay alert and be symptom-free, try a natural remedy.

SAFE SOLUTIONS

A basic, all-purpose hay-fever remedy is to take 500 mg of vitamin C three times a day, and twice a day take 50 mg of pantothenic acid and a teaspoon of grated orange or lemon rind sweetened with some honey. You might not get immediate relief, but chances are you should notice a marked improvement within three days.

Why does this work? Vitamin C is a natural antihistamine, and the bioflavonoids in the citrus peel enhance its bioavailability. Pantothenic acid alone has been known to combat allergy symptoms, and up to 500 mg per day can be taken for this purpose. Experiment for yourself with these substances and you will find just the right combination to keep you from reaching for the antihistamine bottle.

Another solution for hay fever is to figure out what is causing it and remove the item or items from your home. This will work if you are allergic to your cat or the feathers in your pillow, but it might be more difficult to control if you are allergic to the acacia outside your bedroom window.

COLDS AND COUGHS

Cold and cough medications contain a complex variety of active ingredients to relieve the aches, sore throat, coughs, fever, nasal and sinus congestion, runny nose, and sneezing typical of the common cold. The FDA emphasizes that, while these products may relieve symptoms, they cannot "cure" colds.

Most general-purpose cold medications include cough suppressors and expectorants, nasal decongestants, sore-throat medications, and painkillers/fever reducers. Each of these drugs can be purchased also as a separate product to be taken for specific symptoms.

Cough suppressors temporarily inhibit the impulse to cough. Codeine and dextromethorphan act in the brain to depress the activity of the cough center; other drugs alleviate pain and irritation in the throat and bronchial passages to lessen the need to cough. Over-the-counter cough suppressors are intended to be used for periods of less than one week to diminish coughs due to bronchial irritation. People who have asthma, emphysema, and other lung conditions should not take over-the-counter cough suppressors for relief; neither should those who smoke.

The primary danger of cough suppressors that contain **codeine** is the potential for addiction, and in many states they cannot be purchased without a prescription. **Dextromethorphan** can cause stomach upsets, drowsiness, and unconsciousness. Some cough syrups contain very high levels of **alcohol;** a few preparations contain even more alcohol than some alcoholic beverages.

Nasal decongestants constrict swollen blood vessels in the lining of the nose and sinuses, which is the primary cause of stuffy noses. Unfortunately, when the drug wears off, the blood vessels may swell even more than before, making your stuffy nose worse! Decongestants should be used no more frequently than three days in a row, and not without doctor's orders if you have high blood pressure, heart disease, diabetes, or thyroid disease.

Sore-throat medications are designed to provide only temporary relief of minor symptoms and should not be used for more than two consecutive days. Most sore throats are a symptom of an underlying infection or illness that should be treated, not hidden under a cough drop.

SAFE SOLUTIONS

Of course, the first cold remedy that comes to mind is vitamin C, right? Although there is little scientific evidence to show that vitamin C prevents colds, it can significantly shorten the cycle of the cold virus, even if you wait until the first sign of a cold to start taking the vitamin. Start by taking several 500-mg doses throughout the day as soon as you notice the symptoms. You can take up to 4,000 or 5,000 mg each day for the duration of your cold, if you need to.

Also, take lots of hot fluids, chicken soup, and anything spicy. Both cayenne pepper and garlic are germ killers. Among the herbal teas, try chamomile, lemon balm, boneset, elder, vervain, or slippery elm.

To soothe the tickle in your throat, almost any hard candy will work as well as a cough drop. The idea is just to keep you salivating. Your natural-food store probably has herbal drops or hard candies sweetened with honey, rice syrup, or other natural sweeteners.

When I was a child and got really bad sore throats, my parents would make a horrible-tasting concoction of honey and onions. They would slice a whole white onion in a bowl, cover it with lots of honey, then cover the bowl and let it sit. After a few hours, the onion would "sweat" and release its juice. I was given a couple tablespoons of this honey/onion juice, and by the next day I was magically cured.

You could also try hot ginger milk. Heat milk and add two or three slices of fresh ginger (or ½ to ¾ teaspoons ground ginger) and honey to taste. Serve hot.

INSOMNIA

Because many people have difficulty falling asleep or staying asleep, the FDA recognizes the need for safe and effective nonprescription sleep aids. However useful and convenient such a product might be, the FDA has found that most active ingredients used in sleeping pills are unsafe, ineffective, or both.

For many years, the most popular active ingredient in sleep aids was the antihistamine **methapyrilene.** In 1979, products containing methapyrilene were recalled when the National Cancer Institute found that methapyrilene causes cancer in laboratory animals and poses a potential human hazard.

Over-the-counter sleeping pills are intended to be used for no longer than two weeks. Chronic insomnia warrants professional attention.

SAFE SOLUTIONS

First of all, you may not even have insomnia. A good number of "insomniacs" are only insomniacs because they think they need eight hours of sleep every night. Everyone's body is different, and we each require different amounts of sleep. We need only enough sleep to feel rested, and that amount may change at different times in our lives.

The best "medicine" for a good night's sleep is a mug of warm milk. Milk contains the amino acid tryptophan, which aids your body in the production of sleep-inducing serotonin. (Naturally occurring tryptophan in food is fine; however, the food supplement L-tryptophan, which was used by many as a natural sleep aid, was taken off the market as being harmful to health.) Also, a high-carbohydrate evening meal will help you drift off to sleep easily.

Chamomile tea has been shown in scientific studies to have a sleep-inducing effect on ten out of twelve subjects. Other herbs known to have a similar effect are hops, passionflower, catnip, basil, and lemon verbena.

As a former insomniac myself, I can tell you a couple of things that worked for me. First, I changed the sheets on my bed from polyester/cotton to 100 percent cotton. This worked like magic—the very first night I went right to sleep. I later found out that polyester/cotton sheets are heavily treated with formaldehyde, which is known to cause insomnia! After I got that out of the way, I found that what was also keeping me awake was mental tension—although my body was tired, my mind wouldn't relax. It was racing along like an endless tape recorder on fast forward.

So I began learning to quiet my mind by repeating the word *sleep* over and over. At first I couldn't do it because my mind would wander too much, but I just kept at it, night after night, until now I just lie down in bed, close my eyes, think *sleep,* and I'm out.

IF YOU MUST TAKE MEDICATIONS

By the time you have read this far, I hope you are convinced that over-the-counter drugs are not what you want to take for your symptoms, if for no other reason than that they can't cure any of your ills. But if you still want to take them, please use them with good judgment. Here are a few tips for using medications responsibly.

- Prevent accidental poisonings by keeping medications out of children's reach.
- Always check with your doctor to make sure the over-the-counter drug you have chosen is appropriate for your symptoms, especially if you are pregnant. Always tell your doctor *all* the medications you are taking so he or she can assess the possible dangers of mixing medications.
- Take the medication only as directed on the package.
- Do not take any more medications than are absolutely necessary, as the greater the number of drugs taken simultaneously, the greater the likelihood of adverse effects.
- Read package labels and any other information you can find on the drug you have chosen.
- Be aware of how you feel while under the influence of the drug, and watch out for side effects.

Chapter 7

BEAUTY AND HYGIENE

EAUTY AND HYGIENE ITEMS are applied to some of the more sensitive parts of our bodies. We use soap, shampoo, toothpaste, contraceptives, colognes, makeup, toilet paper, and other personal products day in and day out. You would think these products would be tested for safety according to regulations as strict as those for the food we eat. Unfortunately, they are not.

Not surprisingly, the most common complaint associated with personal-care products is skin rash, which can range in intensity from moderately irritating to painful and disfiguring. For many years, people thought that the skin was impenetrable, but now we know that everything we put on our skin goes directly into our bodies. Skin patches are used in some cases to administer drugs, for doctors know that what is absorbed through the skin eventually travels to every part of the body. Since we are applying beauty and hygiene products to some of the more sensitive and thin-skinned parts of our bodies, it makes good sense to use only the purest natural products we can.

Beauty products also have other hazards. Did you know your lipstick may be carcinogenic? Or that an accidental swallow of perfume could kill your child?

At a government hearing in July 1989 on the safety of cosmetics, numerous cosmetologists testified about symptoms such as headaches, loss of balance, memory loss, asthma, and irreparable nervous system and respiratory problems as a result of working with cosmetics. Because of these testimonies, a House subcommittee asked the National Institute of Occupational Safety and Health (NIOSH) to analyze 2,983 chemicals used in cosmetics.

The results were as follows: 884 of the ingredients were found to be toxic. Of these, 314 can cause biological mutation, 218 can cause reproductive complications, 778 can cause acute toxicity, 146 can cause tumors, and 376 can cause skin and eye irritations.

Labeling

Most hygiene products are regulated by the FDA as "cosmetics," a category that includes anything that can be "rubbed, poured, sprinkled or sprayed on, introduced into, or otherwise applied to the human body . . . for cleansing, beautifying, promoting attractiveness, or altering appearance without affecting the body's structure or functions."

The law does not require that cosmetics be tested for safety before they are allowed to be sold. The FDA can take action on a case in which harm is done only after a product is on the market, and only after it has received enough consumer complaints and enough evidence has been collected to prove in court that the product is hazardous. Then the FDA can halt its production and sale.

More than three thousand different ingredients derived from **petrochemicals** or natural animal, vegetable, or mineral sources are used in cosmetics. The FDA requires a complete listing of ingredients on all domestic cosmetics, itemized in decreasing order and expressed in standardized language, yet there is no easy rule of thumb to help you identify the natural ones. (Some commonly used items that we think of as cosmetics are exempt from this labeling requirement. Deodorant soaps, fluoridated toothpastes, antiperspirants, sunscreens, and antidandruff shampoos all claim to affect the body's structure or function and are regulated as over-the-counter drugs.)

"Natural" cosmetics, made primarily from plant, animal, and mineral ingredients, are big business. In the last fifteen years, natural cosmetics have gone from a few poorly formulated items in health-food stores to a wide selection of products that are sold not only in natural-food stores, but in department stores and specialty boutiques as well.

The best advice I can give is for you to start reading labels and looking up the ingredients in books such as *A Consumer Dictionary of Cosmetic Ingredients.* If you've done your homework, it can be a relatively simple task to identify natural cosmetics. Remember, though, that some of these ingredients may be hybrid-natural, containing petrochemicals even though they may say they have a natural source. Two nonrenewable petrochemical derivatives that are practically inescapable—even in natural cosmetics—are **methylparaben** and **propylparaben.** Laboratory tests have proved these common preservatives to be safe; however, I wouldn't call them natural.

Some clever manufacturers create "natural" formulas by adding natural-sounding ingredients such as honey or herbs or aloe vera, instead of actually making a more natural formula by removing unnecessary **artificial colors, fragrances,** and **preservatives.** And frequently I have found ingredients made from petrochemicals—particularly **artificial colors**—in cosmetics marketed "Cruelty-free." Just because a product wasn't tested on animals doesn't mean it's natural, though they are marketed side-by-side with natural cosmetic items.

Here's a good example of an ingredient list on a natural cosmetic product, **Dr. Bronner's Peppermint Oil Soap,** a mainstay that has been sold for years in every natural-food store: Coconut Oil, Olive Oil, Peppermint Oil, Potassium Hydroxide, Water. All these ingredients are easily recognizable except maybe potassium hydroxide, which is a natural mineral salt.

If you are allergic to certain substances, you need to beware of products labeled *hypoallergenic.* Because allergies are so individual, no one product can be truly hypoallergenic for everyone. Hypoallergenic simply means that the more *common* allergens have been removed—fragrance, lanolin, cocoa butter, cornstarch, cottonseed oils—but these products still may contain ingredients to which you are sensitive.

SAFE SOLUTIONS

Start by looking for natural cosmetics in your local natural-food store. Most have a good selection of everything from soap, shampoo, and toothpaste to complete makeup collections. These products can be reasonably relied upon to be made primarily from plant, animal, and mineral ingredients, though few are completely petrochemical-free and the plant ingredients are grown with pesticides. Many department stores are also now selling natural cosmetics. Read the labels very carefully, as I have found a number of petrochemical ingredients in them, particularly artificial colors and mineral oil. If in doubt about an ingredient, look it up. A little extra time is worth the effort, and once you've found brands that you like, you will also have learned to recognize ingredients.

You can also make many beauty and hygiene products yourself at home. It's mostly a matter of getting back to basics and using natural products that are in harmony with your body. I'm not suggesting to you women that you will have to change the way you look, though you may choose to do that when you see the gorgeous colors available in natural cosmetics, or the subtle highlights in your hair when you rinse it with chamomile tea, and how softly your hair stays in place with lemon juice hair spray. A warm, fragrant herbal bath is much more luxurious than any bathtubful of bubbles. Take care of yourself with products that not only make you more attractive, but are good for you too. All the top fashion magazines and the most beautiful women in the world agree that you are the most beautiful you can be when you are healthy and fit and use beauty products to subtly enhance your own beauty, rather than drastically changing the way you look, which hides the real you.

You can also order safe beauty and hygiene products by mail.

Simmons Handcrafts carries some of the purest natural body-care products, including vegetarian olive oil soap they make themselves.

Kettle Care offers body-care products hand made with organically grown herbs from original recipes—herbs come straight from the garden into the products.

Catalogs that have a general assortment of safe, natural, unscented, nontoxic, natural-food-store-type beauty and hygiene products include **Alexandra Avery** (organically grown ingredients), **Allergy Relief Shop, Allergy Resources, American Environmental Health Foundation, Home Health,**

Janice Corporation, Karen's Nontoxic Products, The Living Source, Logona USA (organically grown ingredients), ***Natural Lifestyle, Nontoxic Environments,*** and **Weleda** (biodynamically grown ingredients).

DENTURE CLEANERS

DANGER: Injurious to eyes. Harmful if swallowed. Keep out of reach of children.

Despite the ominous warning, denture cleaners actually are relatively safe to use. Most are made up of a combination of salts—**sodium perborate, sodium chloride (table salt), magnesium sulfate (Epsom salt), calcium chloride, sodium carbonate,** and **trisodium phosphate,** which, while not intended to be eaten, will cause no more than an upset stomach if accidentally ingested by a child.

These salts are very irritating to the eyes, however, so if you leave your teeth sitting around in a glass of denture cleaner and have little ones in the house, make sure to keep the glass out of their reach. Children are inquisitive, and they could reach for the glass and spill it into their eyes. Denture cleaners also can irritate the skin, but again the hazard here is minor.

The only other ingredients found in denture cleaners are **artificial colors and flavors** and various **preservatives,** neither of which pose a real hazard by this method of exposure.

SAFE SOLUTIONS

Now that you know there's very little danger in using denture cleaners, you might want to just go ahead and use them. But you can save some money by making them yourself at home. These recipes use exactly the same active ingredients as the commercial denture cleaners, and so will clean them just as well. Remember to take precautions around children, because these homemade potions also can irritate their eyes.

- The simple method: dissolve ¼ teaspoon trisodium phosphate (TSP) into ½ glass of water and soak dentures overnight. This is the same TSP you may have already purchased at your hardware store to use for nontoxic cleaning. If you want something fancier, shake ⅝ cup of TSP together in a bottle with 7 drops of essential oil of cinnamon or peppermint or whatever flavor you prefer (available at your natural-food store), then proceed as above, using ¼ teaspoon of the flavored TSP to ½ glass of water.

- The complex method: Mix together 1¼ cups TSP (plain or flavored), ⅝ cup sodium perborate (a bleaching agent, available at drugstores), and ⅝ cup salt. Dissolve ¼ teaspoon in ½ glass of water and soak overnight. This combination of salts is very similar to the commercial formulas and has a bleaching action that plain TSP doesn't have.

Of course, you should rinse your dentures well in the morning before wearing them.

FEMININE DEODORANT SPRAYS AND DOUCHES

WARNING: Avoid spraying in eyes. Contents under pressure. Flammable. Do not puncture or incinerate. Do not store at temperatures above 120°F or use near fire or flame. Keep out of reach of children. Use only as directed. Intentional misuse by deliberately concentrating or inhaling contents can be harmful or fatal.

CAUTION: For external use only. Spray at least 8" from skin. Do not apply to broken, irritated, or itching skin. Persistent, unusual odor or discharge may indicate conditions for which a physician should be consulted. Discontinue use immediately if rash, irritation, or discomfort develops.

Feminine hygiene sprays generally contain only a pleasant fragrance; they do not contain antibacterial agents to stop odor. Irritation is common and can range from rashes and discomfort to infection and open sores. Men can also suffer from skin problems if their partners use a deodorant spray prior to intercourse.

A long-term danger to using feminine hygiene sprays on a regular basis is that most feminine deodorants contain **talc,** which can be contaminated with carcinogenic **asbestos.** Studies have shown that there is no safe level for asbestos exposure. Asbestos causes its greatest harm when inhaled into the lungs, and when it is dispensed with an **aerosol spray,** as these products are, it is very likely to end up just where you don't want it.

Similarly, feminine douches often do more harm than good. They generally contain **ammonia, detergents, artificial fragrance,** and **phenol.** Phenol is a very toxic chemical that is easily absorbed by the skin. Douches can cause irritation, allergic skin reactions, and "chemical vaginitis." In addition, toxic chemicals are easily absorbed by the delicate skin inside the vagina, compounding their danger. It sounds to me like a big risk to take for a product most physicians think is totally unnecessary for healthy women.

SAFE SOLUTIONS

A daily rinsing with plain water while bathing should keep the vaginal area odor-free. Do not use soap inside, as it may cause irritation for you or your sexual partner.

If you regularly have a disagreeable odor, consult your physician and check for infection, rather than trying to cover up the smell.

HAIR SPRAY AND STYLING MOUSSE

> **WARNING:** Flammable. Avoid fire, flame, or smoking during application and until hair is fully dry. Avoid spraying near eyes. Contents under pressure. Do not puncture or incinerate. Do not store at temperatures above 120°F. Keep out of reach of children. Use only as directed. Intentional misuse by deliberately concentrating and inhaling contents can be harmful or fatal.

Common ingredients in hair spray include **aerosol propellants, alcohol,** carcinogenic **polyvinylpyrrolidone plastic (PVP), formaldehyde,** and **artificial fragrance.**

Regular users of hair spray run the risk of developing a lung disease called thesaurosis, which causes enlarged lymph nodes, lung masses, and changes in blood cells. Fortunately, the disease is reversible. An FDA report noted that in one study, more than half of the women afflicted with this disease recovered within six months after discontinuing hair spray use.

Also, many people have allergic skin reactions to hair spray that ends up on delicate facial skin instead of on the hair. Eye and nasal irritations are common side effects.

Styling mousse contains almost exactly the same ingredients as hair spray. The only real difference is that it comes in a foam instead of a spray.

SAFE SOLUTIONS

Check your local natural-food store for an unscented natural hair spray in a nonaerosol pump spray bottle. These are much safer than the standard brands in the aerosol can, but still may contain alcohol, perfume, and other ingredients that can cause allergic reactions in some people.

You can make your own hair spray from lemons. I don't use hair spray at all, but I have many friends who use this one, and they tell me it keeps their hair in place and still leaves it feeling soft. No, it doesn't get sticky if the proportions are right, and it smells less than an aerosol hair spray.

Chop 1 lemon (or 1 orange for dry hair). Place in a pot, cover with 2 cups pure hot water, and boil until only half remains. Cool and strain. Place in a fine spray bottle and test on hair. If it's too sticky, add more water. Store in the refrigerator, or add 1 ounce vodka per cup of hair spray as a preservative (with the vodka, you can keep this hair spray unrefrigerated for up to two weeks).

If that seems like too much trouble, you can also make hair spray with honey! Put two to five teaspoons of honey in a spray mist pump dispenser with about a cup of warm water and shake well. You'll have to experiment a bit with the proportions. The more honey it contains, the greater the holding power, but too much honey will make your hair sticky. Store the mixture in the refrigerator.

Even easier is to just pour some beer into a pump spray bottle (this only holds well on fine hair, though).

Now, if you prefer to use mousse, try gelatin instead. Dissolve a quarter-teaspoon of plain, unflavored gelatin in one cup of boiling water, and let it sit at room temperature (do not refrigerate) until slightly set. You can make this in advance and keep it in a jar in the bathroom. To use, just rub it into wet or dry hair with your fingers and blow dry. It leaves no residue but gives lots of body.

SHAMPOO

> **CAUTION:** Not to be taken internally. Keep out of reach of children. Avoid getting shampoo in eyes—if this happens, rinse eyes with water. If irritation occurs, discontinue use.

Dandruff shampoos are the most dangerous of all hair-care products because they contain highly toxic medications to prevent the scalp from peeling. One popular antidandruff agent is **selenium sulfide,** which, if swallowed, can cause vital organs to degenerate. **Recorcinol** is very easily absorbed through the skin and can lead to inflammation of the inner eyelids, skin irritation, dizziness, restlessness, rapid heartbeat, breathing difficulties, drowsiness, sweating, unconsciousness, and convulsions. In addition, dandruff shampoos may contain toxic **cresol,** carcinogenic **polyvinylpyrrolidone plastic (PVP), formaldehyde, detergents, artificial colors,** and **fragrance.**

Regular shampoos also have their risks. Formaldehyde is commonly used as a preservative and may be present in shampoos, hidden under the name **quaternium-15.** In addition to being a potential human carcinogen, formaldehyde can be an irritant to skin, eyes, and respiratory passages, even at very low concentrations. Government regulatory agencies require some products containing this chemical to carry warning labels, but shampoo does not have to.

Another hidden and unpredictable hazard is sometimes found in shampoos—this is the intimidating sounding **2-bromo-2-nitroprone-1, 3-diol (BNPD).** This chemical can create carcinogenic **nitrosamines** when combined in a bottle with **triethanolamine (TEA)** or **diethanolamine (DEA),** two rather harmless ingredients found in most shampoos, or with amines on your skin or in your body. This reaction occurs at random, so one bottle of shampoo might be loaded with nitrosamines and another bottle with the same ingredients sitting right next to it on the shelf may be absolutely safe. And you could take that safe bottle and use it with no ill effects, but it might create nitrosamines when used by another family member. Because nitrosamines are easily absorbed through the skin, you may get a higher exposure to this carcinogen from washing your hair than you would from eating nitrite-cured bacon.

SAFE SOLUTIONS

If this were an advertisement for a new dandruff shampoo, you would read, "At last! You can get rid of dandruff forever!" I, personally, never have had dandruff, and so have never tried this method, but several of my friends swear by it. This sounds strange, I know, but it works.

Instead of using shampoo of any kind, use baking soda (just baking soda and nothing else) to wash your hair. Take a handful of dry soda and rub it vigorously into your wet hair, using the tips of your fingers to massage it into your scalp. Rinse thoroughly and dry hair. Stop using all shampoo, conditioner, hair spray, or any other product on your hair. Wash your hair at the same intervals you normally do, but keep using baking soda and no chemicals on your hair whatsoever.

The first time you do this your hair might look like straw (don't try it right before a hot date), but just stick with it. After a few weeks, old dandruff scales will be gone, your scalp will begin to generate its natural oils, and your hair will get very soft. One of my friends said this made her hair feel better than any conditioner ever did. Once you get to this point, you can use a natural shampoo alternately with the baking soda. You will find your own balance of products to keep your hair beautiful and dandruff-free.

To find a natural shampoo, don't look in the drugstore; go instead to a natural-food store. They are stacked to the ceiling with them. At last count, I could obtain locally more than three dozen different brands that were either all-natural or contained an acceptable minimum of relatively safe petrochemical derivatives. And this doesn't even include the number of natural shampoos available by mail. So there's no excuse for using unhealthful products on your hair.

You can also use any liquid soap for shampoo or rub bar soap into your hair. You will need to rinse thoroughly, and if it leaves a residue, try to rinse with diluted vinegar or lemon juice. I have heard soap works well for dry or normal hair, but I don't find it satisfactory on my oily hair. My hair just doesn't get fluffy enough. However, "shampoo bars" that are specially formulated for hair work very well.

You can make your own shampoo by grating a one-ounce bar of mild soap such as **Kirk's Castile Soap** (sold in all drugstores) and adding it to one cup of boiling distilled water. Simmer for five minutes while stirring occasionally. To this, you can add fragrances or beneficial herbs.

I've read that back in the 1920s, beauticians used eggs for shampoo! Just beat an egg and apply half to your hair as if it were shampoo. Rinse with *lukewarm* water (so you don't end up with scrambled eggs in your hair), then repeat with the other half of the egg. Rinse with the juice of half a lemon mixed with two cups of water.

As long as we're discussing hair, here's a tip about hairbrushes and combs. If you have a problem with static electricity in your hair, it is probably caused by the nylon bristles on your brush or plastic comb. When you switch to a natural bristle brush and a wooden comb (both available at natural-food stores and by mail from ***Janice Corporation, Simmons Handcrafts,*** and ***Traditional Products Company***), the problem will go away immediately.

MOUTHWASH, TOOTHPASTE, AND TOOTHBRUSHES

> **CAUTION:** Keep out of reach of children. For rinsing only. Do not swallow. Do not administer to any child under 6 years of age.

Let's start with mouthwash first, since that's the product with the warning label.

Mouthwashes contain a number of ingredients that could be harmful or fatal if swallowed. I find it interesting that the same germ killers **(phenol, cresol,** and **ethanol)** that are used in bathroom disinfectants are also used (although in a lower concentration) in a product designed for use in the mouth, which could be swallowed. Ethanol is a petrochemical version of the same ethyl alcohol you drink in alcoholic beverages, and can affect the central nervous system and cause nausea and drowsiness. If too much is taken, the body can go into shock or a coma, possibly resulting in death. Mouthwashes might also contain **formaldehyde, artificial colors, ammonia,** and **hydrogen peroxide.**

Mouthwash is one of those products that's easy to make assumptions about. You would think that if a product is intended for use in the mouth, it would also be safe to swallow. I was surprised to see the label warn against this.

Fluoride toothpastes have no warning labels, but may contain **ammonia,** ethanol, **artificial colors and flavors, formaldehyde, mineral oil, sugar,** and carcinogenic **polyvinylpyrrolidone plastic (PVP),** the same plastic resin used in hair spray.

Fluoride mouthwashes and toothpastes are often given to children as added protection against tooth decay. While there is no question that the optimal dose of fluoride will help prevent cavities, there is a possible danger here that with the combination of fluoride in mouthwash, toothpaste, and tap water, children might be getting *too much* fluoride, causing mottling of the teeth and many common ills.

Many mouthwashes and toothpastes, both fluoridated and unfluoridated, are sweetened with **saccharin,** which is known to cause cancer in laboratory animals. Food products and chewing gum containing saccharin require warning labels to this effect, but mouthwash and toothpaste don't.

Nonfluoride mouthwashes and toothpastes formulated to prevent bad breath contain many similar ingredients and pose the same types of hazards.

Another possible hazardous ingredient is **sodium lauryl sulfate (SLS).** Recent research from the University of Oslo in Norway found that when people prone to canker sores brushed with SLS-free toothpaste, their incidence of canker sores fell by 70 percent. Researchers suspect that the canker-sore promoting characteristic of SLS stems from its tendency to dry out protective mucous tissue, leaving the gums and insides of the cheeks susceptible to irritants.

SAFE SOLUTIONS

Check with your dentist to see if your child needs fluoride treatment. It may be safer and more effective to have your dentist give periodic fluoride treatments in the office, where the dose can be regulated, than to apply fluoride haphazardly with mouthwash and toothpaste.

I know of at least one natural toothpaste **(Tom's of Maine)** that contains the natural mineral calcium fluoride. It is widely available at natural-food stores and by mail, as are other natural toothpastes.

If you're not interested in fluoride in your toothpaste, you can brush your teeth with plain baking soda (or baking soda flavored with a few drops of your favorite extract or essential oil), or mashed strawberries. I know this sounds funny, but I have heard good reports about mashed strawberries. They foam up just like toothpaste and seem to contain an ingredient that helps people with gum problems. Brushing without toothpaste works fine too. The point is to get the food out from between your teeth.

Good oral hygiene, including regular brushing and flossing, will prevent bad breath, but if you are one of those people who likes to use mouthwash just because it makes your mouth taste good, you can get the same effect by rinsing your mouth with very strong, cooled mint tea (or any other flavor, for that matter), or with your favorite flavored extract (such as peppermint, anise, or cinnamon) mixed into pure water. You can also buy mouthwash made from natural ingredients at your natural-food store or by mail. You should have no trouble finding one, as there are several popular brands on the market.

If you have a persistent problem with bad breath, consult your dentist.

It seems appropriate to make a comment here about toothbrushes. While it would be difficult to categorize a nylon-bristle toothbrush with a plastic handle as "toxic," if you prefer a toothbrush made from natural materials, it is available. My favorite is the **Brooks Pearwood Toothbrush**, which is sold in many natural-food stores and catalogs. It can be ordered directly from the importer (***Traditional Products Company***) or from ***Allergy Relief Shop, Janice Corporation, Karen's Nontoxic Products,*** or ***Natural Lifestyle.***

ASTRINGENTS AND TONERS

> **CAUTION:** For external use only. Avoid contact with eyes. In case of accidental ingestion, seek professional assistance or contact a poison-control center immediately.

Most astringents are just **alcohol** (denatured to make it undrinkable) with a little **artificial fragrance** and **artificial color** thrown in to make it more interesting, and a bit of glycerin to soften skin. Some astringents are very harsh and can burn skin, and the perfumes can irritate the skin and cause allergic rashes. Accidentally splashed in the eye, astringents can damage delicate membranes. Fumes from the alcohol can irritate nasal passages and cause nausea, drowsiness, and dizziness. If accidentally swallowed, astringents can be deadly, especially to a child.

SAFE SOLUTIONS

As a person with oily skin, I have been using astringents all my life. I remember using a very popular brand once that got rid of the oil all right, but also made my face red and blotchy and burned so much I couldn't sleep at night.

Gentle glycerin and herbal soaps, appropriate for my skin type, seem to work better to balance my skin than any of the fancy department-store skin-care "systems."

For a luxurious treat to pamper yourself, use a clay mask to absorb excess oil. Go to the natural-food store and buy pure clay; don't use a department-store mask, which contains many chemicals. Mix clay with water to form a thin paste, apply, and relax until the clay dries. Adding a little oatmeal to the mask will help make your skin softer. Regular applications of clay masks will reduce the overall oiliness of your skin and will probably eliminate the need for an astringent, though you can find astringents made from natural substances at your local natural-food store. There are several widely distributed brands available.

Because the active ingredient in most astringents is alcohol, you can use a cotton ball dampened with vodka for the same effect. Strong chamomile or mint tea (cooled) also has natural astringent properties and a pleasant aroma. Using buttermilk will not only remove oil, but will leave your skin very soft. Simply apply with a cotton ball, wait ten minutes, then rinse.

You can also use the following formulas to make your own astringents at home. I know they sound funny, but try them and see how well your skin responds. Just process the ingredients as directed, then pour them into a glass spray bottle and store in the refrigerator.

- Boil green lettuce leaves for 10 minutes in enough water to cover. Let cool and strain.

- Mix 1 part vodka with 9 parts strong chamomile or mint tea.

- Combine ⅔ cup pure water, 2 tablespoons vodka, and ¾ cup borax in a blender until borax is dissolved.

- Blend ¼ cup lemon juice, ¼ cup lime juice, ¼ cup pure water, and ⅛ cup vodka. Strain to remove pulp. This works especially well on very oily skin.

NAIL POLISH AND NAIL-POLISH REMOVERS

> **CAUTION:** Keep away from small children. Harmful if taken internally. In case of accidental ingestion, consult a physician or poison-control center. Harmful to synthetic fabrics, wood finishes, and plastics.

Since nail-polish remover is the product that shows a warning label, let's start with that. The primary ingredient in most nail-polish removers is the solvent **acetone,** which can not only dissolve nail polish, but can cause your nails to become brittle and split, and skin rashes to develop on your fingers. When inhaled, the fumes from nail-polish remover can irritate your lungs and make you feel lightheaded. When accidentally ingested, acetone can cause restlessness, vomiting, and ultimately, collapse into unconsciousness.

Nail polish is even more toxic, but, amazingly, doesn't have a warning label. Nail polish contains **phenol, toluene,** and **xylene,** three highly volatile and harmful chemicals, but its basic ingredient in the past was a **formaldehyde** resin, which can cause discoloration and bleeding under the nail. My great-aunt used to own a drugstore, and when I was a teenager wearing nail polish, she used to tell me stories of the women who would come into the store with their nails cracked and bleeding from wearing nail polish all the time. She said their nails "couldn't breathe" and warned me to remove the nail polish regularly to expose my nails to air.

SAFE SOLUTIONS

I haven't any suggestions for making nontoxic nail polish, and as of this writing I don't know of any brands that are any more natural or less toxic than others. However, in recent years, there have been some improvements.

Although many makers of nail polish have removed formaldehyde from their formulas, read labels carefully (bring a magnifying glass with you to the store, as lettering is infinitesimal). Still, even without the formaldehyde, nail polish is loaded with toxic chemicals, so apply it in a well-ventilated place (preferably outdoors).

All major brands of nail-polish remover now have an acetone-free variety, which is easy to find at major drugstores.

HAIR-REMOVAL PRODUCTS

> **CAUTION:** Do not apply near eyes, on inflamed, chapped, broken, or newly tweezed areas, or the vaginal area. If cream gets in eyes, flush thoroughly with lukewarm water.

The most dangerous ingredient in hair-removal products is **ammonium thioglycolate,** which can cause severe skin rashes, swelling, redness, and the breaking of small blood vessels under the skin.

SAFE SOLUTIONS

Instead of using a chemical product, remove unwanted hair by shaving, tweezing, waxing, or electrolysis.

You can remove facial hair with natural beeswax. Buy it in chunks at a natural-food store or hardware store, or an uncolored beeswax candle will work fine too. Just melt a small amount in a pan until it's very warm but still cool enough to touch. Dust your skin with cornstarch and apply the warm wax with a wooden spatula. Allow the wax to dry for a few seconds. Press a clean cloth to the still-soft wax and remove with one quick motion. The hairs will come out with the wax. It hurts about as much as when you pull a Band-Aid off your arm. Soothe your skin with a bit of unscented cream, lotion, or pure aloe.

There are also home-use appliances for hair removal. One permanently removes individual hairs with an electric current. Another keeps skin smooth by removing hair at the root with an electric shaver–type device. Both can be purchased at department stores and from mail order catalogs such as *The Safety Zone* and *Selfcare Catalog*.

Keep in mind that any hair-removal method that removes hair at the root can promote ingrown hairs for some people. Using a loofah daily offers some protection against that.

HAIR COLORS

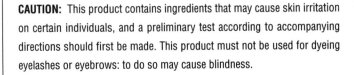

CAUTION: This product contains ingredients that may cause skin irritation on certain individuals, and a preliminary test according to accompanying directions should first be made. This product must not be used for dyeing eyelashes or eyebrows: to do so may cause blindness.

If the FDA had its way, this warning would appear on all packages of hair coloring:

WARNING: Contains an ingredient that can penetrate your skin and has been determined to cause cancer in laboratory animals.

Manufacturers are able to get around the warning labels by just slightly reformulating their products to remove the carcinogen, but then they replace it, quite legally, with another chemical that is just as dangerous. It takes four years or more to test a new chemical for safety before the FDA can propose another warning label, and many manufacturers take full advantage of the lag time.

Unfortunately, the FDA has no jurisdiction over hair dyes, which are mutagenic and suspected human carcinogens. An investigation conducted by *Consumer Reports* magazine revealed about twenty different chemicals used regularly in hair-coloring products that are potential human carcinogens. Hair-dye products also may contain **coal-tar dyes, ammonia, detergents, hydrogen peroxide,** and **lead.** Many hair-dye chemicals, which can easily penetrate the scalp and enter the bloodstream, are not even tested for safety. One study suggests that women over the age of fifty who have used hair dyes for ten or more years have an increased risk of breast cancer. It is recommended also that women avoid hair dyes entirely when pregnant or of child-bearing age.

Regardless of the toxicity of the chemicals used, though, hazardous hair-coloring products cannot be banned from the marketplace because of a 1938 law, still in effect, which was passed when the hair-dye industry persuaded Congress to exempt these products from government regulation. At that time, the synthetic coal-tar dyes used were known to cause serious allergic reactions in some users. Because government regulation of these hazardous products would have been a major threat to the entire hair-dye industry, manufacturers lobbied relentlessly until they won the exemption they needed to stay in business.

SAFE SOLUTIONS

The safest commercial hair color is henna, a powder made from a plant source (available at most pharmacies and natural-food stores). Many different shades are available to darken or highlight your hair. Henna gives hair a semipermanent protein coating, which washes out gradually over a six-month period.

For best results, be sure to use pure henna—without metallic bases, "henna enhancers," or chemical dyes. On henna labels, "100 percent natural henna" doesn't necessarily mean "100 percent *pure* henna." There is some controversy about the different shades of henna. Several sources claim that any shade that is not orange-red also may contain chemical dyes.

You can intensify the color by adding other ingredients. Use paprika, beet juice, or Red Zinger tea to bring out red; for brown, use ginger, nutmeg, or hot coffee instead of water. Gold is accentuated with black tea, chamomile, or onion juice. To tone down the orange-red, add one part chamomile flowers to two parts henna.

Never use henna on eyebrows, eyelashes, or facial hair, or if you already have a chemical dye on your hair or are about to get a permanent.

You can color your hair temporarily with natural rinses made from plant materials. Women used these rinses for centuries before chemical dyes were invented. These natural products will not change your hair color as drastically as chemical formulas, but they can highlight and enrich your hair color in beautiful and subtle ways that no chemical dye can duplicate. When the rinse is used repeatedly, the color will deepen in intensity each time. Once your hair is the shade you like, use the rinse periodically to keep color from fading.

Use the following formulas to make your own plant-based

hair rinses. Process the ingredients as directed, then strain and cool before using. Pour the liquid through the hair fifteen times, catching it in a basin below and rerinsing with the same liquid. Wring out any excess and leave in the hair for fifteen minutes before a final rinse with clear water.

BLONDE

Note: The following rinses will lighten the hair to an even greater degree if you dry your hair in the sun.

- Mix 1 tablespoon of lemon juice in 1 gallon of warm water.

- Simmer 4 tablespoons of chopped rhubarb root in 3 cups of hot water for 15 minutes.

- Steep ½ cup yellow-blossomed flower or herb (try chamomile, calendula, mullein blooms and leaves, yellow broom, saffron, turmeric, or quassia chips) in 1 quart boiling water for ½ hour. (You can also mix this rinse with an equal amount of lemon juice, add a little arrowroot, and stir over low heat until it forms a gel. Apply the gel to your hair and sit out in the sun for an hour.)

BROWN/BRUNETTE

- Rinse hair with a strong black tea or black coffee.

- Cook an unpeeled potato and apply the cooking water to your hair with a cotton ball, keeping the rinse away from your skin to prevent discoloration.

TO COVER GRAY

- Simmer ½ cup of dried sage in 2 cups water for 30 minutes, then steep for several hours. Apply the tea to hair and leave it on until your hair dries; then rinse and dry your hair again. Apply weekly until desired shade is achieved, then monthly to maintain color.

- Cover crushed black walnut shells with boiling water, add a pinch of salt, and soak for 3 days. Add

3 cups boiling water and simmer in a glass pot for 5 hours, replacing water as needed. Strain and simmer the liquid until it has reduced to ¼ of the original volume. Add 1 teaspoon ground cloves or allspice and steep in the refrigerator for a week, shaking the jar every day. Strain and use carefully, as this mixture will stain everything you touch. Wear gloves and try to avoid skin contact.

RED

- Make a strong tea of rosehips or cloves, or use strong black coffee.
- Steep together 1 tablespoon each of henna, chamomile flowers, and vinegar for 15 minutes in boiling water.

I have found three brands of "alternative" hair colors.

- **Vita Wave Cream Hair Color** is less toxic but still contains many chemical ingredients. It is sold at many natural-food stores and by mail from *Allergy Relief Shop, Karen's Nontoxic Products,* and *Natural Lifestyle.*
- **Logona Hair Colors** contain organically grown henna plus finely ground herbs, roots, leaves, seeds, fruits, wood, and bark gathered from the wild. Instead of penetrating the hair, these colors coat each strand of hair with a protective film that both strengthens the hair and creates a color uniquely yours. Also available at natural-food stores or by mail from *Logona USA* and *Karen's Nontoxic Products.*
- **Herbavita Vegetal Color** and **Herbatint** are made from herbal formulas and contain no ammonia. They are available in some natural-food stores.

If you absolutely must use a commercial hair dye, *Consumer Reports* magazine suggests you take the following precautions.

- Don't use hair dyes more often than necessary. Once every 4 to 6 weeks should be frequently enough.

- Don't leave the dye on your head any longer than necessary according to package instructions.

- Flood your scalp thoroughly with water after applying dye.

- Use a technique that involves minimum contact between the dye and your scalp.

- Put off using any hair dyes to as late in life as possible.

PERMANENT WAVES

> **CAUTION:** Keep out of reach of children. Avoid getting waving lotion in eyes. If it does, rinse eyes with water. In case of accidental ingestion, consult a physician immediately.

Ammonium thioglycolate is the most hazardous ingredient in permanent-wave solutions. It can cause skin rashes on your hands and scalp, redness, swelling, and hemorrhages under your skin. Because the scalp is very porous, this substance can easily be carried into the bloodstream.

In addition, permanent waves smell very strongly of **ammonia,** which can cause breathing difficulties and coughing.

Many pregnant women have been told by their doctors not to have perms during pregnancy.

SAFE SOLUTIONS

If you want to perm your hair, use ammonia-free **VitaWave** perms available in natural-food stores or by mail from *Allergy Relief Shop, Karen's Nontoxic Products,* and *Natural Lifestyle.*

TAMPONS AND SANITARY PADS

> **ATTENTION:** Tampons are associated with Toxic Shock Syndrome (TSS). TSS is a rare but serious disease that may cause death.

Toxic shock syndrome (TSS) made headlines back in 1980, when a number of women suffered from fevers of 102°F or more, vomiting, diarrhea, sunburn-type rashes and subsequent skin peeling, and a rapid drop in blood pressure that sometimes led to fatal shock.

The exact cause of TSS still is unknown, but it has been determined that staphylococcus bacteria are present in most cases. Although TSS has been associated with all tampon use, the brands made from superabsorbent fibers seem to pose higher risks.

As of this writing, tampon packages still warn against TSS; however, the Centers for Disease Control reports that currently, the actual incidence of TSS is practically zero.

Of course, you could also use feminine napkins, but if you do, stay away from the deodorant variety. More than 20 percent of the respondents in a survey done by *Consumer Reports* magazine indicated that they had been warned by their doctors not to use deodorant tampons or pads. Even people who are not normally allergic to perfume can, over time, develop skin irritations from these deodorant scents.

A newly discovered danger, which applies to both tampons and sanitary pads, is the presence of **dioxins** in the bleached paper from which both are made. Studies done in Great Britain report 130 parts per trillion (ppt) dioxins remaining in tampons, and 400 ppt in sanitary pads. This sounds like a very small amount; however, one of the dioxins present, **tetrachlorodibenzodioxin (TCDD),** has been called the most toxic chemical ever produced. TCDD, a known carcinogen, causes birth defects and sterility, as well as liver damage and suppression of the immune system. The chemical can be absorbed easily through the skin. Considering that we use these products month in and month out over years, is this a risk we want to take?

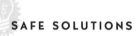

SAFE SOLUTIONS

Choose a brand of tampon that is made with "no superabsorbent fibers." Some brands state this on the label.

A study published in *American Journal of Obstetrics and Gynecology* reported that the presence of superabsorbent fibers significantly increased the rate of growth of staphylococcus bacteria, and that production of the bacteria dramatically decreased when it was grown on cotton fibers.

Materials used in tampon construction are listed on the package, so look for brands that are made of cotton or rayon. First choice among tampons is **Naturacare** (available at natural-food stores and by mail), made from 100 percent cotton whitened without chlorine bleach, and a close second is **Tampax Naturals,** also made from 100 percent cotton (available at supermarkets). Both **Tampax Original Regular** tampons and **o.b.** tampons are made from cotton/rayon blends.

Small, soft sea sponges also can be used as "natural" tampons. Federal regulations prohibit the marketing of sponges "to insert into the body," so you can't go into a store and ask for "tampon sponges." What you want to look for are "cosmetic sponges," which look like fluffy pillows and are used to apply foundation makeup.

Before using a sea sponge as a tampon, first rinse it several times in running water, then sterilize it by boiling it for two minutes in a pot of plain water. Wash your hands before inserting or removing the sponge. After removing it, rinse the sponge well in running water and squeeze it dry. It can then be reinserted. Frequent removal and rinsing is highly recommended. If you have trouble removing your sponge, tie a piece of cotton quilting thread around the sponge to help pull it out.

Sponges should be stored in a clean, airy location when not in use. Do not put a damp sponge in a plastic or airtight container. Resterilize your sponge before each period to prevent bacteria growth.

I have never tried sea sponges for this purpose (I am content with reusable cotton pads), but I have several friends who think they are wonderful. They say they are very comfortable with them and . . . they're never caught without a tampon.

Your natural-food store probably carries reusable menstrual pads made from 100 percent cotton and **Naturacare** "dioxin-free" disposable pads made from bleached paper, or you can order them by mail from *Allergy Relief Shop, Allergy Resources, Gold Mine Natural Food Company, Natural Lifestyle, Nontoxic Environments, Organic Cottons, Seventh Generation, Simmons Handcrafts,* and *Womankind.*

CONTRACEPTIVES

A couple's choice of a contraceptive method is a very personal matter. Because each of our bodies and needs is different, we have to weigh the risks against the benefits individually. Nowadays, in addition to preventing pregnancy, you may also need your contraceptive to protect you against sexually transmitted diseases (STDs). Not all contraceptives do this double duty.

Contraceptive methods for women vary from chemical alteration of hormones to abstinence from intercourse on fertile days. Your gynecologist can help you make a choice that fits your physical needs and lifestyle.

ORAL CONTRACEPTIVE PILLS

> **WARNING:** Cigarette smoking increases the risk of serious cardiovascular side effects from oral contraceptive use. This risk increases with age and with heavy smoking (15 or more cigarettes per day) and is quite marked in women over 35 years of age. Women who use oral contraceptives should be strongly advised not to smoke. The use of oral contraceptives is associated with increased risk of several serious conditions including thromboembolism, stroke, myocardial infarction, liver tumor, gall bladder disease, visual disturbances, fetal abnormalities, and hypertension.

Oral contraceptive pills come in two types: progestin-only "mini-pills" (97 to 99.5 percent effective) and "combination pills," also known as "low dose pills" (99.9 percent effective), which contain both progestin and estrogen. These synthetic hormones prevent pregnancy by altering the chemical balance in your body. They trick the body into thinking it is pregnant, causing the release of eggs to be suppressed. They provide no protection against STDs.

Many women are uncomfortable about taking a hormone-changing medication day in and day out for years on end, and they should be. The list of side effects is lengthy: weight gain, acne, eczema, nausea, dizziness, spotting, breast tenderness, cramping, gum inflammation, inflammation of the optic nerve (leading to loss of vision, double vision, eye pains and swelling, and an inability to wear contact lenses), headaches, vaginal yeast infections, depression, loss of sex drive, formation of blood clots, heart attacks, high blood pressure, stroke, gallbladder disease, liver tumors, birth defects, ectopic pregnancy, cancer of the skin and/or reproductive organs, breast tumors, menstrual irregularities, post-pill infertility, and infections.

According to the FDA, the Pill should not be used by women who have or have had blood clots in their legs or lungs, pains in the heart, heart attack or stroke, unusual vaginal bleeding that has not yet been diagnosed, have known or suspected cancer of the breast or sex organs, or who know or suspect they are pregnant.

BIRTH CONTROL SHOTS

Birth control shots, such as Depo-Provera, are hormones administered by injection every twelve weeks. Like the Pill, the hormones in the shots prevent the woman's egg from leaving her ovaries, thereby preventing pregnancy. It is 99.7 percent effective at preventing pregnancy, but does not protect against STDs.

Because normal hormone patterns are altered, women experience changes in menstrual cycles, tiredness, headaches, abdominal pain, breast soreness, nausea, weight gain, and mood swings. Some problems may not go away until the shot wears off, and women may continue to be infertile for up to eighteen months after the last injection.

IMPLANTS

Implants, like Norplant, are just another way of administering hormones. Six small, soft, thin tubes are placed under the skin in the woman's upper arm, and release hormones over a five-year period. Again, the hormones prevent the woman's egg from leaving her ovaries, thereby preventing pregnancy. It is 99.96 percent effective at preventing pregnancy, but does not protect against STDs.

Side effects can include menstrual changes, headaches, weight gain, depression, and tenderness and infection at the implant site. Use of implants increases risk of ovarian cysts and hair loss.

INTRAUTERINE DEVICES

An intrauterine device (IUD) is a small piece of plastic that is surgically placed in a woman's uterus. It works by preventing the fertilized egg from growing in the uterus. As of this writing, there are only two IUDs on the market. Others have been withdrawn from sale because of negative health effects or because the high cost of defending lawsuits made their sale economically unfeasible for the manufacturer. IUDs provide no protection against STDs.

Side effects include heavy bleeding and increased cramping during menstruation, but the most serious complication associated with IUD use is permanent sterility. The risk is so high that an article in *New England Journal of Medicine* recommends that a woman who has never borne a child use an IUD as a contraceptive only if she does not wish ever to conceive, and that IUD use is appropriate only for women who have borne children, do not want to have more children, and do not wish to undergo sterilization.

SPERMICIDES, DIAPHRAGMS, AND CERVICAL CAPS

Spermicides are foams, creams, jellies, suppositories, foaming tablets, and vaginal films that contain sperm-killing chemicals. Diaphragms and cervical caps are rubber barriers that fit over the woman's cervix, blocking the sperm, and must be used with a spermicide jelly or cream.

Few side effects beyond local irritation have been reported by users of these products, but their use is being connected with cases involving birth defects and spontaneous abortion. In one court case, a mother and child were awarded $5.1 million when the judge ruled that a popular contraceptive jelly caused the child's birth defects, and that the product should have carried a warning label stating that while spermicide is in use, babies conceived may have birth defects. Spermicides do not always kill sperm, and sometimes damaged sperm go on to fertilize eggs, resulting in deformed babies. In addition, United States congressional hearings found evidence to suggest that spermicides might be carcinogenic and mutagenic.

An FDA advisory review panel studying the safety of vaginal spermicides found only a few out-of-date studies that evaluated the safety of spermicides. None of these studies addressed the issues of the effects of spermicides on an unborn fetus, or possible genetic mutation, carcinogenicity, or toxic effects.

Because manufacturers are only required to list active ingredients on the label, it is hard for the consumer to tell exactly what might be in a spermicide product. Additional ingredients could include **alcohol, formaldehyde, methylbenzethonium chloride, perfume,** and **preservatives,** among others.

Diaphragms and cervical caps can cause bladder infections and may be irritating to either partner. They also increase the risk of toxic shock syndrome. Despite these slight risks, both products are relatively safe. However, in order for them to be reasonably effective, they must be used in conjunction with spermicides.

SAFE SOLUTIONS

Unfortunately, the truly safe choices are somewhat limited.

CONDOMS

Condoms are shields of thin rubber that block the sperm from reaching the egg. Most popular are condoms that fit men, but recently a new "female" condom has been introduced. They are 76 to 98 percent effective against pregnancy, and they protect against STDs. Effectiveness increases when used in conjunction with a spermicide.

Condoms are by far the safest commercial contraceptives—the only risk involved is a remote chance of allergic reaction to the latex rubber they are made of, or to the chemicals in the lubricants.

The biggest objection to using condoms is that, obviously, the sexual experience is not quite the same as it is without them. The way around this is for both partners to cooperate, using them only when necessary. With natural birth control, you can have the best of both.

NATURAL BIRTH CONTROL

Many couples today are choosing to use natural family planning (sometimes called the Fertility Awareness Method), which gives them freedom and protection from pregnancy without harmful side effects. It is 80 to 99 percent effective, depending on the type of method used and how well the program is followed.

This method is based on calculating fertile times by monitoring changes in body temperature and vaginal mucus. After using the method, you may also notice subtle changes in mood, skin texture, and weight. Abstinence is required for all the days between the start of the woman's menstrual period and ovulation, approximately two weeks later. It provides no protection against STDs, and works best for couples in a loving, committed, communicative relationship.

This method can be very effective, but it requires diligent practice and a willingness to abstain. Some couples get frustrated waiting for the "safe days," but other couples view the abstinence days as opportunities to explore intimacy in ways that do not involve intercourse. Just the practice of taking responsibility together and monitoring and tracking body changes can bring couples closer, allowing your love life to flow more with nature's cycles rather than using chemicals or hormones to "always be available."

I have purposely not explained the method fully here because you really should research the subject with books and/or classes before relying on natural birth control to be effective. Contact your gynecologist, a women's health clinic, or a local family-planning center about getting more information. Your local library also should have some useful books.

STERILIZATION

Female and male sterilization is 99.9 percent effective at preventing pregnancy, but provides no protection against STDs. Aside from some discomfort and side effects immediately following surgery, sterilization can be a safe option for women and men who do not want to have children.

ABSTINENCE

Abstaining from sexual intercourse is a viable birth control option. Some individuals, for one reason or another, do choose lives of celibacy, and some couples, too, choose abstinence for certain days during the woman's cycle or even for particular periods of their relationship. It is 100 percent effective at preventing pregnancy. Abstinence refers only to intercourse—there are many other ways to express love and affection. Abstinence from intercourse only will not, however, protect you from STDs, as some STDs—such as herpes simplex—can be transmitted even by kissing. If you are sexually active and not in a long-term monogamous relationship, get the facts about protecting yourself from STDs and follow them to the letter.

PERFUMES AND AFTERSHAVES

Perfumes and aftershave lotions are products that should be labeled "keep out of reach of children," but aren't. According to my local poison-control center, because of the high **alcohol** content of these products, it takes only about a tablespoon ingested accidentally for a small child to become intoxicated. This leads to lowered blood sugar, which can cause unconsciousness, and eventually the child could fall into a coma and die, all from one tablespoon of your favorite fragrance.

Perfume consists of a combination of natural essential oils, aroma, chemicals, and solvents in a base of alcohol. Some of these less-than-romantic ingredients include **methylene chloride, toluene, methyl ethyl ketone, methyl isobutyl ketone, ethanol,** and **benzyl chloride**—all designated as hazardous waste-disposal chemicals. According to the EPA, toluene was detected in every fragrance sample collected for a report in 1991. They report that "toluene was most abundant in the auto parts store as well as the fragrance section of the department store."

The FDA acknowledges that the incidence of adverse reactions to perfume and aftershave products appears to be increasing as a result of the rising popularity of stronger, sweeter fragrances. Furthermore, it is difficult for consumers to identify a specific problem ingredient, because the word "fragrance" on a cosmetic label can indicate the presence of up to 4,000 separate ingredients. As many as 600 separate chemicals may be used in a single formulation, many of which are protected by "trade secrecy." Also, many of the chemicals used during the manufacture of perfume are not listed on the label.

Approximately 95 percent of these ingredients are derived from **petrochemicals.** Natural ingredients such as tuberose or jasmine can cost more than $40,000 a pound. By contrast, synthetic ingredients run less than $10 per pound. Eighty-four percent of these ingredients have minimal or no toxicity data, according to the National Academy of Sciences. In 1989, from a list of 2,983 chemicals used in the fragrance industry, the National Institute of Occupational Safety and Health (NIOSH) recognized 884 toxic substances. Some of these are capable of causing cancer, birth defects, central nervous system disorders, allergic reactions, and skin and eye irritations, and of provoking chemical sensitivities.

Although there has been very little scientific study on the health effects of wearing scented products, generally they are recognized as highly allergenic and are notorious for causing mild to severe skin irritation. Fragrances are also a common cause of headaches and nausea. Almost all of us have been in a situation where we have been near someone who was wearing just too much perfume and we felt sick to our stomachs.

SAFE SOLUTIONS

For people to whom fragrance is an integral part of personal expression, I suggest using pleasant natural scents.

Look for essential oils at your natural-food store or order them by mail. When buying essential oils, be sure to find out if the oil has been derived from a natural source. A number of confusing terms are used to describe essential oils, so let's sort them out.

Natural essential oils are derived from plant sources, and the resulting fragrance is that of the plant. A natural lemon scent, for example, would come from a part of the lemon plant.

Synthetic oils also are from plant sources, but the fragrance is not that of the original plant. A synthetic lemon scent might not be from a lemon at all, but from a geranium!

Artificial oils, also called *perfume* oils, are made from petro-chemicals.

Essential oils are labeled according to their dilution. Those labeled *true, absolute,* or *concrete* are pure oils; *extracts* or *tinctures* have been diluted with grain alcohol; and *extended* oils contain plasticizers.

Essential oils are extremely potent and must be used with care. Because they are so powerful, they are very irritating to the skin and should not be applied without dilution. Do not apply to mucous membrane areas at all. Before using, dilute essential oil by adding a few drops to one ounce of vegetable oil or vodka. As with any other perfume product, keep these out of children's reach.

Many people who think they are allergic to perfume find that they can tolerate natural fragrances very well. I used to be allergic to flower fragrances no matter what the source, but could still use citrus and herbal scents; now I can tolerate almost all natural fragrances.

ANTIPERSPIRANTS AND DEODORANTS

Antiperspirants may contain **aerosol propellants, ammonia, alcohol, formaldehyde,** and **fragrance,** but the primary danger is the active ingredient that helps stop wetness: **aluminum chlorohydrate.**

Aluminum chlorohydrate can cause infections in the hair follicles of the armpit, and skin irritations that can be severe enough to require medical attention. There is some concern as to whether the aluminum salts in antiperspirants might contribute to a buildup of aluminum in the body—aluminum from other sources has been associated with various brain disorders—and about the safety of using aluminum in an aerosol spray. Because aerosols produce airborne particles that are likely to be inhaled, there is a good chance that bits of aluminum will enter the lungs and accumulate over time. Because the long-term health effects are unknown, aluminum-containing aerosol antiperspirants are only conditionally approved by the FDA for safety.

Nonantiperspirant deodorants may contain the bacteria-killing ingredient **triclosan,** which can cause liver damage when absorbed through the skin.

Antiperspirants and deodorants historically have a bad track record. In a recent ten-year period, more than eight different ingredients were banned by the FDA or voluntarily removed from products because they posed a threat to users.

SAFE SOLUTIONS

There are a number of natural deodorants on the market (**Tom's of Maine** is sold in most drugstores as well as natural-food stores), but what works best is baking soda—just plain baking soda. I have been using it for seventeen years, and nobody has ever complained. In fact, I have recommended it to a number of people who have suffered for many years with unconquerable body odor, and they say it's the only thing that has ever worked for them. Just take a bit of dry baking soda on your fingertips and pat it under your arms after you've dried off from your shower. Your skin should be slightly damp, but not wet. If the baking soda feels too abrasive to you, you can mix it with cornstarch or white clay.

Another equally nontoxic (but not so inexpensive or simple) alternative is the crystallike "deodorant stones" sold in most drug and natural-food stores. These are nothing more than a combination of minerals crystallized using the same method as that used to make rock candy. If you can't find these in your local natural-food or drugstore, you can order them by mail from *Allergy Relief Shop, Janice Corporation, The Living Source, Real Goods,* or *Seventh Generation.*

BUBBLE BATHS

Bubble baths consist basically of just **detergent** and **artificial fragrance,** but the FDA receives many complaints regarding their use. Skin rashes; irritations; and urinary-tract, bladder, and kidney infections are commonly reported by users. Vaginal irritations and infections also are common, particularly with children, who have extrasensitive skin.

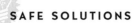

SAFE SOLUTIONS

A long, warm, relaxing bath is one of life's most luxurious experiences. We should be healed and pampered by taking baths, not harmed.

There are many lovely, natural things you can add to your bathwater. Here are some suggestions.

- ½ cup or more of baking soda (this is particularly soothing for a sunburn or skin rash);

- 1 cup Epsom salts;

- 1 quart of whole or skim milk, or buttermilk;

- slices and juice of several lemons or limes, or an orange or grapefruit;

- 5 to 10 peppermint, chamomile, or other herb tea bags, steeped first for about 5 minutes in very hot water, then added to warm bathwater;

- any fragrant dried herbs (try lavender or rosemary) or your favorite sweet-smelling fresh flower petals, or, for an exotic bath, ground or crushed spices (cloves, cardamom seeds, allspice, nutmeg, cinnamon, or ginger);

- to relieve itching, about 1½ cups oatmeal pulverized into a fine powder in a blender or food processor, and stirred into warm bathwater;

- for bubbles, ½ to 1 cup sodium hexametaphosphate (a natural mineral powder you might already have ordered from a chemical supply house to use as a dishwasher detergent) added to warm running water. Sodium hexametaphosphate is the active ingredient used in some popular bath products—it makes the water feel wonderfully soft and slippery. The amount you will use depends on the hardness of your water, and the more you use, the more bubbles you will get. Swish the water around with your hand to dissolve the sodium hexametaphosphate, and then start adding liquid soap, a few table-spoons at a time, right near the faucet where there is a lot of churning water. You will have lots of bub-bles. For fragrance, you can use a naturally scented soap or add slices of lemon, a few drops of essential oil, dried or fresh herbs, or flower petals.

SOAP AND OTHER SKIN-CARE PRODUCTS

Soap has such a "clean" image, it's hard to imagine that it might contain some ingredients that could be harmful to health.

Basically, soap is made from a combination of an animal or vegetable fat and the mineral **sodium hydroxide (lye).** Though, as we have already learned, sodium hydroxide is extremely haz-ardous, don't worry—by the time the soap goes through its process, all the molecules have broken down and recombined into a smooth, safe cleanser. Natural glycerin, a by-product of this combination, is also used as a base for soap. Herbs, scents, col-ors, and other ingredients can be added to either type of soap.

Because soap is not considered a cosmetic, it is not affected by the cosmetic labeling laws requiring ingredients to be listed. Although a few companies voluntarily disclose ingredients, most do not.

The most popular and most heavily advertised soaps are the antimicrobial "deodorant" soaps. An FDA advisory review panel has questioned the safety of using these potent germ killers on a regular day-to-day, year-after-year basis. There is concern about possible dangerous consequences when these substances are ab-sorbed through the skin and accumulate in the liver and other or-gans. As a result, the panel has declared "not safe" or "not proved safe" those deodorant soaps containing **chloroxylenol (PCMX), cloflucarban, phenol, triclocarban,** or **triclosan.** Some other substances that have been banned for over-the-counter sales still are used in prescription soaps.

Despite all the advertising hoopla and questionable bacteri-cides, the panel could find no evidence that these potentially haz-ardous substances actually helped stop body odor any more effectively than did plain soap! They also warned that deodorant soaps should not be used on infants less than six months of age.

In nondeodorant soaps, the most common and troublesome ingredient is **synthetic fragrance.** The fragrances in deodorant and luxury toilet soaps are clearly recognizable, but some of the other soaps commonly regarded as "pure" also contain added synthetic fragrance. Moreover, some soaps represented as "natural" contain synthetic fragrance (of, say, coconut or oatmeal) to enhance the scent of the natural ingredient. Not only are fragrances totally unnecessary to the effectiveness of soap—though they can add aesthetic appeal—they are often irritating and can cause dry skin, redness, and rashes. Scented soaps usually also contain fixatives to keep you smelling "springtime fresh" all day. From an aesthetic point of view, these scents might clash with any natural fragrance you may choose to apply separately.

Other nonsoap skin-care products can also contain unsafe substances. "Cold cream" may contain **artificial colors, ethanol,** synthetic fragrances, and **mineral oil** (a **petrochemical** grease). Cleansing grains and other facial products may contain artificial colors, ethanol, synthetic fragrances, mineral oil, and **talc.** Multiproduct skin-care "systems," as well as the myriad of lotions, creams, and moisturizers sold individually, may be made of these same ingredients, plus **preservatives** such as **BHA/BHT** and **EDTA.**

SAFE SOLUTIONS

Believe it or not, you can have clean, soft skin and a beautiful complexion with just plain soap and an occasional facial made from inexpensive ingredients you probably already have in your kitchen.

You don't need to buy a deodorant soap. Body odor is best prevented by regular bathing with plain soap and hot water. If you have a persistent, strong body odor problem, take it as a symptom that something is wrong with your body and see your doctor. Healthy bodies smell sweet naturally.

Choose the purest soap you can find, preferably one that is unscented and uncolored. Some people feel that soap is "drying to the skin." For some soaps this is true, especially those made from coconut oil. But there are so many mild soaps made from natural glycerin, olive oil, or tallow, and such a variety of scents (or unscented), shapes, and special added ingredients (it would be impossible to list all of them here), that you should have no problem choosing one you like.

You can buy natural soaps at natural-food stores, bath shops, and drugstores, or you can order them by mail. Have fun, and find your personal favorites.

Remember, you can also make your own soap. It's not hard. Check your library for one of the many soapmaking books, and you may discover an enjoyable new hobby!

If you'd like to treat yourself to a facial, try one of these homemade recipes.

Facial Steam Bath

Boil 2 quarts water with 2 tablespoons fresh or dried herbs of your choice for 5 minutes. Pour into a large bowl. Drape a large towel over your head and put your face over the bowl, so that the towel forms a tent over you and the bowl. Allow the steam to penetrate your skin for 5 to 10 minutes, then rinse with very cold water to close the pores.

Masks

There are many recipes for facial masks. Check your natural-food store for books on making your own products and herbal recipes, or mix any of the following groups of ingredients. Prepare for the mask by cleansing your face and taking a facial steam bath (see above), or by moistening your face and neck with warm water. Apply mask to skin, avoiding area around eyes; allow to dry for the specified time, then rinse with warm water, followed by cold water to close the pores.

- Peel and slice half a cucumber. Place in blender or food processor and puree. Mix in 1 tablespoon yogurt. Leave on for 20 minutes.

- Puree ½ cup fresh mint leaves and 3 ice cubes (made from pure water) in blender. Strain liquid and apply. Leave on until dry.

- Puree 1 ripe avocado in blender or food processor. Apply as is or combine with an equal amount of sour cream or yogurt, or ½ cup honey and 2 tablespoons peanut or olive oil, or 1 teaspoon honey and the juice of ½ lemon. Leave on for 15 to 30 minutes.

- Make a smooth paste of oatmeal and water. Apply and leave on until it dries completely. Remove by rubbing off with your fingers. Rinse.

- Mix 1 tablespoon raw wheat germ with 2 tablespoons pure warm water, adding 1 egg yolk to form a heavy dough. Leave mask on for 10 to 15 minutes.

Masks should be freshly made for each use; if necessary, however, larger quantities of those masks containing produce items may be made in advance, then frozen into cubes and thawed as needed.

A NOTE ON SKIN LOTIONS

Skin that is in balance will be naturally soft and supple. However, there are circumstances where skin can be damaged or dry out and we need to add some moisture or a healing substance.

Mineral oil, in fact, *dries* the skin, so you have to keep applying the cream. Plain lanolin, an oily substance taken from sheep's wool, is best if you want this kind of skin treatment. You can buy it in a natural-food store.

Moisturizing creams and lotions replace moisture your skin has lost. Those containing natural glycerin act as magnets to draw water out of the atmosphere and hold it until the skin needs more water. You can make your own moisturizing lotion by mixing equal parts of vegetable glycerin (available at drugstores) and water.

If you have a regular skin problem, such as "dishpan hands," wear rubber gloves to protect your skin. One trick I learned from a prep chef in a gourmet restaurant, whose hands were in water scrubbing vegetables every day, is to use a little honey for lotion (honey also makes skin heal faster if you have a cut).

Plain vegetable oils (such as sweet almond) are also good for dry skin. Skin absorbs the natural oil more easily, and it is more healing than mineral oil.

Your natural-food store carries a variety of skin-care products made from plant-based ingredients.

COSMETICS

Let's start with lipstick, because it's the most toxic. First, lipstick may contain several substances known to cause cancer in animals: **polyvinylpyrrolidone plastic (PVP), saccharin, mineral oil,** and **artificial colors.** These are not yet scientifically proven to cause cancer in humans, but it is known that almost all substances that cause cancer in animals also cause cancer in humans. So it's logical to assume there is a danger here. Are you surprised to see mineral oil on that list? There is enough evidence supporting its danger to make it forbidden as a food coating in Germany, even though its use in food products is still allowed in the United States. Lipsticks also frequently contain **artificial fragrance,** which can be very drying to the lips. Unlike other cosmetics, lipstick poses a double danger; in addition to absorbing it into their skin, women who wear lipstick often ingest a good deal of it when they speak, lick their lips, drink, and eat throughout the day. While I was unable to find studies on the health effects of lipsticks, I am concerned about the possible long-term effects of everyday exposure to these chemicals.

The next most dangerous cosmetic is mascara. It can contain **formaldehyde, alcohol,** and various **plastic resins.** Here, the primary dangers are eye irritation, redness, burning, and swelling. We want to enhance our eyes, not hurt them.

The greatest danger from eyeshadow, powdered blush, and face powder is **talc.** Talc may be contaminated with carcinogenic **asbestos,** and as we apply these powders, they float through the air and end up in our lungs. Of course, many contain artificial fragrance also, which is a common cause of allergic reactions to cosmetics. Many liquid foundation makeups contain mineral oil, which is, as I mentioned before, a suspected human carcinogen.

SAFE SOLUTIONS

Yes, you can still wear makeup. There are a number of good brands of more natural cosmetics on the market (such as **Logona, Dr. Hauschka,** and **Paul Penders**), and as the demand increases, they look more and more like the department-store brands. Look for natural cosmetics in your local natural-food store, but if they don't carry them, you can order them by mail from the catalogs listed at the beginning of this chapter.

Most "natural" brands, however, will contain artificial colors, so read labels carefully. At the very least, use unscented "hypoallergenic" cosmetics.

My favorite cosmetics are made from colored clays, which are available at most natural-food stores. Unless I am having my picture taken or have a television appearance, I don't generally wear foundation. I just brush a little rose-colored cosmetic clay onto my cheeks with a big fluffy brush, put a little charcoal gray, blue, or brown clay around my eyes, brush on the least toxic mascara I can find, and put on a little lip gloss that is tinted with natural carmine red. It gives me a finished look and enhances my natural coloring with other natural colors. Instead of lipstick, you could get also a clear gloss from your natural-food store and apply it to your lips over a bit of cosmetic clay, or after you've "stained" your lips with beet or berry juice. Try it. I was surprised to see how beautiful the colors come out. I had been looking for a certain shade of reddish lipstick for years, and finally found it in my 100-percent natural lip gloss.

SUN PROTECTION

Exposing our skin to natural sunlight is a vital part of maintaining good health. The interaction of sunlight with skin produces vitamin D, a vital nutrient that is not found in foods that are common in our modern diet. (Vitamin D does occur naturally in egg yolks, liver, yeast, shrimp, salmon, tuna, and fish liver oils, and is added to fortified milk and enriched bread. However, sunlight is still needed to help the body synthesize vitamin D from these sources.) Since ancient times, sunbathing was recommended as a restorative for health. Modern studies have shown that exposure to the sun can increase energy levels, lower blood pressure, enhance the immune system, and have other good effects.

But with the thinning of the ozone layer, we also need to protect our skin from the sun. The ozone layer acts as a shield in the upper atmosphere that absorbs most of the harmful types of ultraviolet radiation from the sun that would be harmful to humans, animals, and plants. As more CFCs and other chlorine-based chemicals reach the upper atmosphere and interact with ozone molecules, more ultraviolet rays pass through.

In 1991, scientists reported that ozone levels had declined 4 to 8 percent over the northern hemisphere in the last decade. A wave of studies released in 1991 indicated that the ozone layer was thinning twice as fast as previously expected over highly populated regions.

Also in 1991, scientists preparing an assessment of ozone damage for the United Nations Environment Programme revealed that, for the first time, ozone over midlatitude regions like North America and Europe had thinned during the spring and summer. Depletion during these warmer seasons is more dangerous because the hole allows the sun's rays to penetrate when they're at their strongest and when people more often are outdoors.

Meanwhile the major ozone hole over Antarctica has been growing larger and persisting longer. In 1992, the World Meteorological Organization reported that the ozone hole over Antarctica covered a record area, stretching over 9 million square miles, about three times the size of the continental United States. The hole, about 25 percent larger than in past years, spread over the southern part of Tierra del Fuego, a populated island on the tip of South America. Researchers attributed the increased severity in part to weather, but primarily to higher levels of man-made chemicals. In the Northern Hemisphere, stratospheric ozone declined sharply over parts of Western Europe, and areas of depleted ozone have been found as far south as the Caribbean.

A 10-percent reduction in ozone is likely to lead to about a 20-percent increase in harmful ultraviolet radiation. Increased ultraviolet radiation leads to increased skin cancer and aging and wrinkling of the skin. A 10-percent depletion of the ozone layer could result in almost 2 million additional instances of skin cancer each year. It also appears that increased ultraviolet radiation damages the human immune system at much lower doses than are required to induce cancer.

Ozone depletion also can cause eye damage. The United Nations Environment Programme has estimated that a 1-percent reduction in ozone could cause 100,000 to 150,000 additional cases of blindness worldwide, and a 10-percent reduction could cause up to 1.75 million cases of blindness.

We are already seeing the effects of ozone depletion—they are not just theoretical. Skin cancer and cataracts are increasingly common in Australia, New Zealand, South Africa, and Patagonia. In Queensland, Australia, more than 75 percent of people older than sixty-five now have some form of skin cancer, and children are required to wear large hats and neck scarves to and from school to protect themselves from ultraviolet radiation. In Patagonia, blind rabbits and fish have been caught. Parents in Punta Arenas, Chile's southernmost city, keep their children indoors between ten A.M. and three P.M. The Australian government issues alerts—like Los Angeles smog alerts—when especially high UV levels are expected, and public-service campaigns warn of the dangers of sunbathing like our American ads warn against the dangers of drugs.

Sun damage to your skin is irreparable. It breaks down collagen and elastin fibers in the skin, and its effects may not show up for thirty years.

Sunscreens are widely recommended, but there is some concern that regular use of even natural sunscreen can interfere with your skin's ability to produce vitamin D. The *Journal of Clinical Endocrinologic Metabolism* reports that scientifically controlled studies of skin untreated with sunscreen versus skin treated with sunscreen (SPF-8) demonstrated a large difference in vitamin D production. The sunscreened skin showed no change in vitamin D, while the untreated subjects had blood-level increases of 1,600 percent.

Many sunscreens also contain **ethanol, fragrance,** and **mineral oil,** which is drying to the skin.

SAFE SOLUTIONS

Enjoy the sun, but take precautions to protect yourself from both UVA and UVB radiation. UVB rays have shorter wavelengths and are the principal cause of sunburn, skin cancer, and premature aging of the skin. UVA rays have longer wavelengths and penetrate more deeply into the skin, contributing to skin cancer and aging.

Start by exposing your skin to the sun only a few minutes

each day, and take care not to burn. Minimize your exposure to the sun between ten A.M. and three P.M., when the sun's rays are most intense.

PROTECTIVE CLOTHING

The most prudent way to shield your skin from the sun's harmful rays is to wear protective clothing such as windbreakers, scarves, gloves, and wide-brimmed hats. *After the Stork* carries SunSkins™ clothing for babies, children, and adults made of Solarweave® nylon fabric, which blocks 99 percent of the UVB rays when dry, and 96 percent of the UVB rays when wet (cotton typically is SPF-7, blocking 50 percent dry and 35 percent wet).

Another new brand of sun-protection fabric is Solumbra®, which has received FDA clearance to claim SPF-30 for its products (blocks more than 97 percent of both UVA and UVB radiation). The *Sun Precautions* catalog carries a wide variety of stylish clothing and hats for men, women, and children (you'd never know it was protecting the wearer from the sun), including shirts, pants, leggings, jackets, and skirts, plus a parasol, headwraps, and such unusual items as handflaps and full head to-toe gear for serious protection. Although these fabrics are made from synthetic fibers, you might choose to wear them as a trade-off to getting skin cancer.

SUNSCREENS

There are many lotions and creams on the market, with a wide variety of natural and synthetic ingredients, offering protection that ranges from little or none to complete blockage. Some sun-protection products, like zinc oxide ointment, are physical barriers that reflect or scatter all light. Other sunscreens are chemical barriers that absorb ultraviolet light.

Sunscreen products are rated with a Sun Protection Factor (SPF), which indicates how much longer you can remain safely in the sun while wearing the sunscreen than if you were to go unprotected. For example, SPF-2 would allow you to stay out twice as long; SPF-30 allows you to stay in the sun thirty times as long.

SPF-2–4: minimal protection, and permits tanning

SPF-4–6: moderate protection and permits some tan

SPF-6–8: extra protection and permits a limited tan

SPF-8–15: maximum protection, with little or no tan

SPF-15+: ultra protection, and no tan at all

The general recommendation is to choose a sunscreen with an SPF-15. Other brands are offered for those who tan easily or, at the other end of the spectrum, have very fair skin that needs extra protection. The average fair-skinned person begins to burn after twenty minutes in full sun. Wearing SPF-15 sunscreen allows that person five hours in the sun before burning. Reapplication of the sunscreen may be necessary, as it can be diluted by sweat or washed off by swimming. Reapplication doesn't extend the time of protection, but helps maintain the protection. The SPF system measures only UVB, not UVA rays, so it is important to check the labels for ingredients that block both types of radiation.

All sunscreens use the same FDA-approved list of active ingredients. Most popular now are the cinnamates (cinoxate, diethanolamin p-methoxycinnamate, and octyl methoxycinnamate), derived from cinnamon and coca leaves. These and para-aminobenzoic acid (PABA) offer good UVB protection. Ingredients ending in "benzone" (such as dioxybenzone and glyceryl aminobenzone) also offer good UVB protection, but are derived from petroleum.

Perusing the sunscreen aisle at my local natural-food store, I found more than a dozen sunscreen products with cinnamate sunscreens and other natural ingredients with a range of SPFs, but none that offered both UVA and UVB protection. At a local discount drugstore, I found an assortment of **Coppertone** products all clearly marked to protect against both UVA and UVB. So it's a toss-up. If you're going to be out in the sun, you can choose between natural ingredients or more broad spectrum protection. (Note: The FDA cautions parents not to apply sunscreen to babies until they are six months old.)

If you want to give your skin a darker tan color, try this concoction:

Boil ¾ cup pure water and brew strong tea with 3 black-tea bags. Put ¼ cup tea into a blender with ¼ cup lanolin and ¼ cup sesame oil. Blend at low speed. Add remaining tea steadily, and spread sparingly on your skin.

SUNGLASSES

In the sunglass department, the darker the lens, the more protection.

> Light tint: protects your eyes against 70 percent UVB and 20 percent UVA
>
> Medium tint: protects your eyes against 95 percent UVB and 60 percent UVA
>
> Dark tint: protects your eyes against 99 percent UVB and 60 percent UVA

Maximum protection is provided by sunglass styles that wrap around or have additional side protectors that block sun from creeping in around the edges.

Remember, though, that with all this protection, we do need exposure to some natural light for good health. Try to spend some time each day outdoors without sunglasses, sitting in the shade or under the protection of a wide-brimmed hat.

TALCUM POWDER

 The danger associated with the use of talcum powder is simple—it may be contaminated with carcinogenic **asbestos** fibers. As you pat it on your body, you generally surround yourself with a good cloud of the stuff, and a certain portion ends up in your lungs. There is *no* safe level for asbestos exposure.

SAFE SOLUTIONS

If you wish to use a body powder, there are a few available at your natural-food store and by mail, but it might be just as easy and a lot less expensive for you to make it at home.

The simplest thing to use is just plain cornstarch, rice starch, oat flour, arrowroot, or white clay, all available at your natural-food store. You could also use eggshell powder, although this is a bit more trouble to make. You have to save your eggshells for a while, rinse and dry them thoroughly, and then crush them into a fine powder in a blender or food processor.

You can also add ground herbs to your body powder for a fresh and natural fragrance.

TOILET PAPER AND TISSUES

Three are three main hazardous ingredients in toilet paper and tissues: **formaldehyde, artificial fragrance,** and **dyes.** I have not seen any formal studies on the health effects of toilet paper, but several years ago, "Dear Abby" ran a number of letters describing complaints.

One woman went to her family doctor with symptoms and was sent to a gynecologist, who told her she had genital herpes. For ten years she had periodic flareups, typically after her periods or after sexual activity. She described the emotional strain and frustration this experience caused her. As a last resort, she saw another gynecologist. This doctor accurately diagnosed that she was allergic to the dye in her colored toilet paper. She's been happily symptom-free ever since.

Another reader wrote that for a year the itching and burning were unbearable. She was told she had some kind of infection, but no one would specify what kind. Finally, a nurse suggested the problem might be her colored toilet paper. One week after changing to white toilet paper, the symptoms disappeared.

Yet another letter was written by a man, who stated that shortly after his wife switched to a scented toilet paper, he and his young daughter experienced pain in the genital area. Luckily, they put two and two together and have had no problems since returning to unscented toilet paper.

Recently another danger has been discovered in toilet paper: **dioxins,** about ninety parts per trillion, according to British studies. This is one of the most toxic chemicals ever produced.

SAFE SOLUTIONS

The best you can do with toilet paper is to buy it plain white and unscented. It still will contain formaldehyde, as all wet-strength papers do, but I can't think of any substitute.

The new toilet papers made from recycled papers are a good buy. Not only are they not bleached and therefore dioxin-free (instead they use a de-inking process), but you'll also help save trees and other resources, and reduce environmental pollution.

For tissues, again, buy them plain white and unscented (and recycled), or use cotton handkerchiefs, which are inexpensive and easy to find.

White, unscented, recycled toilet paper and tissues are available in all natural-food stores and some supermarkets, or you can order them by mail from **Real Goods** or **Seventh Generation.**

LUBRICANTS

Generally, petroleum jelly is considered harmless, but it is a petrochemical product and should be approached with caution by anyone who is sensitive to petrochemical derivatives.

SAFE SOLUTIONS

Vegetable oil–based lubricants are available in most natural-food stores. I've even seen one brand, **Autumn Harp Un-Petroleum Jelly,** at a chain drugstore.

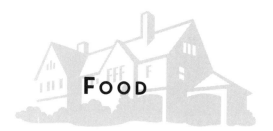

Chapter 8

FOOD

FINALLY, THE CHAPTER ON FOOD. Are you surprised there are so many other household items that are more harmful? With all the emphasis on pesticides and chemical contaminants in foods today, you would think that the food we eat is the source of the most dangerous exposure we have to toxics. Although I don't want to diminish the importance of hazardous substances in foods, in relation to other types of products, foods are so well regulated that the immediate risks are fairly low, but the long-term dangers must be considered.

The quality of our food supply is intimately connected to our health. Generally we think of food as something that tastes good, something to socialize over, or something that supplies nutrients, but food plays a vital role in our lives, for the cells and organs of our bodies are literally made from the foods that we eat. Our body health reflects the quality of the food we put into it. If we eat fresh, live, uncontaminated foods, our health will be vibrant; if we eat undernourished, contaminated, heavily processed, and refined foods, then our health will be less than optimal.

So much has changed in the world of food in the last dozen years since I wrote the first edition of *Nontoxic & Natural*. In that book, I listed pages and pages of brand-name foods that were additive-free, because that was the next step toward pure food that was available at the time (I have to smile when I read that I listed things like 7-Up soda and Godiva chocolates simply because they didn't contain artificial colors and flavors). By the time I got to *Nontoxic, Natural & Earthwise* in 1990, there was only room to list packaged foods with ingredients grown without pesticides (organically grown), because *that* was the next step. Now the availability of organically grown foods has increased so dramatically that to list all the brand-name organically grown packaged foods and mail-order suppliers of organically grown foods would require a book in itself.

Despite this improvement, the majority of our food supply today still is made up of malnourished plants fed limited nutrients from artificial fertilizers, and sprayed with toxic pesticides.

Pesticides and Fertilizers

In 1988, 270 billion pounds of artificial fertilizers were used in agriculture. Not only do they lack adequate nutrition, artificial fertilizers often destroy topsoil and leach into groundwater instead of feeding the plants the limited nutrients they do contain. Nature then sends in insect predators to destroy these weakling plants and return them to the ecosystem, but agribusiness sprays the plants with pesticides to halt the natural cycle and "protect" the weak plants so there will be a crop. It may look like our modern agricultural methods are producing more food, but the quality of that food is lacking. We may have big, juicy tomatoes at the supermarket, but they can't compare to home-grown tomatoes, because the growing practices are specifically designed to build size and shelf life rather than nutrition and flavor.

Nationwide, almost 2 *billion* pounds of pesticides are applied to our land. More than 200 million tons of pesticides containing more than 1,000 active ingredients are used annually on croplands in California alone. In 1987, an EPA report ranked pesticides in food as one of the nation's most serious health and environmental problems. Pesticides are among the more deadly chemicals: according to a report from the National Academy of Sciences, 30 percent of commercially used insecticides, 50 percent of herbicides, and 90 percent of fungicides are known to cause cancer in animal studies.

Ironically, pesticides aren't even doing their job. Since pesticides were first developed after World War II, their use has increased ten times; during that same period, crop loss due to insects has doubled. Often less than .1 percent of the chemicals applied to crops actually reach target pests, although according to independent laboratory tests done in 1983 for the Natural Resources Defense Council (NRDC), 44 percent of produce tested had detectable residues of nineteen different pesticides. Almost half had residues of up to four different pesticides.

Pesticides used in agriculture have contaminated nearly all the air, water, soil, and living beings of the entire planet. According to an article in *The Des Moines Register,* the soil of America's bread basket is so saturated with pesticides that "our clouds are laced with pesticides . . . that have actually evaporated out of the ground along with the water, and rain down on us from the sky." Almost all of us carry residues of toxic pesticides in the fat of our bodies.

The long-term human health effects of chronic, low-level exposures to pesticides currently used on our food are not known, but there are many reports of farmers and their families being poisoned by pesticides, and common sense tells us that to put such substances continuously into our bodies can't possibly be good for us.

Three major classes of chemicals are used as pesticides on food: **organochlorines, organophosphates,** and **carbamates.**

Organochlorine insecticides work by attacking the central nervous system of the agricultural pest, resulting in convulsions and death. Many organochlorines cause cancer, birth defects, and genetic damage in animals. In addition, they are stored in human body fat and can accumulate to high levels over time. Although these pesticides were used predominantly in the 1940s and 1950s, many still are in use today. Three organochlorines have been banned: DDT in 1972; aldrin in 1974; and endrin in 1979, although endrin still is allowed on apple and wheat crops. These poisons can remain in our soil and water supplies an average of fifty to seventy-five years, adding dangerous contaminants to our food without offering any positive agricultural benefit. In the NRDC study mentioned on page 216, DDT residues were found in more samples than any other pesticide, *eleven years* after the chemical was banned from use.

Organophospate insecticides are the most widely used insecticides today. Unlike organochlorines, organophosphates break down into harmless chemicals within several weeks, so they do not pose such a long-term threat. In pest protection, they work by blocking the action of the chemical that aids in the transmission of nerve impulses; as a result, those impulses are transmitted continuously, leading to convulsions and death. Some organophosphates have been found to cause genetic damage in animals, and others are believed to cause serious changes in animal brain activity.

Carbamates also are widely used today. Their toxicity and persistence lie somewhere between the organochlorines and organophosphates. One of the carbamates is suspected of causing birth defects, and a review of its safety has only just begun.

As we have learned already in chapter 4, two federal agencies are responsible for protecting us from pesticide residues in food: the Environmental Protection Agency (EPA) and the Food and Drug Administration (FDA). Under the Federal Insecticide, Fungicide, and Rodenticide Act (FIFRA), manufacturers of new pesticides are required to submit information about which crops they will be used on, their effectiveness and toxicity, and the nature and levels of residues. The EPA then sets a tolerance for each pesticide that sets the amount allowed to remain on crops.

This sounds like a pretty good system, but it has several flaws. Many pesticides now in use were granted tolerances *before* safety tests were required to determine whether the pesticide causes cancer, birth defects, genetic damage, or reproductive disorders. A study done by the National Academy of Sciences reports that 64 percent of pesticides now in use have not even been minimally tested for their toxic effects. Very little information is available on the potential long-term health effects, the possibility of synergistic effects resulting from exposure to more than one pesticide, and the range of individual sensitivities among the human population. Of the nineteen pesticides detected in the NRDC survey to leave residues on produce, eight are suspected of causing cancer, five may induce birth detects, and the others could produce genetic mutations. But, for some of the pesticides used on food, no information is publicly available to enable us to assess for ourselves the possible health hazards.

The EPA sets acceptable pesticide residue tolerances for each individual crop or food type on which the pesticide will be used. The same pesticide might have a different tolerance for each separate fruit and vegetable. Tolerances are determined by considering both the safety of the pesticide and how much the EPA estimates you will eat of that food over the course of your lifetime, based on an estimate of how much an average person eats of that particular food in a year. But currently, new tolerances are set in accordance with a household survey taken in 1966, despite the fact that we have clearly increased our intake of fresh fruits and vegetables since that time. The EPA assumes each of us eats only about *half a pound per year* of almonds, artichokes, avocados, barley, blackberries, blueberries, cantaloupes, eggplants, filberts, figs, garlic, leeks, mushrooms, nectarines, parsley, papayas, pecans, plums, radishes, rye flour, summer squash, and walnuts. Supposedly, we eat only about 1½ pounds of broccoli, 7½ pounds of carrots, 33 pounds of oranges (that's only about 66 oranges in 365 days), 20 pounds of lettuce, 84 pounds of potatoes, 3 pounds of strawberries, and 44 pounds of tomatoes. These figures make me wonder if the EPA has read the *Dietary Guidelines for Americans* recommended by the U.S. Department of Agriculture. I exceeded my year's quota for mushrooms at dinner last night.

Under the Federal Food, Drug, and Cosmetic Act, the FDA tests samples of food crops for pesticide residues. Again, this sounds good, but the tests commonly used by the FDA can detect only 107 of almost 300 pesticides that have established tolerances. As many as 20 pesticides in the food supply that are suspected of causing cancer are not even monitored by the FDA.

Further, although the monitoring system seems well intended, some highly toxic pesticides that are actually banned for use in the United States can be found in our food supply. Organochlorines such as **DDT, 2,4,5T, aldrin, dieldrin, heptachlor, chlordane, endrin,** and **BHC** are illegal here but are shipped to other countries for use. They then return to us on imported foods—coffee, chocolate, bananas, rice, tea, sugar, and tapioca, for example. During the winter months, summer-season vegetables in supermarkets may be imported from Mexico, where pesticide use is not as tightly controlled as in the United States. These include zucchini, summer squash, yellow squash, garlic, string beans, okra, asparagus, bell peppers, cucumbers, eggplant, green peas, snow peas, and tomatoes. Even seasonally, if American crops fail or supplies aren't sufficient, green onions, radishes, parsley, corn, brussels sprouts, spinach, leafy lettuce, watermelons, cantaloupes, honeydew melons, pineapples, and strawberries may also be imported.

Horrible as the pesticide problem is, it is not the only chemical concern we have regarding fresh produce. Bananas, pineapples, guavas, mangos, and other tropical fruits from Hawaii are fumigated with toxic substances before being allowed onto the mainland.

Also, another category of chemicals is introduced for "cosmetic purposes," to make our produce more attractive to the eye. Some oranges are dyed orange with the **coal-tar dye Red No. 32,** known to cause cancer in laboratory animals. And, before green oranges are dyed to look ripe, they are "degreened" with **ethylene gas** to remove the chlorophyll from the rind. The colorless oranges then pass through a vat of hot dye for tinting. Almost all Florida citrus that reaches the marketplace before January 1 has been treated. Other produce that may be dyed are some "new" potatoes (regular potatoes dyed red) and some red yams (actually dyed sweet potatoes).

Concerns about packaging materials are by no means limited to processed foods. Citrus fruits generally are wrapped in papers treated with a potent **fungicide.** The first time I smelled an orange without this fungicide, I was shocked to find that the smell I had associated with "citrus" all these years was not citrus at all; real citrus has a lovely, delicate fragrance, much different from the biting chemical odor of fungicide. With fungicides, not only might you be harmed by eating the food, but you could be affected by smelling it, too.

Some potatoes and onions are treated with **malesic hydrazide,** a potential human carcinogen, to inhibit sprouting and make old onions and potatoes appear fresh. It really doesn't inhibit sprouting at all, but causes the onions and potatoes to sprout *inside* instead of outside where you can see it! I stopped buying supermarket potatoes when I cut a half dozen of them open one day and they all were sprouted inside.

In addition, carrots, oranges, lemons, limes, apples, pears, plums, peaches, melons, parsnips, tomatoes, green peppers, ruta-bagas, turnips, cucumbers, grapefruits, and tangerines may all be coated with **paraffin,** a petrochemical wax that may contain car-cinogenic impurities.

Mushrooms might be grown without pesticides, but fre-quently they are fumigated with **formaldehyde** as a perservative.

Here's a final depressing warning: There is no way to tell what sort of chemical contaminants may be present in any super-market produce, as they have no labels.

Processed Foods and Food Additives

After agribusiness grows unhealthy, toxic plants, most of these are sent to a factory to be processed. There they are stripped of many of their nutrients, bleached, colored, flavored, preserved, and packaged with attractive labels. For example, if you buy peas in a can, 30 percent of the vitamins have been lost in cooking at the canning plant, and 25 percent have been lost in the sterilization process; 27 percent are discarded with the cooking liquid, and 12 percent are lost when you heat the peas after you open the can. What's left? Squishy, tasteless little green balls with only 6 per-cent of their nutritional value. Frozen peas, after processing and cooking, are left with about 17 percent of the original vitamins. White flour loses up to ninety nutrients by milling, and only six nutrients are artificially added to "enrich" it.

Yet, such processed foods are routinely assumed to be as safe and nutritious as fresh, whole foods. Consider the production of apple juice, which is probably the icon of a healthy beverage. After the apples have been grown with **pesticides** and fed with **artificial fertilizers,** they are harvested and trucked to a nearby processing plant, where they are run through a trough of **chlori-nated water** to wash off dirt, pesticide residues, and other unde-sirables. Some plants also run the apples through a bath of **carnauba wax** (also used in car wax) and **preservatives.** Before the apples become juice, they are peeled by running them through a "bath" of hot **sodium hydroxide (lye),** which penetrates beneath the skin and loosens it from the pulp. High-velocity jets of cold water then blast off the skin, and a machine punches out the cores. The peeled, cored apples are crushed in a high-pressure juicer. To keep the juice from turning too dark, some processors add **sulfiting agents,** which inhibit the browning enzyme (if sulfites are added, they must be noted on the label). Then it is **pasteurized** with heat (from 200 to 400 degrees for four or five seconds) to kill any bacteria that might be present, which also reduces the vitamin content. Hardly the same as biting into a crunchy organically grown apple or running the apple through a juicer at home.

Research suggests that a primary contributing factor to many of our modern diseases is our eating of processed, low-fiber, low-nutrition foods. Before 1900, degenerative illnesses like cancer and heart disease were relatively rare. Now heart disease is the leading cause of death in the United States, and cancer hits one out of every three people during their lifetime. Together, cancer and heart disease cause 50 percent of all deaths in this country. Obesity was a problem that generally affected only the wealthy in eighteenth-century Europe, while today half of our population is overweight to some degree.

Studies of other cultures that eat traditional, whole, unrefined, unprocessed foods show a remarkable lack of illness. Yet study after study has found that people who switch from their native diet to a Western one gradually develop Western degenerative diseases.

Food also loses nutrition when it is stored. Yes, we have the convenience of apples all year long in the supermarket, but apples are kept in cold storage and brought out as they are needed. The apple you eat in June was probably harvested the previous October. This is true for many other fruits and vegetables as well.

Food additives (artificial and natural) are those substances or mixtures of substances, other than the basic foodstuffs, which are present in food as a result of any aspect of production, processing, storage, or packaging (not including chance contaminants). Additives in food are nothing new—salt was used as a preservative for raw meat centuries ago. But modern chemistry has given us many new, unnatural, and often unsafe ways to preserve or alter food. We now have more than 8,600 food additives approved for use, of varying safety and toxicity.

All food additives, synthetic or natural, must serve one or more of the following purposes:

- improve nutritional value;
- enhance quality or consumer acceptability;
- improve the keeping quality;
- make food more readily available;
- facilitate food's preparation.

The majority of food additives are used for purposes other than improving nutritional value. Those that are added for nutritional purposes simply attempt to replace nutrients lost in processing; rarely do they make food more nutritious than it would be in its whole, natural state (with the exception of certain breakfast cereals, whose nutrition labels read more like vitamin pills).

Food additives are regulated by the Food and Drug Administration (FDA) under the Food Additives Amendment to the Pure Food and Drug Act, passed in 1958. The Amendment also contains the Delany Clause, which states that "no additive shall be deemed safe if it is found to induce cancer when ingested by man or animal." Exempt from regulation are those additives Generally Recognized As Safe (GRAS). In the late 1950s, the FDA compiled a list of additives they assumed to be safe, and sent it out with a questionnaire to about 900 scientists. Of the one-third who responded, only about 100 offered substantive comments. The GRAS list was finalized from these comments.

Ten years later, the FDA began to review the scientific literature to determine the safety of GRAS substances.

Since 1972, thirty-five widely used food additives have been found to be unsafe and have been removed from the FDA-approved list. Many of these cause cancer. In 1980, the National Toxicology Council contracted with the National Research Council and the National Academy of Sciences to investigate substances from a list of 8,627 food additives. Of these, it was possible to assess completely the health hazards of only 5 percent.

Because the names of many additives do not identify whether their source is natural or synthetic, it is often impossible to know from reading a label if a food contains artificial additives. In general, if the label says "artificial," or if you don't recognize an ingredient as a food, or if it doesn't say "natural" (as in "natural flavor" or "natural color"), you probably shouldn't buy it.

But regardless of the results of the toxicity tests for single food additives, the real issue is how they interact, because that is how we consume them. Food additives can have a synergistic effect and become more harmful when they combine. This was clearly demonstrated in a study by Dr. Benjamin Ershoff at the Institute for Nutritional Studies in California. Rats were given different combinations of three common food additives: sodium cyclamate, Red Dye No. 2, and polyoxyethelene sorbitan monostearate. At first the rats were fed only one of the three additives, and nothing happened. Then the test animals were given sodium cyclamate and Red Dye No. 2; they stopped growing, lost their hair, and developed diarrhea. When the rats finally were given all three additives they lost weight rapidly and died within two weeks.

SULFITES

Sulfites pose the most immediate danger of all additives. Used primarily to reduce or prevent spoilage and discoloration, they can trigger severe allergic reactions in sulfite-sensitive individuals. These reactions include breathing difficulties, wheezing, vomiting, nausea, diarrhea, unconsciousness, abdominal pain, cramps, and hives. In some cases, anaphylactic shock can result in immediate death. Asthmatics are the primary group at risk, and it is estimated that about 10 percent of all asthmatics are sulfite-sensitive. However, one-fourth of the complaints received by the FDA involved individuals who have no history of asthma. Since the FDA considers this additive to be safe for consumption by the general public, it is not banning its use, and you must take the responsibility for controlling your intake.

Sulfites appear on package labels as **sulfur dioxide, sodium sulfite, sodium and potassium bisulfite,** and **sodium and potassium metabisulfite.** They are more commonly found in dried fruits, shellfish (fresh, frozen, canned, or dried), soups, wine vinegar, vegetables (fresh, peeled, frozen, canned, or dried),

packaged lemon juice, avocado dip, maraschino cherries, potatoes (fresh, peeled, frozen, dried, or canned), salad dressings,
sauces and gravies, and corn syrup. Sulfites almost always are
used in wine and beer production, and are *not* always listed on
the labels of alcoholic beverages. The most common exposure to
sulfites, however, is in restaurants, where the kitchen may use
them to keep foods looking fresh when they're really not. Sulfites
are frequently used in salad bars, on fresh fruits and vegetables,
precut potatoes, seafood, cooked vegetable dishes, and bakery
products without informing the customer.

NITRATES

Nitrates are the next-most dangerous, because they can cause
cancer. Nitrite is added to 60 to 65 percent of all pork produced
in the United States, as well as some other meats, poultry, fish,
and cheese. It is especially prevalent in processed meats, such as
bacon, sausage, luncheon meats, and hot dogs, to preserve the
pink color and inhibit the growth of the bacteria that cause botulism food poisoning. Nitrates themselves are not particularly
harmful, but when they combine with amines in the food, they
form carcinogenic **nitrosamines.**

ARTIFICIAL COLORS

Artificial colors also pose a cancer risk—almost all have been
shown to be carcinogenic in animal studies. According to the
National Cancer Institute, "We should assume that agents that
cause cancer in animals are likely to cause cancer in humans. To
prevent cancer, we cannot afford to wait for absolute proof of carcinogenicity in humans. Instead, we must heed the warnings provided by laboratory animal experiments and reduce or eliminate
human exposure to probable cancer-causing agents."

But cancer, though certainly a major concern, is not the only
problem. For, along with artificial colors, **BHA, BHT,** and **artificial flavors** have been linked to hyperactivity and behavioral
disturbances in children by Dr. Benjamin Feingold of Kaiser-
Permanente Medical Center. While it has been very difficult to
substantiate this claim with scientific studies, the observations of
parents and doctors over the past twenty years confirm that avoiding artificial additives has significantly improved their children's
conditions, making this evidence hard to ignore.

MSG

MSG is a popular additive that gained widespread use as a flavor enhancer before its healthfulness came into question. However, many users probably wondered privately about the safety of this additive, since its most well-known side effect is Chinese Restaurant Syndrome—a condition characterized by numbness, weakness, heart palpitations, cold sweat, and headache. Not everyone has the reactions, and not everyone experiences symptoms of the same intensity, but I have heard from several friends who have been to China that when you eat MSG three times a day, every day, you really start to feel it. In addition, animal studies show that MSG can cause brain damage, stunted skeletal development, obesity, and female sterility. It is on the FDA list of additives that need further study for mutagenic and reproductive effects.

EDTA

Also on the EPA list for further study is the preservative ethylenediaminetetraacetic acid (EDTA). Toxicology books list many possible symptoms associated with large exposures, including dizziness, sneezing, headaches, nausea, and asthma attacks. The effects caused by the amounts ingested in food are still being investigated.

SUGAR AND SALT

Most processed foods contain sugar or salt. Although moderate amounts of either of these substances are not particularly harmful for most people, the amounts of sugar and salt in your everyday diet can add up quickly if your diet is composed primarily of packaged foods. People with high blood pressure need to be particularly cautious about their intake of salt, and may find that a diet of processed foods goes beyond the level of salt intake recommended by their doctors.

PACKAGING

Many packaged foods also wind up being contaminated by their packaging. In the past, all canned foods were packed in cans made with lead solder, which can leach into the food, doubling or tripling its original lead content. Continuous low-level exposure to lead has been found to produce permanent neuropsychological defects and behavior disorders in children, including low IQ, short attention span, hyperactive behavior, and motor difficulties. Low-level exposure also may be carcinogenic, mutagenic, and teratogenic. There is no demonstrably safe level for lead.

Today, however, virtually all canned natural foods come in lead-free cans, and most conglomerate food producers also have switched. Lead-soldered cans are now the exception instead of the rule, but still they are common enough to watch out for. Once you know what to look for, the different cans are very easy to identify. You can find them at supermarkets as well as natural-food stores.

Soldered cans have a top and bottom rim with a side seam that peeks out at the edge of the label. A lead-soldered can has an obvious, protruding side seam, and traces of solder also may be visible on the outside. If you run your finger around the top or bottom of the can near the rim, you'll be able to feel the lumpy seam of a lead-soldered can. These you should avoid. A *lead-free* soldered can has a flat, thin, neat seam with a characteristic narrow black or blue line running down the middle. You will recognize such a can as different from the lead-soldered variety right away. The lead-free aluminum can also is distinctive. Formed from one piece of metal, it has a rounded bottom, a rim at the top, and no seam.

Other packaged foods (such as cheese spreads, whipped cream, or no-stick pan coatings) come in **aerosol** or pressurized containers. When inhaled, aerosols are known to cause lung diseases from normal use, and death from high concentrations. Because aerosol spray containers are a form of packaging, aerosol propellants are not considered an additive and their safety is not discussed in literature on food additives. It's up to us to learn about these food contaminants and limit our intake.

Plastic frequently is used to package processed foods, and many times can leach into the food. The health effects are unknown.

Labeling

Food labeling has some inconsistencies that would actually seem amusing, if they weren't so tragic. Fresh produce that is full of pesticides, for example, requires no labeling, whereas if you want to sell uncontaminated produce, you must label it very carefully to describe what it *doesn't* contain. On the other hand, once you turn that raw pesticide-laden food into a processed food product, labeling laws require that you list additives the product *does* contain (with the exception of the pesticides, of course)!

In addition, the presence of many other additives in food products may be *legally concealed*. Food processors may use ingredients already containing additives without being required to list these additives on the label. Ham included in processed foods, for instance, will contain nitrates and nitrites, and the shortening used may contain BHA and BHT, but only "ham" or "shortening" will appear on the product label.

SAFE SOLUTIONS

Although many additives are hazardous, some additives with strange-sounding names come from natural sources and are safe or even beneficial to use. To find out the derivation and safety of almost any food additive, see *A Consumer Dictionary of Food Additives*. Here are some safe food additives that are often used in natural foods.

Acetic acid: another name for plain vinegar

Agar-agar: derived from seaweed

Albumin: derived from egg whites

Alginates: derived from seaweed

Annatto: taken from a rain-forest tree

Beta-carotene: vitamin A derived from carrots

Carrageenan: derived from seaweed

Citric acid: vitamin C from citrus fruits

Dextrose: corn sugar

Dulse: derived from seaweed

Guar gum: made by grinding the seed of a plant cultivated in India

Gum tragacanth: the dried gummy exudate from a Middle Eastern plant

Lactic acid: made by fermentation of whey, cornstarch, potatoes, and molasses

Lecithin: isolated from eggs, soybeans, and corn

Pectin: taken from lemon or orange rinds

Sodium chloride: common table salt

The optimal plan for minimizing your exposure to added toxic substances in food is based on a diet of fresh, whole foods.

- Fresh raw, dried, and home-cooked vegetables and fruits
- Whole grains and legumes
- Eggs from free-range hens
- Lean meat or poultry from free-range animals
- Nonfat milk and low-fat cheeses
- Ocean fish
- Honey and other natural sweeteners (in small quantities)

Ideally, these all would be organically grown.

ORGANICALLY GROWN FOODS

Organically grown foods are those grown or raised without synthetic fertilizers, pesticides (including herbicides, insecticides, and fungicides), artificial ripening processes, growth stimulators and regulators such as hormones, or antibiotics and other drugs. In addition, organically grown foods also must be processed, packaged, transported, and stored without the use of chemicals such as fumigants, artificial additives, and preservatives, and without food irradiation.

While this is the general philosophy, there are many different methods of organic agriculture, which are specific to the site, the foods being grown or raised, the problems with pests, and the philosophy of the farmer. In general, though, organic growers maintain a program of reintroducing organic matter back into the soil by using compost, green manures, cover crops, animal manures, and fish meal. Minerals and other soil-building amendments such as seaweed and bonemeal often are added to balance the soil to a healthy fertility. Crop rotation is used to manage weeds and plant disease, and natural predators, such as ladybugs and other beneficial insects and microorganisms, are introduced. Some organic growers plant unusual varieties of foods to help maintain biological diversity. And most organic growers are small family farmers who are concerned about developing regionally self-reliant food production systems, though larger growers are also starting to go organic.

The Organic Food Production Act of 1990 required the U.S. Department of Agriculture (USDA) to establish an organic certification program for producers and handlers of organically produced agricultural products. Since October 1993, it has been a violation of federal law to sell or label an agricultural product as organically produced, or to affix a label or provide other market information that implies directly or indirectly that a product is organically produced, unless the product is produced and handled in accordance with the requirements established by the program.

The act also requires all producers and handlers of organically produced agricultural products to be certified by a state or private certifier accredited by the USDA—so if it's not certified, it can't be called "organic," even though a farmer might use organic methods (if you come across food not labeled *organic,* which describes organic methods, use your best judgment—there are many reasons why small growers choose not to be certified, even though their products meet, or even exceed, organic standards).

Growers and processors who want to be certified have to submit a written plan of their organic practices. Then, as was common in previous certification programs, the national certification requires a three-year waiting period, during which the land is free from synthetic chemicals, before the harvest of a certified crop. At this time, the grower is issued a "pending" or "transitional" certification, which will change to "full" certification once all conditions are met. After harvest, processors are not allowed to add any synthetic ingredients or ingredients that haven't been produced organically unless those ingredients are approved by the program or represent less than 5 percent of the finished product. They also cannot add sulfites to wine or foods, or nitrates and nitrites to processed meats or other foods. Fungicides, preservatives, and fumigants are forbidden in packaging, and even any water used has to meet federal standards for safety.

While fully certified organically grown plants are somewhat healthier and contain fewer pesticide residues from the soil, buying organic foods pending certification is just as important. Many farmers have some fully certified fields and some in transition, and as more and more farmers go organic, the number of fields with certification pending will far outnumber those that have full certification. Whether the field is fully certified or transitional, both use the same organic methods with the only difference being that the fully certified fields have not used pesticides and artificial fertilizers for at least three years. Transitional is just that, being in transition to organic, and needs to be supported as a midway step between chemical agriculture and organic agriculture. What is most important is that organic methods are used.

Livestock (including wild game, poultry, fish, and other forms of nonplant life) also is covered under the Organic Food Production Act of 1990. To be called "organic," only organically grown feed can be given—no growth promoters, hormones, antibiotics (except to treat illness), or other synthetic substances that are used routinely in this country. Dairy cattle have to be raised in this way for at least one year before their milk and products made from their milk are certified.

For processed foods, if 50 percent or more, by weight, of the ingredients are organic (excluding water and salt), the product as a whole can be labeled organic. If less than 50 percent of the ingredients are organic, the word *organic* can be used on the ingredient list only next to those ingredients that are organic.

Certification organizations for organically grown food, which have sprung from within the industry itself by especially caring and dedicated growers, have been in place for more than a decade, and both local and national organizations exist across the country. There are thirty-two certifying organizations in the United States (national organizations are listed in Resources). Each state is allowed to develop its own certification program, as long as it is at least as strict as the national program. Certifying organizations must be accredited by the Secretary of Agriculture.

More than one third of the states have passed state legislation governing the use of the term *organic* for growing or labeling foods: California, Colorado, Connecticut, Idaho, Iowa, Maine, Massachusetts, Minnesota, Montana, Nebraska, New Hampshire, New York, North Dakota, Oregon, Rhode Island, South Dakota, Texas, Vermont, Washington, and Wisconsin. Since more states pass such legislation every year, it is likely that soon every state will regulate the use of this term. Because space does not permit details on the requirements of each of these laws, if your state has a law, get a copy and study it. Your local natural-food store or any place that sells organically grown food should have a copy.

The state of California has one of the oldest laws regarding labeling of organic food, originally written in 1979 and revised in 1990. Many states have used the California standards over the years, and products all over the country are labeled "Grown and processed in accordance with section 26569.11 of the California Health and Safety Code."

Unfortunately, although much of our supply of organically grown food has increased, there isn't enough organically grown food to go around for everyone quite yet. As with any other product that is in short supply, often you have to be willing not only to make an extra effort to find it, but also to pay a little more.

Organically grown food is now available through many outlets, more or less depending on where you live. Here in northern California, I can buy fresh organic produce at my local independently owned supermarket, natural-food stores, food co-ops, and the farmers' market.

For most of the year I get my produce from my own backyard, or from three local organic farms through a program called a CSA. Short for Community Supported Agriculture, a CSA offers local residents the opportunity to purchase shares in the harvest of a farm for the growing season. For a flat fee, you get a share of whatever is produced. Some weeks there is little in the basket, and other weeks it is overflowing, but it is a good plan that keeps a direct connection between the farmer and the consumer. We can even work on the farm anytime we want, as if it were our own.

Now, what I'd really like to say is, "Make all your meals from fresh, organically grown ingredients," but realistically I know that's not going to happen. Even I will buy the occasional jar of pasta sauce, condiments and potato chips. What you can do is purchase packaged foods with organically grown ingredients. Again, in northern California, I can buy these at the supermarket as well as at the natural-food store.

If you have difficulty finding organically grown foods in your area, they are available by mail. Though it may sound silly to order food through the mail, many people do and find that even with the shipping, they have considerable cost savings. Some general organic-food catalogs to order are **Allergy Resources, Deer Valley Farm, Gold Mine Natural Food Company, Jaffe Brothers,** and **Natural Lifestyle.** Each of these carries basic bulk staples and/or packaged products you would find in a natural-food store.

There are two exceptional organic-food catalogs I want to mention—one has been around forever, and the other is fairly new. The old-timer is **Walnut Acres.** For three generations, one family has been farming organically on the same land—their soil has been free of synthetic fertilizers, pesticides, and herbicides for nearly fifty years. Their fifty-plus-page catalog carries every food you can imagine, almost all organically grown. In addition to fresh produce, whole grains, and other basic foods, they sell soups, stews, cookies, and baking mixes, all made from these raw, organically grown ingredients. They even have a holiday fruitcake made with unsulphured dried fruits instead of artificially colored red and green candied cherries. If you wanted to, you could order all your food from this one catalog.

The newcomer is **Diamond Organics.** They specialize in overnight delivery of the most gorgeous organically grown produce, straight from the field to your door, so it is fresher than if you bought it at your local store.

At the very least, take the step from buying packaged foods with additives to buying those with additive-free, organically grown ingredients. Read the labels carefully. Don't forget to compare prices—some large corporations actually are removing artificial ingredients from selected items, and these are available at a lower cost than some natural brands with identical ingredients. On the other hand, supermarkets with natural-food departments frequently sell the same foods found in natural-food stores at greatly inflated prices. Also, instead of having separate natural-foods departments, some supermarkets shelve the natural-foods brands with the supermarket brands and sell them at competitive prices. I shop mainly at a locally owned supermarket because they carry organically grown produce and the same brands of organically grown packaged foods and recycled paper products as the natural-food store *across the street* . . . but at lower prices. A little comparison shopping is well worth the effort.

BIODYNAMICALLY GROWN FOODS

A special type of organic agriculture is called "biodynamic." Biodynamically grown food comes from farms designed to be self-contained, sustainable ecosystems, which bring together the complex interrelationships of plants, animals, and soil, with the warmth of the sun, the seasonal energies of the earth, and the rhythms of the cosmos. It meets or exceeds all other organic growing standards. Biodynamic concepts were introduced by philosopher Rudolph Steiner more than sixty years ago. Less known in this country than in Europe and other parts of the world, biodynamic foods can be found in some natural-food stores and in mail-order catalogs.

NUTRICLEAN FOODS

The NutriClean program, run by Scientific Certification Systems, does not certify foods to be organically grown. Instead, their certification is for a different standard they call "clean food"—food certified to contain no detectable pesticide residues.

The purpose of the NutriClean system is to screen produce for pesticides that have the greatest health concern to the public, measuring final crop performance against a strict "no detected residue" standard. Their comprehensive audit and review process includes complete disclosure of the pesticides used by the grower, on-site inspections, field sampling of products, and extensive laboratory tests for each and every pesticide used.

NutriClean standards for pesticide use are stricter than government and some organic standards, because they do not allow residues either of synthetic pesticides or of the natural pesticides sometimes used in organic agriculture. The certification is limited, however, because it addresses pesticide residues only, and not the fertility of the soil or the overall sustainability of the farm.

WILDCRAFTED FOODS

Wildcrafted is another term used to identify pesticide-free foods, particularly herbs. Wildcrafted plants are, as the term suggests, gathered from their natural, wild habitat, often from pristine areas. Sea vegetables, wild rice, and some wild fruits also are wildcrafted.

When wildcrafting is done sustainably with proper respect, generally only the branches or flowers from plants are gathered, and the living plant is left. If it is necessary to take the whole plant, seeds of the plant are placed in the empty hole from which the plant was uprooted. Care is taken to remove only a few plants, flowers, or branches, so plenty remain to continue the supply.

Wildcrafted plants are regulated by the Organic Food Production Act of 1990. Harvesters must designate the area they are harvesting and provide a three-year history of the area, which shows that no prohibited substances have been applied there. A plan for harvesting must indicate that the harvest will sustain the wild crop. No prohibited substances may be added by processors.

NATURAL FOODS

In response to our concern about the safety of food additives, more and more "natural" foods are introduced to the marketplace every day. Ironically, though, the growth of the industry has resulted in much confusion and some downright deceit regarding what is *really* natural.

Unfortunately, there is no legal definition of the word *natural* as it appears on food labels. If a label says "100% Natural," technically it should contain no artificial colors, flavors, preservatives, or other synthetic additives in the food product at all. However, just because something is labeled "100% Natural" does not necessarily mean pesticides or other chemicals were not used in processing.

In general, a food may be called natural only if it contains no artificial ingredients and had no more processing than it would normally receive in a household kitchen. Minimal processing includes washing or peeling fruits or vegetables; homogenizing milk; freezing, canning, or bottling foods; grinding nuts; baking bread; and aging meat.

Because of the large demand for natural products, many large corporations are now marketing their unnatural products in a way that misleads you into thinking they are natural. Don't be confused by pictures of farms on the label or big letters announcing the absence of one particular additive. Read the ingredients carefully, and if it contains ingredients that you don't recognize as food, don't buy it.

Food patterns are hard to change, because we have so many emotions tied to them. We remember our favorite dishes from childhood; we want to socialize with friends. We have a basic instinct to eat certain foods, and it's difficult to stop and think about the potential hazards of the foods we are putting into our bodies.

Changing your eating habits needn't be drastic—you don't have to do it overnight. The idea is to start choosing fresh, whole foods more often, and choose packaged foods less often. You might start simply by eating more fresh fruits and vegetables each day, or by drinking low-fat or nonfat milk instead of whole milk. Substitute fresh fruit for desserts. Buy whole-grain breads instead of white bread. And whenever possible, buy organically grown foods and let your local merchants know you want them to continue to carry more. Even if you change just your brand of pickles, it's a good place to begin.

COFFEE

As I write this, coffee seems to be gaining ground as the most popular drink in America. Specialty coffee boutiques seem to be opening on every street corner in major cities, so I thought it deserved a few words.

Most coffee sold in the United States is grown in foreign countries that often use **pesticides** so toxic they have been banned here in this country. Coffee drinking may contribute to a higher incidence of cancer of the pancreas, the fourth most common cause of cancer death in America. Although no physiological studies have been done, scientists at the Harvard School of Public Health have made a statistical link to support this theory.

The **caffeine** in coffee is responsible for many ills, including increased incidence of heart attacks, headaches, indigestion and ulcers, insomnia, anxiety, and depression. Pregnant women should limit their intake of caffeine; in large quantities it has contributed to the incidence of miscarriages, premature births, and birth defects.

In addition, bleached white coffee filters may release trace amounts of **dioxin** into your cup of coffee. And, if you drink it in a **polystyrene** cup, you're probably drinking a few molecules of plastic as well.

Instant gourmet coffees additionally may contain **artificial flavors** and **sugar.**

SAFE SOLUTIONS

Limit your consumption of coffee and avoid instant and flavored coffees, which contain many chemical additives. Instead, use freshly ground coffee beans (preferably organically grown, available at natural-food stores or by mail from *Walnut Acres* and others) and brew in a nonplastic container. If you prefer decaffeinated coffee, drink steam- or water-processed varieties to avoid the **hexane** and **methylene chloride** used in the decaffeinating process. Purchase unbleached brown paper coffee filters, cotton cloth filters, or invest in a French "press pot" that self-filters the coffee grounds. Some companies manufacture "permanent filters" as well. These are reusable and eliminate paper waste.

As an alternative to coffee, try herb tea (again, preferably organically grown) or noncaffeinated hot beverages with flavors similar to coffee, such as those made from roasted grains (sold at natural-food stores). Remember that tea bags contain small amounts of dioxin, too, so if you are going to drink tea—herbal or otherwise—brew loose tea or choose a brand that advertises their tea bags as "dioxin-free."

Recently I've discovered the joy of drinking organically grown green tea. Fragrant and delicate, it seems to have a calming effect while at the same time it gives me a little pick-me-up. Green tea comes from the same leaves as black tea, but because it is not fermented, it retains its healthful ingredients. Chemical analyses of green tea have revealed that it contains significant amounts of water-soluble vitamins and minerals. In Japan, green tea consumption goes up in winter, when fruits and fresh green vegetables are scarce. Medical researchers have discovered that green tea is effective in preventing cavities, bad breath, flu, some types of cancer and heart disease, and helps regulate blood-sugar levels and blood clotting.

MEAT, POULTRY, AND EGGS

This product was prepared from inspected and passed meat and/or poultry. Some food products may contain bacteria that could cause illness if the product is mishandled or cooked improperly. For your protection, follow these safe handling instructions.

- Keep refrigerated or frozen. Thaw in refrigerator or microwave.
- Keep raw meat and poultry separate from other foods. Wash working surfaces (including cutting boards), utensils, and hands after touching raw meat or poultry.
- Cook thoroughly. Keep hot foods hot. Refrigerate leftovers immediately or discard.

You're going to need a strong stomach to read this section. After you read this, you may become a vegetarian forever.

Most meat, poultry, and animal products on the market today come from factory farms that raise animals as "biomachines." The animals are confined in dark, crowded quarters, fed diets high in drugs and chemicals and low in nutrients, and deprived completely of exercise and fresh air. The results are highly stressed, deformed, and diseased animals, which hardly qualify as high-quality foods.

In today's market, many of the animals offered to us to eat are not the same kinds of animals even our grandparents ate. Thanks to the modern science of genetic manipulation, we are sold animals that grow faster (for efficient, high-yield production), but are of poorer quality. Hens are laying more eggs than ever before, but these eggs are smaller, with more white and less yolk, and they are paler and more watery than eggs from barnyard chickens.

The greatest source of contamination in factory animals comes from their feed. Farmers want to feed their animals something cheap that will make them grow heavy fast. Although some animals are fed soybeans, corn, barley, and other grains, others may be fed **ground cardboard, old newspapers, sawdust, and recycled animal wastes.** Researchers are even studying **human sewage** for ways to process it into animal feed.

Commercial feed may contain **growth-stimulating hormones, coloring agents, fungicides and pesticides, drugs and medicines** to treat diseases, and **flavoring agents** to make it more appealing to the animals. Fully 100 percent of all poultry, 90 percent of pigs and veal calves, and 60 percent of all cattle are fed **antibiotics** as a regular part of their diets. More than 40 percent of all the antibiotics produced in the United States are used as animal-feed additives. And 75 percent of all hogs are given **sulfa** drugs. In all, more than 1,000 drugs and another 1,000 chemicals are approved by the FDA for use in feed. And many of these substances wind up in our bodies via burgers, chicken dinners, and bacon breakfasts.

Many chemicals in the feed alone are likely to leave residues in meat and poultry. **Organochlorine** pesticides used on feed grains can accumulate to very high levels in animal fat. The General Accounting Office of the U.S. government has identified 143 drugs and pesticides that are likely to leave residues in raw meat and poultry. Of these, 42 are known to cause or are suspected of causing cancer, 20 can cause birth defects, and 6 can cause mutations.

Calves raised for "milk-fed" veal are fed a "milk replacer" formula containing dried skim milk, dried whey, starch, fats, sugar, mold inhibitors, vitamins, and antibiotics. No iron is allowed in their diet, because iron discolors their meat. Farmers must choose exactly the right time to take them to the slaughterhouse—when they've reached a minimum weight, but before they die from anemia. Typical farms lose 15 to 50 percent of their calves to disease.

Many chickens, ducks, and turkeys suffer from retarded

growth, eye damage, blindness, lethargy, kidney damage, disturbed sexual development, bone and muscle weakness, brain damage, paralysis, internal bleeding, anemia, and physical deformities as a result of vitamin deficiencies. Chicken feed contains **artificial color** to make their skin look healthier. After slaughter, carcasses are washed in a **chlorine** solution to kill salmonella bacteria. Chlorine residues may remain when the birds go to market.

Egg-laying hens also get artificial color in their feed—to brighten the pale yolks of their eggs. Some egg producers add chemicals to the feed. The chemicals pass through the digestive tract and into the manure, where they kill fly larvae. Of course, these chemicals probably also end up in the eggs. **Arsenic** frequently is added to feed to speed maturation and stimulate egg production. These speedy hens may produce more eggs in a shorter amount of time, but a barnyard hen lays eggs for fifteen to twenty years, and factory hens last only about a year and a half before they are made into soup and other processed foods.

U.S. Department of Agriculture (USDA) meat and poultry inspection programs were established in 1906, before modern farming methods increased production to more than 10 billion pounds of animal carcasses each year. An inspector is allowed about three seconds to examine each carcass. Random samples of residues from carcasses are taken and sent to a laboratory for analysis. By the time the results are back, the meat is already in the stores. The USDA does not even test for ninety-seven drugs and pesticides likely to leave residues, or twenty-four known or suspected carcinogens. Fully seventeen of the chemicals in meat and poultry are suspected of causing birth defects.

Despite inadequate facilities, however, USDA inspectors do ferret out hazards. Animals are examined before slaughter for obvious signs of disease or abnormality. Each year about 116,000 mammals and nearly 15 million birds are condemned before slaughter. After killing, another 325,000 carcasses are discarded and more than 5.5 million major parts are cut away because they are determined to be diseased. Shockingly, 140,000 tons of poultry is condemned annually, mainly due to cancer. The diseased animals that cannot be sold are processed into . . . animal feed.

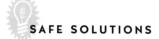

SAFE SOLUTIONS

Considering current growing practices, it's not surprising that diets heavy in meat and animal fats have been associated with higher incidences of heart disease, colon cancer, stroke, and other degenerative diseases.

Many Americans eat much more protein than they actually need. Without ever eating animal products, we can fulfill all our protein needs with amino acids from grains, legumes, nuts, and vegetables.

If you continue to keep meat in your diet, check your natural-food store for fresh or frozen chicken, beef, or lamb from farms that raise their stock organically—the animals have been pasture grazed, and their diets contain no drugs, antibiotics, hormones, or other chemicals to stimulate or regulate growth or tenderness. Also look for game that has been hunted in its natural habitat and "contaminated" only by those chemicals found in the natural environment. A whole variety of uncontaminated wild meats is available by mail.

> *Allergy Resources:* organic buffalo, venison, and other meats
>
> *Czimer Foods:* wild game meats and birds, including pheasant, duck, partridge, quail, wild turkey, Canada goose, squab, venison, buffalo, elk, bear, wild boar, moose, reindeer, antelope, camel, hippopotamus, water buffalo, lion, mountain sheep, wild goat, llama, kangaroo, zebra, giraffe, alligator, rattlesnake, beaver, raccoon, and rabbit. They also have some smoked meats and unusual fish and seafoods.
>
> *Deer Valley Farm:* beef, pork, and poultry products, including non-nitrate-cured sausage, ham, and bacon, processed in their own plant
>
> *Walnut Acres:* raises their own natural beef, chicken, and turkey.
>
> *Whippoorwill Farm:* sells free-range beef, pork, lamb, and veal raised organically on a farm that has been in the same family for more than 100 years.
>
> *Wolfe's Neck Farm:* organically grown beef.

If your only source of meat is the supermarket, you can reduce your exposure to toxic substances by avoiding liver, sweetbreads, and other organ meats, which contain the greatest concentration of toxics. Remove fat before cooking other cuts, as toxics tend to accumulate in the fat rather than in the muscle flesh. Also, ask your butcher for fresh cuts wrapped in butcher paper rather than meats and poultry in heat-sealed plastic packages.

Buy eggs from your natural-food store—they were laid by free-running hens that are not fed antibiotics or stimulants. These growing practices will be stated on the carton. Check your supermarket, too, as many supermarket chains are realizing that uncontaminated eggs sell very well. "Fertile" eggs are often produced with natural methods, but the word *fertile* alone on the carton does not guarantee the eggs are natural; it simply means that the eggs can be hatched into baby chicks. Some people believe that fertile eggs have added health benefits.

MILK AND DAIRY PRODUCTS

Milk can contain residues of any of the chemicals or drugs used in the feed. Nearly all milk sold in the United States today contains pesticide residues because almost all grazing lands still are contaminated with residues of banned pesticides such as **DDT.** Fortunately, the contaminants tend to accumulate in the fat molecules, so the lower the fat content of the milk product, the lower the contamination. Nonfat milk would have very low concentrations; butter would be highly contaminated.

Most milk on the market has been pasteurized, homogenized, and fortified. Pasteurization is simply a heating process that destroys bacteria. Homogenization mixes milk under pressure to reduce fat particles to a uniform size in order to improve taste, color, and the tendency to foam. Neither of these processes adds chemical contaminants, but it is very rare to find pasteurized and homogenized milk that has not been fortified with vitamins A and D, a process that adds **propylene glycol, alcohols,** and **BHT.**

There is evidence, however, that the process of homogenizing milk, wherein a substance called **xanthine oxidase** is released, may contribute to heart disease in humans. When humans consume the milk, xanthine oxidase passes through the intestine into the circulatory system, where it deposits in the artery lining and destroys a substance called plasmalogen. People who have heart attacks or serious arteriosclerosis have a marked decrease in plasmalogen, and the increased incidence of heart attacks in the United States and other countries very closely parallels the increased use of homogenized milk.

A new additive of questionable safety in milk is **bovine growth hormone** (**BGH,** also known as **BST, rbGH,** and **rbST**). It is one of the first products of bioengineering that the FDA has approved to enter our food supply. BGH is a hormone naturally produced by cows. Four companies have learned how to isolate the strand of cow DNA that codes this hormone, insert it into the DNA of bacteria, grow the bacteria in vats, and then extract large quantities of BGH from those vats. Dairy cows that are injected with BGH can produce milk for nearly twice as long after calving.

The FDA doesn't require the treated milk to be labeled, so again, as with pesticides, what labeling there may be indicates the lack of something as a benefit, rather than the presence of something that may cause harm.

SAFE SOLUTIONS

If you drink milk, buy organic; check around for an organic dairy in your area. At my local supermarket, we have our choice of two brands of organic milk—one shipped in from Arizona packaged in paper cartons, and the other from California in a plastic bottle. The one they don't carry is the one in glass bottles produced right here in our own county(!)—the best choice for their customers, but they don't want to deal with the glass bottles. To buy this requires a trip to the natural food store.

Your natural-food store may have some local milk without BGH.

If possible, buy milk in glass bottles. Some local dairies will deliver milk in glass right to your door. Milk in paper cartons would be a second choice. Avoid milk in plastic containers, because it can absorb plastic, which then goes straight into your body when you drink. Also, paper cartons contain traces of toxic **dioxins,** which have been known to migrate into milk samples.

Some people like to drink "raw" milk. It has its advantages, mainly that it has not been processed in any way and therefore contains no additives. Health-food advocates say that raw milk is more healthful because the pasteurization process destroys vitamins and enzymes. However, the safety of this milk is a controversial subject, because raw milk has been linked with a number of cases of salmonella poisoning. Also, according to an article in the *Journal of the American Medical Association,* pasteurization affects only three vitamins, for which milk is a minor source: thiamine, B_{12}, and C, and none of these losses exceeds 10 percent.

I prefer raw milk because it is closer to the milk that actually comes out of the cow. If you are more concerned about salmonella than about the lost nutrients, you could boil the raw milk yourself—you would have a much purer product than standard pasteurized/homogenized/fortified milk.

You also could try soy milk, which you can make yourself from organic soybeans, or buy at your natural-food store.

There are some cheeses made with organic milk. Again, your natural-food store should carry them, or try an upscale food store or specialty cheese shop. We have nearby what you might call a "gourmet supermarket," which stocks at least 200 varieties of cheese, including some raw-milk and organic-milk cheeses made by small producers, which the natural-food stores (who tend to buy everything from natural-foods industry distributors) don't carry. If you can't otherwise find organic cheese, order by mail.

Dutch Mill Cheese Shop sells Amish cheese made with milk from traditional Amish farms, clotted with a vegetable enzyme and colored with vegetable color.

Shelburne Farms makes their own farmhouse cheddar from fresh milk produced by their herd of Brown Swiss cows. Descended from stock raised for cheesemaking in the Swiss mountain villages, these cows are noted for their high-protein, moderate-fat milk. The cheese is made in small batches by hand and ripened at cool temperatures.

If you can't get organic cheese, choose fresh, natural low-fat or nonfat cheeses, as pesticide residues tend to concentrate in the fat. Avoid processed cheese, flavored specialty cheese, and cheeses in aerosol cans. Choose fresh, natural cheese instead. Raw-milk cheeses usually do not contain any additives.

FATS AND OILS

The primary safety concern regarding fats and oils is **pesticide residue.** Pesticides are stored in the oils of plants and the fat of animals, and separating the oils concentrates the pesticides (and in the case of animal fats, residues of **antibiotics, hormones, tranquilizers,** and other **chemicals** used in milk production), making them more potent. A cup of corn oil, for example, would have more concentrated pesticides than a cup of whole corn. Most common oils found in supermarkets, which are virtually indistinguishable from one another, have been extracted using **hexane,** a petrochemical solvent, then bleached, filtered, and deodorized—each step leaving yet another residue of chemicals.

But there are also other health concerns associated with fats and oils, depending on their type. Reacting to studies linking fat intake to obesity, heart disease, and cancer, Americans seem to be on a frenzy of living "fat-free," even to the point of developing artificial fat substitutes.

The idea that we should consume no fat at all is far from a healthy one. Our bodies need some fat for nutrient absorption, for proper cell function, to create body heat, and for the general health of our whole body organism. The problem is that in our standard diet of processed foods, we eat way too much of the wrong fats. We need to *lower* our fat intake, not eliminate it entirely. So let's straighten out which fats to use in moderation, and which to minimize or avoid.

First off, I'm skeptical about the safety of the new fat substitutes. As I write this, Olestra (developed by Procter & Gamble) has been approved by the FDA, but is not yet on store shelves. Olestra, which will be marketed under the name Olean, is made from eight fatty acids attached to one molecule of sucrose; natural fats are made from three fatty acids attached to one molecule of glycerol. Inside your small intestine, enzymes attack the molecules of fat, breaking them down into smaller molecules which then can be absorbed by the intestine. Because the masses of fatty acids that create Olestra are so big, the enzymes cannot break them down, and they pass right through the intestine.

Though the FDA endorsed Olestra's safety after an eight-year investigation, the approval came with a caveat to customers:

Olestra may cause abdominal cramping and loose stools in some individuals, and it inhibits the body's absorption of certain fat-soluble vitamins and nutrients. The FDA has asked Procter & Gamble to monitor consumers for adverse health reactions.

Then there is the debate about saturated and unsaturated fats. Saturated fats, found in butter, eggs, fish, chicken, and meats, are high in cholesterol; unsaturated fats, such as sunflower, sesame, corn, and olive, are low in cholesterol. Most of us need a certain amount of both kinds of fat in our diet to be healthy. More than 8 percent of our brain's solid matter is made of cholesterol. Our hormones, skin, and even the membranes of our cells use cholesterol as an essential building block in their basic production and structure.

It is widely accepted that saturated fats may encourage heart disease, whereas unsaturated fats may discourage and perhaps even reverse it. On the other hand, other research shows a possible link between *processed* polyunsaturated vegetable fats and cancer. A high overall total fat intake seems to be linked to cardiovascular disease and breast and colon cancer.

So the question seems to be not saturated or unsaturated, but how refined or processed the fat or oil is.

Margarine is a processed polyunsaturated vegetable fat, sold as a "healthier" alternative to butter. It is hydrogenated oil, which means that hydrogen gas is bubbled through a tank of liquid polyunsaturated oil in the presence of nickel. The process turns cheap polyunsaturated fats such as corn or safflower oil into saturated fats. So when you think you are getting a polyunsaturated fat in your margarine, you are actually getting the very saturated fats the margarine sellers claim they are helping you avoid.

I strongly suspect that diseases associated with fats are caused more by the concentration of pesticide residues in the fats and oils rather than by the fats and oils themselves. In the high-fat diets of traditional peoples, the incidence of cancer appears to be small—the greater cancer risk is found in populations with industrialized, processed diets.

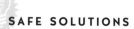

SAFE SOLUTIONS

The better fats and oils for human consumption are those which are closest to their natural state, least processed, and organically grown to be free from pesticides.

In my kitchen, we use primarily butter made from local organic milk, and organically grown olive oil. There are many varieties of oil to choose from in natural-food stores and gourmet-food shops.

Purchase *unrefined* "pressed" or "expeller pressed" oils, squeezed from organically grown vegetables, nuts, and seeds by a mechanical process that does not use chemicals. These oils retain colors, flavors, and aromas from the original sources, so take care to use an oil compatible with whatever food it is being used to prepare.

Pressed olive oils are designated as "extra virgin" (from the first pressing) or "virgin" (from the next pressing). So-called "pure" olive oil, however, has been solvent extracted from either the pit or the remaining fruit pulp.

Beware of labels that say "cold-pressed." This has become meaningless health-food-store jargon. Often cold-pressed oils are solvent extracted, and should be avoided unless the label clearly states that the oil has been pressed at a temperature less than 100°F.

If you prefer a refined oil, choose one that does not contain preservatives.

FISH AND SEAFOOD

 Fish and seafood commonly contain high levels of the **water pollution contaminants** present in the area from which they are taken. Fish can concentrate pollutants to levels up to 2,000 times more than the surrounding waters. Two water pollutants of grave concern found in fish and seafood are toxic **mercury** and carcinogenic **PCBs. Radioactive materials** also are found in fish and seafood harvested near marine dump sites.

Once the seafood is harvested, **chemical preservatives**

may be added to keep it fresh. **Sulfites** are sometimes used on clams, lobster, crab, scallops, and shrimp. **Sodium benzoate, polytrisorbate,** and **polyphosphates** also may be used.

SAFE SOLUTIONS

Select species of fish that spend most of their lives in deep water, far out at sea and away from the human population: herring, sardines, anchovies, small salmon (pink, coho, sockeye, and Atlantic), scrod, hake, haddock, pollock, mackerel, pompano, redtail and yellowtail snapper, striped bass, butterfish, squid, and octopus. Tuna, bluefish, swordfish, and king salmon are best when taken from nonindustrialized coastal waters. Avoid coastal and freshwater fish, which are more likely to have encountered polluted waters.

Shellfish is a little more difficult to buy. All the commonly eaten shellfish live in coastal waters, and since a great deal of water passes through their systems during their normal bodily functions, they are natural collectors of high levels of contaminants. It's best to eat these infrequently.

If you like to eat fish as a regular part of your diet, find a local fresh-fish market where you can become acquainted with the manager and find out the source of the fish you buy and if it has been treated with chemicals.

SWEETENERS

> **WARNING:** Use of this product may be hazardous to your health. Contains saccharin, which has been determined to cause cancer in laboratory animals.

Let's face it. We all know sweet things aren't good for us, but we're going to eat them anyway. Right? So all we have to do is choose the sweet that is least harmful and eat it in moderation.

To begin with, let's discuss the most dangerous sweets: artificial sweeteners.

Used as an artificial sweetener since 1879, **saccharin** was accepted as safe until the 1960s, when tests showed that it caused bladder cancer in laboratory rats. In 1972 it was removed from the GRAS list, and in 1977 the FDA announced it would be banned from food and beverages. After intense lobbying by saccharin manufacturers and users, saccharin still is allowed to be sold, though it must carry a warning label. Currently it is on the FDA list to be tested for mutagenic and reproductive effects. Check labels carefully, particularly on diet foods.

Aspartame (NutraSweet, Equal) is the new favorite; it's a "natural" sweetener made of phenylalanine and aspartic acid, containing "nothing artificial." In the body, these naturally occurring substances break down into the same amino acids found in any protein food. Sounds harmless, but it isn't.

The problem with aspartame lies in overconsumption and the fact that phenylalanine alone (without its companion amino acids) is not a normal part of the diet. Large doses of phenylalanine are toxic to the brain and can cause mental retardation and seizures in people with phenylketonuria (PKU), a genetic disorder. For others, the sweetener may cause chemical changes in the brain that could contribute to headaches, depression, mood swings, high blood pressure, insomnia, and behavior problems. In addition, it could cause your appetite-control center to malfunction, so your diet drinks could be causing more harm than good. Aspartame may also cause birth defects and is not recommended for use by pregnant women.

Because aspartame is found in so many products, it is very easy to overdose without realizing it. A child meets the FDA maximum safety limit by drinking only 5 cans of diet soda per day; a 150-pound adult would exceed the limit by drinking 16 cans. This sounds ridiculous (how many people drink 16 cans of diet soda each day?), but when you take a vitamin pill with aspartame, eat your breakfast cereal and hot cocoa with aspartame, have some aspartame-sweetened gelatin and a soft drink for lunch, chocolate pudding with aspartame for dinner dessert, and maybe another soda, it adds up very quickly. Children could easily consume twice the FDA limit every day and possibly develop learning impairments and behavior problems. Part of the problem with the current labeling for aspartame is that the actual amounts used do not have to be listed, so you really have no idea how much aspartame you are consuming.

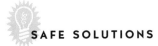

SAFE SOLUTIONS

So when the sweet tooth strikes, what do you do?

SUGAR

Teaspoon for teaspoon, eating white sugar (sucrose) *in moderation* as part of a diet that is based on fresh whole foods probably is safer than using any artificial sweetener. Moderation is the key word here, for a high-sucrose diet can contribute to significant nutritional deficiencies, lower resistance to disease, tooth decay, diabetes, hypoglycemia, heart disease, ulcers, and high blood pressure. It also can stimulate your appetite and make you fat. Steer away from processed foods with high amounts of hidden sucrose (it has many names, including sugar, corn sugar, corn syrup, dextrose, and glucose syrup). Buy unsweetened products such as breakfast cereal, and add sugar with discretion. Here's where reading labels can really pay off.

As a food, refined white sugar is highly contaminated, having been sprayed with multiple pesticides, processed over a natural gas flame, and chemically bleached (an exception is **Sucanat,** evaporated sugar-cane juice that can be substituted cup for cup for sugar). With this in mind, and considering the health effects of sugar, you may want to choose one of the sweeteners offered at your natural-food store that are less contaminated and owe their sweetness to sugars other than sucrose.

HONEY

When one thinks of a "healthy" sweetener, the first one that comes to mind, of course, is honey. It is composed of glucose and fructose and is generally the least chemically contaminated sweetener because bees don't come back to the hive if they've been exposed to pesticides.

Legally, for a bottle to be labeled "Honey," it must contain "the nectar and floral exudations of plants gathered and stored in the comb of honeybees." Honey is always honey, regardless of how it is labeled. "U.S. Grade A" or "Fancy" refers to the level of filtration and does not give any indication of quality or freedom from chemical contamination.

The best processing is the least processing; avoid honey that has been subjected to heat or chemicals or that comes from bee-hives that are sprayed with antibiotics or other chemicals. Since some honey is diluted with corn syrup, choose a brand whose label states that it is undiluted.

There are many different types of honey. The lighter-colored honeys usually are more delicate, while darker-colored honeys have a very strong, distinct flavor. For sweetness without too much flavor, try clover, star thistle, mountain wildflower, or orange blossom honey. Iron bark tree honey tastes like butter-scotch. Tupelo is best for baking. Other types of honey include alfalfa, black-eyed bean, buckwheat, cabbage, conifer, grapefruit, Hawaiian wild lava plum, hawthorne, heather, lime, lemon blos-som, manzanita, mesquite, rosemary, safflower, and thyme. Your natural-food store will have a good selection.

Honey is 40 percent sweeter than sugar, so replace each cup of sugar with one-half to three-fourths of a cup of honey and re-duce the liquid in the recipe by one-fourth cup for each three-fourths of a cup of honey used.

One problem you may encounter is that the flavor of the honey sometimes comes through in the finished product even when a light honey is used. By using less honey than is called for in the recipe, you will get the sweetness without as much of a honey taste.

A new product called Honey Sweet (order by mail from **Home Health**) is 100 percent natural honey in a powdered form. It dissolves instantly in hot or cold beverages and can be substituted one-to-one for sugar in baking.

FRUIT SWEETENER

Fructose (fruit sugar) is a popular sweetener now used in many "natural" products as a sugar replacement. It is the sweetest sugar, so you get more sweetness per calorie and you can use less. The problem with fructose is that as a commercial product, it is about as close to the natural sugar found in fruits as white sugar is to the sugar cane. Like aspartame, it is an isolated form of a chemical component usually found in combination with other components that help our bodies assimilate it. Another problem with fructose is that often it is made from corn syrup and can con-tain up to 55 percent sucrose, so if you're trying to avoid the lat-ter, fructose won't help much.

Real fruit sugar is available in the form of a thick syrup, made from a blend of fruits that are concentrated by removing water, natural fruit acids, and strong flavors. It can be used as a syrup like honey, or substituted cup-for-cup for sugar (reduce liquid in recipe by one-third).

MAPLE SYRUP

Maple syrup, another natural sweetener, is nothing more than boiled-down maple-tree sap—real maple syrup, that is, not the artificially flavored corn syrup called "pancake syrup." It's not hard to find. If your supermarket doesn't carry it, your natural-food store will.

Maple trees are grown without fertilizers or pesticide sprays, but in America, the law permits injection of the trees with formaldehyde pellets to increase the flow of sap and does not require this to be stated on the label. The Canadian Food and Drug Directorate, on the other hand, does not allow this practice.

Government regulations stipulate that all maple syrup be maple-sap syrup, free from foreign material, and weigh no less than eleven pounds per gallon. The syrup is then graded by color according to U.S. color standards; the lighter the syrup, the higher the quality and the more delicate the flavor. Grade Fancy—Light Amber is the highest quality, the first syrup made each season. Grade A—Medium Amber is produced in greatest quantity, with a medium maple flavor. Grade B—Dark Amber has the strongest maple flavor, which really comes through in recipes.

Maple syrup is a sucrose sweetener, however, and has all the same health risks as white sugar, so you may want to limit your intake to a trickle over your Sunday waffle rather than use it as an all-purpose sweetener.

DATE SUGAR AND FIG SYRUP

Two wonderful, delicious, and easy-to-use sweeteners are date sugar and fig syrup. Because they are made from real foods, they are among the few sweeteners that have some nutritive value. Date sugar is made by dehydrating dates and grinding them up into a rather coarse, granulated-type sugar. Fig syrup is made simply by boiling figs in water. Although date sugar will not dissolve very well in your cup of coffee, it works very well, substituted cup-for-cup, in any baked-goods recipe that calls for brown sugar. Substitute fig syrup cup-for-cup in recipes that call for molasses. Here's a recipe in which you can try them both.

Gingerbread Cookies

¼	cup butter	¼	teaspoon ground cloves
½	cup date sugar	½	teaspoon ground cinnamon
½	cup fig syrup	2	teaspoons powdered ginger
3½	cups whole wheat flour	¼–⅓	cup water
1	teaspoon baking soda		

1. Blend together butter, date sugar, and fig syrup.
2. Sift together flour, baking soda, and spices.
3. Combine butter and flour mixtures together alternately with water. You probably will have to use your hands to mix near the end. For softer cookies, add more water.
4. Roll out dough to about ¼ inch and cut out shapes. Cookies can be decorated with bits of dried fruits.
5. Bake at 350°F for 8 to 10 minutes, or until lightly browned.

BARLEY MALT AND RICE SYRUP

You will find these natural sweeteners at your natural-food store, but they are more difficult to use and almost impossible to substitute in regular recipes.

Barley malt, composed mainly of maltose, is made by soaking and sprouting barley to make malt, then combining it with more barley and cooking this mixture until the starch is converted to sugar. The mash is then strained and cooked down to syrup or dried into powder.

Barley malt syrup is only about 40 percent as sweet as sucrose, so you would need to substitute about two cups of syrup for one cup of sugar. This can really throw off the moisture balance in a recipe. On the other hand, barley malt powder is 2,000 percent sweeter than sucrose, so it can be very difficult to measure.

Rice syrup, also a natural sweetener composed mainly of

maltose, is made by combining barley malt with rice and cooking it until all the starch is converted to sugar. The mash is then strained and cooked down to a syrup that is only 20 percent as sweet as sugar.

Barley malt and rice syrup are best used for a bit of sweetness on toast, whole grains, or in tea, or to sweeten salad dressings, rather than as a substitute for sugar in baking.

And remember, just because these sweeteners are natural or organically grown doesn't mean they are foods. Use them sparingly.

FOOD POISONING

Not all harmful contaminants in food are chemical or added by human beings. Nature has its own toxins that occasionally show up, too.

Salmonella, Clostridium perfringens, Staphylococcus, and *Clostridium botulinum* are bacterial organisms that multiply by dividing. They can contaminate all types of foods, causing stomach upset, abdominal pains, diarrhea, vomiting, headaches, and, in extreme cases, death.

Salmonella is one of the more common causes of food poisoning. Fortunately it is not often fatal—more than 2 million cases of *Salmonella* poisoning are believed to occur in the United States each year. *Salmonella* is commonly found in raw meats, poultry, eggs, milk, fish, and products made from these foods. Chocolate, yeast, and spices also have been known to carry these bacteria. Symptoms of *Salmonella* poisoning are fever, headache, diarrhea, abdominal discomfort, and vomiting. These symptoms appear in twenty-four hours, and most people recover in two to four days. Children younger than four, elderly people, and people already weakened by disease could become seriously ill from these bacteria.

Clostridium perfringens is more widely distributed over the earth than any other disease-causing microorganism—in the soil, dust, on food, and in the intestinal tracts of humans and other warm-blooded animals. Large numbers of these bacteria will cause diarrhea and abdominal pain about twelve hours after the contaminated food is ingested.

Staphylococcus organisms are in your respiratory passages and on your skin. They usually enter food by way of human contact and can multiply in meats; poultry and egg products; egg, tuna, chicken, potato, or macaroni salads; cream-filled pastries; and sandwich fillings. If staph germs are allowed to multiply to high levels, they form a toxin that cannot be boiled or baked away. Symptoms of poisoning include diarrhea, vomiting, and abdominal cramps that occur one to seven hours after eating, and subside within twenty-four to forty-eight hours.

Clostridium botulinum poisoning is rare—fortunately, for it is often fatal. Spores are found throughout the environment and are harmless until they divide in the proper environment and produce a poisonous toxin. Symptoms begin twelve to thirty-six hours after eating and include double vision, inability to swallow, speech difficulty, and progressive paralysis of the respiratory system. If botulism is suspected, call a doctor immediately—medical help must be obtained at once.

Another kind of poisoning comes from aflatoxin, the product of two common molds, *Aspergillus flavus* and *Aspergillus parasiticus*. Aflatoxin has been detected in corn, wheat, barley, rice, figs, grain sorghum, cottonseed, certain tree nuts (such as Brazil nuts), and peanuts, and is known to cause hepatitis and liver cancer in humans.

SAFE SOLUTIONS

These bacteria can enter food in any stage of growing and processing. In some cases, food you buy may already be contaminated, but you are the one who is responsible for safe handling practices from the supermarket or natural-food store to the dinner table.

Don't buy any foods in packages or cans that are outdated, broken, bent, or leaky. Especially avoid bulging cans, as these could contain *Clostridium botulinum*. Make sure meat, poultry, and frozen foods are kept cold. Buy them last, so they don't warm up or defrost in your cart while shopping. Make the grocery store your last stop while shopping so you can go right home with perishables. Put meat and poultry in the refrigerator at 40°F or the freezer at 0°F immediately when you get home. Also put frozen foods in the freezer right away. Refrigerating or freezing foods prevents any existing bacteria from multiplying.

Thaw frozen foods in the refrigerator before cooking, or cook them while still frozen. To thaw foods quickly, use a watertight plastic bag submerged in cold water. Never thaw frozen food uncovered on a kitchen counter at room temperature. There are bacteria everywhere that could quickly multiply.

When preparing foods, take care that cross-contamination does not occur. After cutting up raw meat, poultry, or fish, wash your hands, knife, and cutting board thoroughly with hot water and soap before preparing other foods with the same equipment. Better yet, keep a separate cutting board for meat and poultry. I have a large wooden cutting board I use for vegetables, and a smaller one for meat and poultry, which I can submerge in a sinkful of hot soapy water. Bacteria from the meat, poultry, or fish can be transferred easily to other foods and then multiply later, when conditions are favorable.

If you have cuts or sores on your hands, use rubber gloves when preparing foods to keep both the bacteria from the food out of your sores, and the bacteria from your sores out of the food.

Because bacteria can grow rapidly at room temperature, don't keep cooked dishes at room temperature for more than two hours before serving, and refrigerate leftovers as soon as the meal is over.

Pets also are carriers of bacteria. After handling pets, wash your hands before preparing food. Keep pet-feeding dishes, toys, and bedding out of the kitchen. Don't let pets touch food, utensils, or work surfaces where food is prepared.

Most bacteria are destroyed by heat, so always use a meat thermometer and cook food thoroughly. Also, heat leftovers completely before serving; don't just "warm them up."

The most common cause of botulism poisoning is home canning. Be sure to follow proper procedures for sterilizing and sealing jars, and to cook the food thoroughly. Botulism also can develop in foods that are slightly warm and stored in an oxygen-free environment. This condition sounds almost impossible, but such situations may happen frequently—for instance, consider a leftover baked potato or sauteed vegetables wrapped in foil and kept at room temperature overnight.

There is little we can do to protect ourselves from aflatoxin, since it can be present and invisible in foods when they are purchased. If nuts are a part of your diet, store them in a cool, dry place, and take care not to eat any that are discolored or moldy. Otherwise, all you really can do is avoid those foods most likely to contain aflatoxin.

FOOD IRRADIATION

 When I wrote about irradiated food in *The Nontoxic Home* in 1986, it was not yet on supermarket shelves. Irradiated foods themselves still aren't, to my knowledge; however, they may be hidden as ingredients in processed foods.

The FDA proclaims that irradiation of foods is safe, and has already authorized the irradiation of fruits, vegetables, pork, herbs, spices, teas, and seeds. The Department of Energy and the Pentagon, however, have refused to release their research into the long-term effects. Some researchers suspect that a regular diet of irradiated food may cause leukemia, other forms of cancer, and kidney disease. At this point, I don't think we really know the health effects. As with some other products that initially appeared to be safe, such as cigarettes, pesticides, asbestos, and CFCs, I believe we may not learn the dangers of irradiated foods until they become widely used.

Food is irradiated by zapping it with a dosage of radiation almost 60 million times that of a chest X ray. Gamma rays (radioactive by-products of the nuclear industry) or X rays are used to kill insects and bacteria, prevent sprouting, and slow rotting. While the process does not make the food itself radioactive, the chemical structure of the food is altered, and there are a number of animal studies that show negative health effects.

The facilities where irradiation takes place also pose health and environmental risks to workers and the general population.

Besides potential problems with transportation of radioactive materials, there already have been in existing plants several radiation leaks and contaminations, as well as numerous safety violations.

And, like other harmful food practices, irradiation may not even be effective. Researchers reported in the British medical journal *Lancet* that "irradiation confers no advantage over heat processing in respect of bacterial toxins." Another study in *New Scientist* examined irradiated coconuts and found that while the process killed fungi that affect the taste of the coconut, other bacteria had flourished, including a variety that can cause food poisoning.

So far, spices are the mostly widely irradiated food in the United States. The FDA requires whole foods that have been irradiated to display on the label an international logo of a flower in a circle and the words "treated by [or "with"] irradiation." However, when irradiated food is used as an ingredient in processed foods or in spices, the fact that it has been irradiated does not have to be indicated on the label.

SAFE SOLUTIONS

The only advice I can give you is to watch for the irradiated logo on food products. I have never actually seen one on a food product, but by law they should appear on whole foods that have been irradiated.

Because irradiated ingredients in processed foods need not be mentioned on a label, we can assume that some irradiated ingredients may be present in processed foods without our knowledge—another reason to eat fresh whole foods we prepare ourselves at home.

COOKWARE

Copper and **aluminum** cookware should not be used if the cooking surface that comes in contact with the food is made from either of these metals. Foods cooked in aluminum can react with the metal to form aluminum salts. Little research has been done on the amount of exposure we may receive from food cooked in aluminum cookware or its health effects, but aluminum salts from other sources of exposure have been connected with brain disorders such as dementia, Alzheimer's disease, behavior abnormalities, poor memory, and impaired motor-visual coordination. One British study showed that foods cooked in aluminum cookware may cause indigestion, heartburn, intestinal gas, constipation, and headaches. And a study in Sri Lanka showed that the amount of aluminum that leaches into food increases 1,000 times when fluoridated water is used for cooking.

In the past, the connection between exposure to aluminum and Alzheimer's disease has been controversial; however, recent research has strengthened the connection. In an interview in the Rodale Press publication *Men's Health*, Theodore Kruck, Ph.D., a member of a leading team of aluminum-investigating scientists at the University of Toronto, said, "we have progressed to the point where we now have a smoking gun [aluminum] lying beside a dead body [the Alzheimer's victim]. Although we still can't prove *conclusively* that the bullet came from that gun, we now believe there is *very strong* circumstantial evidence that aluminum *is* the murder weapon." Dr. Kruck and his colleagues recommend limiting your intake of aluminum to less than 10 milligrams per day, including not using aluminum cookware for acidic foods such as tomatoes, vinegar, and applesauce. Dr. Kruck no longer uses aluminum foil even under meats when cooking or for wrapping foods for the freezer.

Stainless-steel cookware also may be harmful. It seems that if stainless-steel cookware is scoured only once with an abrasive powder or steel wool, small amounts of highly toxic metals such as **chromium** and **nickel** may leach into every food cooked in it thereafter. But if stainless-steel cookware always is soaked clean and no abrasives are used, it should be harmless.

Pots and pans with "no-stick" finishes, such as **Teflon** or **Silverstone,** should not be used, period. They can scratch easily and contaminate foods with bits of plastic during cooking.

SAFE SOLUTIONS

So what's left? Glass, cast iron, porcelain enamel–coated cast iron or stainless steel, or terra-cotta clay (check to make sure the glaze doesn't contain lead, particularly if the item is imported). Cookware made from all these materials is available at most department stores and kitchen shops. The *Williams-Sonoma* catalog carries a variety of clay pieces.

Anodized aluminum is another possible choice. Aluminum is

a favored metal for cookware because it distributes heat evenly. Though there are health problems associated with aluminum cookware, if a label says the cookware is made from "anodized" aluminum, it is safe to use. This means that the aluminum was dipped into a hot acid bath that seals the aluminum by changing its molecular structure. Once anodized, the aluminum will not leach into food.

For a no-stick finish, season cast-iron cookware before using by covering the bottom of the pan with cooking oil and placing the pan on a warm burner or in a warm oven for one hour. Wipe out excess oil, leaving a thin film of oil in the pan. Each time you use it, the pan will become more seasoned, if you don't allow the food to stick. Maintain the seasoning by wiping the pan with a clean towel after cooking or rubbing the bottom of the pan with coarse salt.

For an instant no-stick finish, heat the pan first, then add the oil, then add the food to the hot oil. If you're on a diet, spread a film of liquid lecithin over the cooking surface before using it. Lecithin is the active ingredient in no-stick aerosol cooking sprays and can be purchased at your natural-food store.

Line baking pans with parchment paper (available at most cookware stores) for no-stick baking and easy cleanup.

DISHWARE

The hidden danger in dishware is the **lead** used in glazes. And it's not just brightly colored dishware from other countries that is a problem—most major manufacturers of dinnerware sold in department stores and home-decorating shops still use lead glazes, without labeling them as such. The federal government prohibits the sale of dinnerware that releases lead in amounts greater than 2,000 ppb (which prevents direct cases of lead poisoning), but the state of California requires warning labels on any dishware that releases lead in amounts greater than 224 ppb, to protect against long-term health risks.

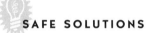

SAFE SOLUTIONS

Before you buy dishware, ask the salesperson and verify with the manufacturer whether or not a lead-free glaze was used on the particular style you are interested in. Often local potters use lead-free glazes, and with them you have the advantage of being able to ask the person who made the dish what kind of glaze was used.

You could also purchase clear glass dishware, which has no glaze at all. Or you might want to consider wood. ***Karen's Nontoxic Products*** has solid wood bowls, plates, and utensils.

If you have dishware that you suspect may have a lead finish, you can test it using **Lead Check Swabs,** available by mail from ***Air Check, Allergy Resources, Lead Check,*** and ***Nontoxic Environments.***

FOOD STORAGE

The main problem with food storage is **plastic,** which may migrate into the food being stored.

SAFE SOLUTIONS

Use glass jars instead of plastic containers to store food on shelves and in the refrigerator. You can either purchase decorative glass containers at import shops, or simply save glass jars from food products.

Instead of plastic bags, use cotton bags. These are handy for storing grains, potatoes, onions, produce, and bread. Inexpensive cotton bags are often sold at natural-food stores, or you can order them by mail from ***Clothcrafters*** or ***Real Goods.***

A disposable alternative to plastic bags is cellophane bags. Some natural-food stores carry them. If yours doesn't, order from ***Janice Corporation, Karen's Nontoxic Products,*** or ***The Living Source.***

MICROWAVE OVENS

The safety or danger of exposure to **microwaves** from microwave ovens has not yet been established one way or the other. There is some concern because even microwave ovens that are functioning perfectly emit microwaves. FDA safety standard limits allow microwave emissions of up to one milliwatt per square centimeter ($1mW/cm^2$) when the oven is purchased, and up to $5mW/cm^2$ after the oven has been in use.

Animal studies done by Bell Telephone Laboratories convinced this company to establish tighter safety regulations than those required by the U.S. government. They recommend only "incidental exposure" from one to ten milliwatts, and that daily exposure should not exceed one milliwatt. Russian safety regulations prohibit exposure at one milliwatt for more than one minute, and then only with goggles to protect the eyes. Clearly, these regulations apply to microwave exposure well within the range that might be encountered while using a microwave oven.

Workers who are subjected to exposure to microwaves on the job complain of headaches, fatigue, irritability, sleep disturbances, weakness, increased incidence of viral infections, low heart rates, changed EEGs, and increased thyroid functions. There is also some concern that microwaves may cause birth defects and possibly cancer.

The Food Safety and Inspection Service (FSIS) of the USDA warns against using foam trays and plastic wraps when heating or thawing the food in microwaves. Also, you should avoid using such cold-storage containers as margarine tubs, whipped-topping bowls, and cottage cheese cartons. These containers "are not heat stable at high temperatures. They can melt or warp from the food's heat, possibly causing chemicals to migrate into the food," says the FSIS flyer "A Microwave Handbook."

SAFE SOLUTIONS

How about going back to cooking the old way, in the oven and on top of the stove?

If you have a microwave oven and you really love the convenience of it, you may not have to give it up. *Consumer Reports* magazine suggests that you can minimize your risk by keeping a reasonable distance from the oven while it is in operation (the farther, the better), and try to operate and maintain the oven in such a way that will minimize leakage. Make sure the oven door closes properly and that no damage occurs to the hinges, latches, sealing surfaces, or the door itself. Make sure that no soil or food residue accumulates around the door seal, and avoid placing any objects between the sealing surfaces. You could also test the oven for leakage. And when you're cooking, heat-resistant glass is safest.

BARBECUED AND BROILED FOODS

Most barbecued and broiled foods contain **benzo(a)pyrene,** a proven cancer-causing substance.

The cooking temperature, type of fuel used, and the fat content of the meat all affect the amount of benzo(a)pyrene that is formed. Cooking methods that create the most benzo(a)pyrene are charcoal grilling and gas grilling, when the gas flame is *below* the meat. Grilling meats closer to the coals produces more of the carcinogen than grilling farther from the heat source. Benzo(a)pyrene seems to form most rapidly when a fatty meat is cooked over gas or charcoal close to the heat source for a long period of time.

SAFE SOLUTIONS

For some unexplained reason, broiling with a gas flame or electric coil *above* the meat produces *no* benzo(a)pyrene. So slather on the barbecue sauce and stick your meats under the broiler!

One of my favorite foods is good barbecued *anything,* and broiling just isn't the same. Besides, humans have been cooking over fire for millennia, so I don't think a few barbecued steaks are a major cause of cancer. University of Hawaii researchers have found you can reduce the danger of carcinogens in grilled meat by eating lots of green vegetables—the chlorophyll in vegetables binds with the carcinogens during digestion, limiting their absorption. My personal solution: we have a barbecue every couple of weeks in the summer months and include a big green salad.

ALCOHOLIC BEVERAGES

> **WARNING:** According to the Surgeon General, women should not drink alcoholic beverages during pregnancy because of the risk of birth defects.
>
> **WARNING:** Consumption of alcoholic beverages impairs your ability to drive a car or operate machinery and may cause health problems.

Alcoholic beverages are regulated by the Bureau of Alcohol, Tobacco, and Firearms (BATF), not the FDA. Although the Food, Drug, and Cosmetic Act of 1938 does not exempt alcoholic beverages, no agency is enforcing this law, and ingredients are not listed on labels.

One or two drinks a day may not be harmful and, indeed, may be beneficial, but once this limit is passed, problems begin. Alcoholism can cause heart disease, hepatitis, cirrhosis of the liver, decreased resistance to disease, shortened life span, nutrient deficiencies, cancer, fetal alcohol syndrome, brain damage, stroke, phlebitis, varicose veins, and a reduced testosterone level in males that can cause sexual impotence, loss of libido, breast enlargement, and loss of facial hair.

Unfortunately, the harmful effects of alcohol do not stop with the body of the drinker. Alcohol is responsible for many needless deaths caused by drunk drivers and is a factor in more than half of all the homicides, rapes, and sexually aggressive acts in this nation. Many alcoholics also die from falling, inability to escape during a fire, drowning, and suicide.

A nonalcoholic danger found in most wines and beers is **sulfites.** Sulfites in wines have caused many unsuspected allergic reactions.

SAFE SOLUTIONS

Since the law does not require ingredients of alcoholic beverages to be listed, look for brands that voluntarily reveal the purity of their ingredients.

BEER

I know of no beers that use organically grown hops or malt, but there are many natural beers. All German beers are protected by a law called the *Reinheitsgebot* ("law of purity"), which makes it a crime to brew beer with ingredients other than hops, malt, and water. In addition, many popular beers, such as Coors, Budweiser, and Pabst, are additive-free, and you might want to look for beers from small local breweries, which generally use the finest of natural ingredients. Brewing beer at home also has become a popular pastime—if you want to try your hand at this, you can order supplies from **Great Fermentations.**

WINE

Many natural-food stores now sell some very nice wines made from organically grown grapes. Some are imported from France, Germany, and Italy (order by mail from **The Organic Wine Company**), quite a few are made in California, and wineries in other states also are going organic.

A few small producers have made organic wines since the early 1980s, and most have been carefully labeling and advertising their special growing practices. Now, larger companies—including Gallo, Fetzer, Sutter Home, and Buena Vista—also are using organic grapes (don't assume, though, that all wines made by these companies are organic). More than sixty California wineries (10 percent of the total) now have vineyards certified by California Certified Organic Farmers, and many others are using organic practices but choose not to be certified for a variety of reasons (many winemakers see just going organic as the responsible thing to do, but are not certified so as to maintain flexibility and the ability to use pesticides occasionally).

One major problem with wines, whether made from organically grown grapes or not, is the presence of sulfites. Sulfite, generally considered a food additive to be avoided, is formed naturally in the process of fermentation. Virtually all wines contain some sulfites; however, some winemakers also add sulfites to inhibit oxidation and spoilage (a practice that has been used for centuries). If a wine contains more than ten parts per million (ppm) sulfite, the statement "Contains sulfites" must appear on the label. Most wines contain 30 to 150 ppm.

By law, in America, a wine can be labeled "organic" only if it is made without the use of added sulfites (other than the sulfites that are formed naturally). Otherwise, a proper label could say "Made with organically grown grapes" so long as "Contains sulfites" also is included. A few wines are completely sulfite-free, but most vintners think sulfites are necessary to make a good wine.

The Organic Grapes into Wine Alliance has its own standards for organic wine, which include being made from certified organic grapes, having low sulfite levels, using no toxic materials in packaging (including no tin-lead capsules), and using recycled glass bottles.

For those who wish to avoid alcoholic beverages entirely, a number of delicious nonalcoholic drinks are available at your natural-food store. Try one of the no-alcohol beers, a varietal grape juice made from wine grapes, or a sparkling apple cider or other fruit juice instead of champagne. Read labels carefully, though, to watch for sulfites. Because juice is a *food,* and not an alcoholic beverage, any sulfite in the product must be listed on the label.

Beware of "dealcoholized" wines. Because they begin as wines and then have their alcohol removed, they still may contain the same sulfites and other additives used in winemaking. The National Council on Alcoholism also warns that "nonalcoholic" or "dealcoholized" on a wine bottle or beer can does not necessarily mean completely free of alcohol. Under federal law, these beverages may contain up to 0.5 percent alcohol, without stating so on the label.

VITAMIN AND MINERAL DIETARY SUPPLEMENTS

The only vitamins and minerals you need to watch out for are the heavily advertised, brightly colored, high-potency multivitamins with clever names. They may contain **BHA, BHT, artificial colors, artificial flavors, mineral oil, sugar, sulfites,** and **talc.** The brightly colored coatings may be made not from food, but from **plastic;** those in gelatin capsules may be preserved with **formaldehyde.**

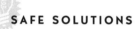

SAFE SOLUTIONS

If you are going to take vitamins, at least take ones that are additive-free. Your natural-food store probably is full of them, so you should have no problem finding them.

Should you take supplements at all? Do you need them? This is a very controversial subject, and the answers range from "No, you get adequate nutrients in your daily diet" (if you eat a variety of fresh, whole, organically grown foods) to "Yes, you need mega-amounts to compensate for poor food choices, the nutrients missing in our modern food supply, our high level of daily stress, and our exposure to environmental chemicals." Your individual need probably falls somewhere between the two. Also, when you are under extra stress or your body defenses are down when you are ill, you may need specific nutrients to help your body come back into balance.

The next question, regardless of why you might want to take nutritional supplements, is: Should you take vitamins and minerals made from natural sources, or synthetic vitamins made from petrochemicals?

Even though many people claim that natural and synthetic supplements are chemically identical, natural supplements do have molecular, biological, and electromagnetic differences that produce greater levels of biological activity and are therefore better utilized by the body than synthetic forms.

In some cases, synthetic vitamins have entirely different chemical structures than their natural counterparts found in food. In his book *The Body Electric,* Robert O. Becker, M.D., states, "All organic compounds . . . are identified by the way they bend light in solution. The dextrorotatory (D) forms rotate it to the right, while levorotatory (L) isomers refract it to the left. All artificial methods of synthesizing organic compounds yield roughly equal mixtures of D and L molecules. However, living things consist of *either* D *or* L forms, depending on the species, but *never both.*"

There are twelve pharmaceutical manufacturers in the world (five in the United States) that make vitamins. Almost all the distributors of the more than three thousand vitamin products you see on the market buy their vitamins from these giant companies, which produce them according to internationally accepted standards. In most cases they all are synthetic and artificial. Most "natural" vitamins on the market today either are fortified (a *very* small amount of low-potency natural vitamins mixed with high-potency synthetic vitamins) or are synthetic vitamins in a *very* small amount of natural base (the label will say something like "in a natural base containing . . .")

The only truly natural vitamins are those that come from foods. They are available in nutritional supplements as highly nutritious, concentrated foods; powdered concentrates of foods and herbs with the moisture removed; and an isolated component of a food. Sources of these include alfalfa- and barley-juice powder, bee pollen, bone meal, brewer's yeast, chlorophyll, wheat-grass juice or powder, cod-liver oil, desiccated liver, kelp, flaxseed oil, lecithin, freshwater algae (blue-green algae, chlorella, spirulina), sea vegetables such as kelp, enzymes, wheat-germ oil, and minerals from ancient sea, clay, or vegetation beds.

Herbs also are becoming an increasingly popular natural way to cleanse, nourish, and strengthen the body to maintain good health. Many people take herbs, either individually or in certain combinations, as nutritional supplements for preventive health care, as herbs often are good sources of minerals, vitamins, and other nutrients. If they are organically grown, biodynamically grown, or wildcrafted, all the better.

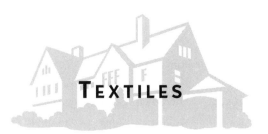

Chapter 9

TEXTILES

THE FABRICS FOUND IN A "chemical closet" are made from **synthetic** fibers—**nylon, polyester,** and **acrylic** are among the more popular. Though these fibers may look like the natural fibers they attempt to imitate, they are actually very soft **thermoplastics** (see chapter 3), made from **petrochemicals.**

Very little research has been done on the possible toxic effects of wearing plastic fibers. Still, these are plastics containing **polyvinyl chloride** and **formaldehyde**-based finishes, and they continuously give off minute plastic vapors as the fiber is warmed against your skin. Many people experience irritating skin reactions. While this certainly isn't life threatening, anyone who has ever spent an entire day itching all over knows how annoying it can be.

Perhaps a more practical reason for not wearing synthetic fibers is that they just aren't very comfortable. None of them absorbs moisture very well, and they can leave you feeling hot, sticky, and clammy during warm weather. They're not much better for winter wear, because they don't hold the heat of your body very well.

Plastic fibers also have maintenance problems. They tend to absorb oil from your skin and hold oily stains that can be removed only with specially developed synthetic detergents. And static cling is a condition unique to synthetic fibers, caused by an electric charge created by the friction of the synthetic fiber against your body. Even more synthetic chemicals are used in fabric softeners and **aerosol** antistatic agents in an attempt to solve this problem.

FORMALDEHYDE FINISHES

Many textile products are treated with **formaldehyde.** Even if not stated on the label, all polyester/cotton-blend fabrics have formaldehyde finishes. Polyester/cotton bedsheets have a particularly heavy finish because of their continuous use and frequent laundering. Formaldehyde is also used on nylon fabrics to make them flameproof, and some pure-cotton fabrics also have been treated with formaldehyde finishes for easy care.

The finishing process combines formaldehyde resin directly with the fiber, making the formaldehyde irremovable. At the end of processing, new textile products often contain free-formaldehyde levels of 800 parts per million (ppm) to 1,000 ppm. Simple washing can lower these levels to 100 ppm, but formaldehyde continues to be released as the resin breaks down during washing, ironing, and wear.

Formaldehyde vapor inhalation can cause tiredness, insomnia, headaches, respiratory problems, coughing, watery eyes, excessive thirst, and many other common symptoms. Exposure also can aggravate asthma attacks. Contact with formaldehyde finishes can result in mild to severe skin rash. Remember, we spend one-third of our lives in bed, with our noses next to the pillowcases and our skin rubbing against the sheets; perhaps the formaldehyde resin might explain mysterious nighttime symptoms.

FLAME RETARDANTS

According to the Consumer Product Safety Commission, thousands are hurt each year in fire accidents caused by playing with matches, smoking while cleaning paintbrushes with combustible solvents, reaching over lighted gas burners, and falling asleep while smoking in bed. The Flammable Fabrics Act, passed in 1953 to protect consumers from injuries and deaths associated with highly flammable fabrics, has been amended over the years, and at this point, standards have been set for general wearing apparel, carpets and rugs, mattresses and mattress pads, and children's sleepwear.

Each category has its own standards for allowed flammability. The standard for general wearing apparel is easy to meet; it does not require testing of individual garments, and bans only extremely flammable items. Children's sleepwear is another matter. Each individual garment design must pass strict performance standards, as even the type of fiber used in the thread can affect the garment's ability to burn.

There are three types of flame resistant fabrics: (1) synthetic fabrics made from fibers for which the flame resistance is inherent in the fiber; (2) synthetic fabrics made from fibers to which flame-retardant chemicals have been added during manufacture; and (3) fabrics to which flame-retardant chemicals are added after the fabric is woven.

Nowadays, most children's sleepwear is made from polyester that is inherently flame resistant. Just out of curiosity, I looked up "polyester" in a textile book I have called *Understanding Textiles,* by Phyllis G. Tortora, to see what its combustibility is in relation to natural fibers. The book states: "Polyester shrinks from flame and will melt, leaving a hard, black residue. The fabric will burn with a strong, pungent odor. Some polyesters are self-extinguishing. Melted polyester fiber can produce severe burns." I am assuming that the polyester fibers used to make children's sleepwear are the self-extinguishing sort.

The use of chemical flame-retardant finishes (such as **TRIS,** which was banned for use in children's sleepwear because of its carcinogenicity) has, in the words of an employee of the Consumer Product Safety Commission, "pretty much gone by the wayside." It's very unlikely that you would encounter a chemical flame-retardant finish on general wearing apparel, either. But it is still used legally in adult sleepwear, hospital gowns, industrial uniforms, wigs, and other textile products we use daily.

DYES

In the past, direct **dyes** used on cotton fabrics contained highly carcinogenic **benzidenes.** One of them, **dichlorobenzidene,** is very easily absorbed through human skin. These are no longer used in the United States, but they may be on fabrics imported from other countries.

Now, you may wonder how the dye is released from the fabric onto the skin. Dyes are sometimes remarkably unstable. Look under the arms of an old shirt you have been wearing for a long time, and see how the color has faded. Have you ever had the experience of wearing a dark-colored shirt under a light-colored sweater, and the dark dye soaks right through the sweater when you perspire? If the dye is released, it can be absorbed by the skin. These direct dyes are the same type used in do-it-yourself dyes, which can be purchased at any supermarket or hardware store.

Other dyes in natural and synthetic fibers also can be harmful, but the primary danger with these is limited to skin irritation.

Labeling

Fortunately, the Textile Fiber Products Identification Act, passed in 1960, requires that all textile products, all yarns, fabrics, household textile articles, and wearing apparel be labeled with the generic names of the fibers from which they are made. The generic names, established by the Federal Trade Commission (FTC), include twenty-one man-made fiber groups, plus the natural fibers. Imported goods also must adhere to this law, and the labels must reveal the country of origin as well. This labeling appears along with the name of the manufacturer, the size of the garment, and cleaning instructions, and is usually attached to the seam of a garment near the waist or hemline.

The act states that

- fibers must be listed in descending order according to percentage by weight (e.g., "80% polyester, 20% cotton");
- trademark names are permitted but must be capitalized if listed ("100% Fortrel polyester");
- if a fiber makes up less than 5 percent of a fabric's total weight, it must be listed as "other fiber" unless it has a specific purpose ("4% spandex added for elasticity");
- fibers of unknown origin (miscellaneous scraps, rags, textile by-products, secondhand materials,

and waste materials) be listed as "undetermined fiber"; and

- fibers making up less than .5 percent of the total weight need not be revealed. Technically, this would allow a manufacturer to make a fabric labeled "100% cotton" that is actually .5 percent polyester, but the National Cotton Council feels that no manufacturer would go to the trouble of making a fabric containing .5 percent polyester because an amount of synthetic fiber that small would not affect the performance of the fabric. So we can safely assume that fabrics labeled 100 percent natural fiber probably are.

Label information seems to apply only to the fibers used in the *body* of the garment or item. Sometimes labels will read, "100% natural fiber, exclusive of decoration," without revealing the fabric of the decoration. Sweaters labeled "100% cotton" often have nylon threads running through the bottom edge and sleeve cuffs to help retain their shape. Cotton chamois shirts sometimes have nylon interfacings behind the buttons. Polyester thread may be used in natural-fiber garments, as well as synthetic zippers, elastic, trims, linings, and interfacings, and plastic buttons and hooks. Many less-expensive cotton undergarments have synthetic elastic and trim.

Also, upholstery stuffing; outer coverings of furniture, mattresses, and box springs; linings, interlinings, stiffenings, or paddings incorporated for structural purposes and not for warmth; sewing and handicraft threads; and bandages and surgical dressings are exempt from the TFPIA.

Often, independent textile organizations sell logos to manufacturers, which give information about the fiber content or performance of the textile products that bear them. The use of these logos is regulated, and products are tested to make sure they live up to their claims.

- The brown-and-white *Seal of Cotton* logo, a trademark of Cotton, Inc., created in 1973, indicates that an item is made from 100 percent domestic cotton. It can be used on fabrics, garments, bed linens, and towels only by permission.

- The *Natural Blend* seal, also a trademark of Cotton, Inc., and in use since 1974, can be used only on fabrics that contain at least 60 percent cotton.

- *Woolmark* is a registered certification owned by the Wool Bureau, Inc., a division of the International Wool Secretariat. Labels are purchased by manufacturers for apparel, knitwear, floor covering, upholstery materials, blankets, and bedspreads. Since 1964, more than fourteen thousand companies in more than fifty-seven countries have been licensed to use it. Items bearing this logo must be of pure wool and be labeled "100% pure wool," "100% virgin wool," "All pure wool," or "All virgin wool."

- The *Woolblend Mark* was introduced in 1972 by the Wool Bureau, Inc. Products displaying this logo must contain at least 60 percent wool and identify all nonwool components by their generic names.

- *Superwash* is a registered certification mark used in conjunction with *Woolmark* and *Woolblend Mark.* This logo indicates that the wool product has been chemically treated to make it felt resistant.

Fabrics treated with formaldehyde resins are not required by law to be labeled as such; however, they will usually be easy to spot. Look for the terms *crease resistant, permanent press, durable pressed, no-iron, shrinkproof, stretchproof, water repellent, water-proof,* or *permanently pleated* on the label. I have noticed that the term *no-iron* is now being used on cotton flannel sheets as well, but don't be concerned about this. I have purchased several sets with this labeling and have found them to be free of finishes. It's true, they are naturally no-iron; cotton flannel doesn't wrinkle because of the weave of the fabric, not because it has been treated.

Manufacturers are not required to label garments as flame resistant, but they may identify their garments or fabrics as flame resistant as a selling point. They *are* required, however, to label flame-resistant fabrics with precautionary instructions regarding treatments that may cause their flame resistance to deteriorate. If you are concerned about a chance encounter with a rare flame-retardant chemical, a good clue would be to look for labels warning against washing the fabric with nonphosphate detergents in hard water, washing the fabric with soap, or using bleach during laundering.

SAFE SOLUTIONS

There are a number of wonderful, natural fibers and stuffing/insulation materials that can be used in place of synthetic fibers. And it is possible to purchase ones without harmful finishes or dyes.

Fibers and stuffing materials that come from natural plant or animal sources are cotton, linen, silk, all the various types of wool, ramie, down, feathers, kapok, and natural-fiber blends: cotton/silk, linen/cotton, and wool/cotton (commonly known as Viyella).

A second choice would be to wear rayon, a man-made fiber that, unlike other synthetic fibers, is composed of cellulose, a substance found in all plants. Cellulose used in making rayon is taken from cotton linters, old cotton rags, paper, and wood pulp. The cellulose is broken down with petrochemicals and then re-formed into thread resembling cotton or silk.

Here's a quick review of natural fibers, their origins, and their processing, to help you choose those that best suit your needs.

COTTON

Cotton is a natural cellulose fiber, taken from fibers that develop around the seed pod of the cotton plant. After it is picked, the pod is placed in a cotton gin, which separates the seed, the lint, and the linters. The lint is then spun into yarn, and the shorter linters are used for cotton batting, in making rayon, and in the production of paper.

Cotton quality is determined by the length of the fiber around the seed pod. Long-staple varieties, such as Sea Island, Egyptian, and Pima, are higher quality.

Two terms that you will find frequently on labels of cotton items are "sanforized" and "mercerized." Sanforized fabrics have been precompressed to the size to which they would shrink after washing by way of a mechanical process that controls shrinkage, involves no chemicals, and is considered harmless. Mercerized fibers have undergone a nontoxic process by which they have been immersed under tension in a strong solution of lye, which is then washed off. This permanently improves the strength, absorbency, and appearance of the fabric, and provides excellent colorfastness.

Most cotton-growing methods, however, present environmental problems. Cotton is the most contaminated of all the natural fibers; seeds are treated with fungicides, and herbicides and pesticides are used repeatedly and heavily worldwide. Whatever pesticide residues might remain in cotton fabrics after processing seem to be harmless, but we must consider also the environmental contamination of our air, land, and water, and the illnesses these pesticides cause to the cotton growers and their families.

The good news is that now there are quite a number of acres of cotton being organically grown without pesticides or chemical defoliants. In 1991, because of the increasing numbers of organic cotton claims, the Texas Department of Agriculture began to certify organically grown cotton, and now has a full-scale program. They certify all phases of production from the growing through the ginning process. Manufacturers of organically grown cotton textiles often use less toxic dyes, and many eliminate the finishing process as well.

The most innovative organic cotton by far is **FoxFibre,** developed by Sally Fox. In 1982, while trying to breed insect resistance into cotton plants, she noticed that occasionally a cotton plant produced green or brown cotton, just as occasionally a flock of white sheep has a few black lambs. So far she has commercialized green and brown cottons, and says that light pinks and blues probably will be possible after years more breeding work. The colors deepen with age rather than fade, as dyed fabrics do. While Sally's breeding nursery is certified organic, unfortunately not all the colored cotton grown on contract is grown using organic methods; pesticides are used, but no defoliants. If the label says **FoxFibre Colorganics,** the fiber has been organically grown.

Another safer cotton is "green cotton." Though not organically grown, it has no dyes, bleaches, or formaldehyde finishes. There has been a rumor going around that bleaching cotton creates toxic dioxins in a similar way to bleaching paper; however, I have been unable to confirm this. I doubt that this is the case, as the dioxins in paper are created by the interaction of chlorine with the lignin in wood, an organic substance that is not present in cotton or other fibers. I have heard also that many bleached cottons are bleached with hydrogen peroxide instead of chlorine, so there is no formation of dioxin.

These unbleached cottons can be trusted to be formaldehyde-free, as these fabrics are diverted from the manufacturing process before dyes or finishes are applied.

LINEN

Linen is made from fibers from the inner bark of the flax plant and is possibly the first fiber used by man. The bark is removed from the plant and left in the field so natural bacterial action can loosen the fibers. The stems are then crushed mechanically, and the fibers removed. At the mill, the fibers are combed to separate the different lengths and align them in preparation for spinning.

Flax has relatively few insect pests, but if they are present, they are controlled with harmful pesticides such as **parathion, dieldrin,** and **heptachlor.**

Linen often is used in its natural beige shade or bleached to make it a lighter color, but it can also be dyed.

RAMIE

Ramie is a stingless nettle indigenous to mainland China. Most ramie is grown in Asia, where the fiber is extracted by hand. The usual procedure is to hand-cut green plants, remove the leaves, then pull ribbons of fiber from the woody stem. If the fiber is to be exported, sometimes it is exposed to sulfur fumes to bleach it to a uniform light-straw color.

Ramie is used as a textile fiber in Asian countries. In America, it is generally blended with cotton for use in knit sweaters.

HEMP

Hemp fibers are taken from the stems of the *Cannabis sativa* plant. Not to be confused with marijuana, this variety of cannabis has practically none of the THC for which marijuana is valued. Even so, it is illegal to grow hemp in this country, so the fabrics are imported from China, Hungary, Chile, Germany, and England. Much more durable than cotton, it can be used to make anything from lace to rope.

SILK

A protein fiber, silk is taken from the cocoon of the silkworm caterpillar. Each cocoon is spun from one continuous silk filament extruded from the caterpillar's body.

Most silk is produced by cultivated silkworms. The cultivation process begins with the laying of eggs by silk moths. After incubation, young silkworms are fed mulberry leaves until they are ready to begin spinning their cocoons. The cocoons are made of silk filaments and a gummy substance that holds them together. After the cocoons are harvested, the gum is softened with warm water, allowing the silk filaments to be separated and formed into strands of yarn. The gum is then removed entirely with a soap solution.

WOOL

The term *wool* is a general one, referring to protein fibers spun from the fleece of more than two hundred different breeds of sheep and from the hair of the angora rabbit, the cashmere goat, the camel, the alpaca, the llama, and the wild vicuña.

The higher-quality sheep's wool and exotic wools are generally taken from the animals by seasonal shearing or by combing the animal and collecting the hair as it naturally sheds. However, much lower-quality sheep's wool is removed from slaughtered animals with chemicals or natural bacterial action.

After shearing, the wool fleece is washed a number of times in a soapy alkaline solution. This "scouring" removes the lanolin, a natural oil that keeps the fleece soft and waterproof. "Unscoured" wool retains the natural water repellency of the lanolin.

If significant amounts of dirt, burrs, sticks, and other vegetable matter remain after scouring, the fleece is carbonized with sulfuric acid to remove the extraneous matter. The wool is then carded and combed, the fibers separated with fine wire teeth in preparation for spinning.

Because wool is highly susceptible to attack by moths, many companies treat their woolens with chemical mothproofing. Because this is considered to be a positive selling point, the fact that an item has been mothproofed is likely to appear on the label. For your health, though, it is best to buy unmothproofed products.

Most wool imported from the British Isles, South America, Iceland, and Greece is unmothproofed. Domestic stores and distributors often treat woolens on the premises to prevent problems with moths. Check with the retailers before purchase to see if mothproofing has been done. Often, by advance request, retailers will hold for you an unmothproofed garment from a future shipment.

If you consider yourself allergic to wool, try a softer, unbleached, variety; your allergy may be to the bleaches and dyes.

One special advantage of wool is that it is naturally fire resistant and can be used to make beds and sleepwear, which by law are required to be fireproof.

LEATHER

Most leathers are taken from animals that have been slaughtered for meat, and are treated with toxic tanning agents and dyes. Although some people prefer not to use leather for these reasons, it is much more comfortable and less toxic than plastic.

DOWN AND FEATHERS

All down and feathers are taken from the bodies of ducks and geese (goose down is the highest quality and most expensive) and are processed only by washing and sanitizing, as chemicals would break down the proteins in the feathers and destroy them.

Ducks and geese raised for down and feather production are plucked four or five times during their lifespan; then they are butchered for meat, and their final feathers are removed by machine.

KAPOK

Kapok is a fiber taken from the seed pod of the tropical kapok, or silk-cotton, tree, and is used as a natural stuffing material.

CLOTHING

Need I say it again? Clothing made from synthetic fabrics contains plastics—**acrylic, nylon, polyester** and **polyvinyl chloride.** And more **formaldehyde**-based no-iron finishes.

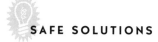

SAFE SOLUTIONS

Purchase clothing made from natural fibers, and wash them before wearing to remove excess finishes and dyes. Switching to natural fibers will be a gradual process; as much as you might like to, you probably won't be able to discard your entire wardrobe and buy all new clothes. Start by sorting through your existing clothing to determine which of the pieces you already own are made from natural fibers. Since natural fibers have been in fashion over the last decade, you may have, even unintentionally, quite a few. Wear these most often, and next time you buy new clothes, look for natural fibers.

You should be able to find clothing made from natural fibers almost anywhere, in every kind of store that sells clothing. Just read labels carefully, as I often find surprises—plastics mixed in with natural fibers. Unfortunately, the fashion pendulum seems to be swinging back to synthetics, with all the shiny vinyls and stretchy clothes. But there will always be natural-fiber "classics," which last longer and hold their styles year after year.

Take a look at these catalogs for a variety of natural-fiber fashions.

> ***American Environmental Health Foundation:*** organic-cotton basics for men and women
>
> ***Barbara Coole Designs:*** an "odd collection" of colorful natural-fiber clothing (sizes XS–3X) in styles you won't find in the mass market, including basic items like cotton sweats in every possible style and size, blouses, vests, and capes. Items are custom-dyed in small batches, so it is possible to get virtually all the styles in natural cotton. Inexpensive prices, good selection, and custom sewing are available.
>
> ***Casco Bay Fine Woolens:*** beautiful hooded capes for women, handcrafted from jewel-toned wools
>
> ***Castle Gray:*** hemp and hemp-blend basic clothing items for men and women
>
> ***ChiPants:*** homemade cotton pants, shorts, shirts, and jackets with "a unique gusseted design that gives

you total comfort without tightness or binding," for men and women; organic cotton/hemp walking shorts, too

The Cotton Place: cotton lounge wear, undergarments, sleepwear, and basic sportswear for men and women

Cotton Threads Clothing: flowing designs made of solid-color, batik, Indian-print, or organic-cotton fabrics for larger-size women

Decent Exposures: cotton and organic-cotton bras in 150 styles and 15 colors; all elastic is covered for comfort

Eddie Bauer: natural fiber casual sportswear for men and women

Garnet Hill: a small selection of nice natural-fiber clothing for women; fine cotton undergarments and lingerie in many styles; silk slips

J. Crew: a large catalog of natural-fiber clothing for men and women, including casual wear and dress attire; simple, elegant designs; reasonable prices

J. Jill: homemade dresses and women's separates, mostly cotton, with generous fit and detailing; many exclusive designs with loose, flowing styles; larger sizes

Janice Corporation: cotton pajamas, robes, and undergarments for men; cotton undergarments, lingerie, and dresses for women; unisex cotton knit caps, scarves, mittens; and organic-cotton undergarments, knit shirts, sweatclothes

Karen's Nontoxic Products: organic-cotton sportswear for men and women

L. L. Bean: traditional selection of basic cotton and wool outdoor wear

Land's End: fiber sportswear and casual wear for men and women

Natural Lifestyle: organic-cotton unisex basics

The Ohio Hempery: basic clothing made from hemp and hemp/natural-fiber blends (some with natural dyes) for men and women

Organic Cottons: a good selection of comfortable sportswear and undergarments for men and women in organic cotton only; great prices.

Pueblo to People: hand-loomed cotton clothing in bright South American colors for men and women

Reflections Organic: organic-cotton basic clothing items—T-shirts, sweats, jeans, undergarments, etc.— for men and women (some in colors)

Seventh Generation: organic- and natural-cotton casuals and undergarments for men and women

Tweeds: elegant natural-fiber clothing for men and women

Winter Silks: everything to keep you warm all winter—long johns, undergarments, pajamas, sweaters, turtlenecks, scarves, gloves—made from silk and silk/cotton or silk/wool blends

BEDS AND BEDDING

One of the most intimate exposures you have to plastics is the bed you sleep in night after night.

If you're like most Americans, you sleep on a mattress made of **polyurethane foam** plastic (even if you have an innerspring mattress, it still is wrapped with foam), sprayed with chemical **fire retardants,** and covered with **polyester** plastic fabric. As I stated before in Plastics in chapter 2, exposure to polyurethane foam can cause bronchitis, coughing, and skin and eye problems. Polyurethane foam also releases **toluene diisocyanate,** which can produce severe lung problems—hardly something you'd want to breathe for one-third of your life.

On top of this mattress, you probably have a polyester mattress pad, covered with pretty polyester cotton sheets, treated with a **formaldehyde**-based permanent-press finish for easy care. Your pillow is probably polyester, spun to make it light as feathers, and you may have a polyester comforter, too—if not, probably a few **acrylic** plastic blankets keep you warm at night.

Amid this cloud of plastic vapors, is it any wonder that millions of Americans take drugs to get to sleep at night?

SAFE SOLUTIONS

Back in 1980, when I first started looking for a safe bed, I had few choices. There were no cotton innerspring mattresses or even futons that I knew of. Finally, out of desperation and using all the creativity I could come up with, I bought the metal springs to a roll-away bed and piled up ten folded cotton thermal blankets on top. I rolled up cotton towels and stuffed them in a pillowcase. Fortunately, I found one out-of-the-way linen shop that carried the one available brand of those "old-fashioned" 100 percent cotton sheets that need ironing. It wasn't the most comfortable (or beautiful) bed I'd ever had, by a long shot, but it was safe and I could sleep. For the first time in my life, I didn't have insomnia.

Today the availability of natural beds and bedding has changed dramatically. Now I sleep on several layers of three-inch-thick organic-cotton and wool futon mattresses, which rest on a wood-slat frame. They are covered with a fuzzy wool mattress pad and soft, untreated-cotton flannel sheets. I have pillows filled with feathers and organically grown cotton and wool, and little wool neck rolls to keep my spine aligned. I *love* sleeping in this bed and always miss it when I have to stay in a hotel even for one night.

While you may not be able to find natural beds in your local stores, you should be able to find pieces. Most major department stores now sell untreated-cotton sheets at reasonable prices, because more manufacturers make them now. Also, it is easy to order a complete natural bed by mail. Here are only some of the choices.

> ***Allergy Relief Shop:*** cotton mattresses and box springs, cotton futons, natural-cotton bed linens, cotton blankets, cotton comforter covers, natural-cotton quilted mattress pads, and cotton pillows

Allergy Resources: organic-cotton innerspring mattresses and box springs, cotton pillows, cotton bed linens, and cotton mattress pads

American Environmental Health Foundation: cotton bed linens, cotton pillows, quilted cotton mattress pads, and cotton blankets

Barbara Coole Designs: natural-cotton flannel-sheet blankets and open-weave blankets that can be custom dyed

Bright Future Futon: natural- and organic-cotton futons and wooden platform bed frames; natural- and organic-cotton pillows and bolsters and buckwheat-hull pillows that can be custom made to any size and shape

Chambers: luxurious natural-fiber bed linens from around the world

The Cotton Place: cotton innerspring mattresses and box springs, cotton futons, cotton pillows, and cotton and linen bed linens

Cuddle Ewe: mattress pads made from layers of thick wool batting sewn between cotton ticking

Environmental Home Center: cotton/wool mattresses and box springs, cotton and wool futons, wool "mattress toppers" and comforters, wool- and organic cotton–filled pillows, and cotton bed linens

Garnet Hill: a breathtaking selection of beautiful cotton percale and flannel bed linens in many unusual styles and colors (some have formaldehyde-based "easy care" finishes, so read copy carefully); and thick English flannel, natural-cotton, and Italian linen bed linens; coordinating bedskirts, coverlets, and duvet covers that make complete bed ensembles; cozy cotton and wool blankets, and cotton-, wool-, or silk-filled comforters; solid-wood bed frames with coordinating bedside tables; pillows filled with cotton, wool, or down, and cotton pillow protectors; cotton mattresses and box springs, and natural-fiber mattress covers; and many exclusives and European imports

Grateful Threads: colorful and creative decorative throws woven of organic cotton (low-impact dyes)

Heart of Vermont: completely organic wool/cotton and all cotton futons, cotton futon covers, cotton- and wool-filled comforters, cotton "top mattresses" (very thick mattress pads) filled with cotton or wool, washable cotton flannel mattress pads, wool/cotton innerspring mattresses and box springs, cotton and wool pillows, cotton flannel and chambray bed linens

Janice Corporation: cotton innerspring mattresses and box springs; felt mattress pads; cotton and organic-cotton percale bed linens; cotton flannel sheet sets; cotton sleep pillows, throw pillows, and neck rolls; cotton and organic-cotton zippered mattresses, box springs, and pillow protectors; cotton bedspreads and blankets; custom quilt/comforters (cotton, wool, or down fill, with washable-cotton and organic-cotton covers)

Karen's Nontoxic Products: organic-cotton and cotton pillows, organic-cotton futons, organic buckwheat-hull pillows, cotton percale and flannel bed linens; and handmade cotton quilts with custom-embroidered heart designs

Land's End: cotton bed linens

The Living Source: untreated white-cotton bed linens, cotton blankets, and cotton pillows

The Natural Bedroom: homemade cotton/wool and cotton/wool/latex (from the rubber tree) mattresses and box springs; components for "the layered bed"— cotton and wool futons to mix and match to create an airable sleeping surface suited to your needs; wool "mattress toppers"—wool- and organic cotton–filled pillows and neck rolls; wool comforters; and cotton and linen bed linens in plain and elegant styles

Natural Lifestyle: organic-cotton and organic-cotton/wool innerspring mattresses and futons, natural ash hardwood bed frames, organic-cotton (cover and batting) and organic buckwheat-hull pillows; untreated-cotton sheet sets; and organic-cotton afghans colored with low-impact dyes

Nontoxic Environments: cotton and cotton/wool innerspring mattresses and box springs, organic-cotton and wool futons, wool pillows and neck rolls, organic-cotton pillows, organic-cotton futon covers and mattress pads, wool mattress pads, and wool comforters

Organic Cottons: completely organic wool futons, cotton futons, futon covers, wool comforters, wool pillows, cotton pillows, and duvet covers

Real Goods: wool and natural-cotton pillows, wool neck rolls, and natural-cotton bed linens

Royal-Pedic: natural-fiber innerspring mattresses and box springs in many styles and custom sizes

Sajama Alpaca: blankets made from alpaca yarns hand spun and dyed with plants indigenous to the highlands of Bolivia. The wool comes from animals who live on the open range, kept by local people who spin the yarn themselves

Seventh Generation: a good selection of natural and naturally colored cotton bed linens in attractive styles and patterns, naturally colored cotton blankets, cotton and wool mattress pads, organic-cotton and cotton innerspring mattresses and box springs, organic-cotton and cotton futons, wool and down comforters, organic-cotton and down pillows

Testfabrics: untreated 180-inch unbleached cotton muslin sheeting, also available in bleached 180-thread-count percale cotton

Vermont Country Store: cotton bedspreads, cotton percale and flannel sheets, waterproof cotton flannel/rubber sheets, overstuffed featherbeds, cotton and down pillows, cotton pillow covers, and cotton and wool mattress pads

SHOWER CURTAINS

The problem with shower curtains is that they are made of soft **vinyl** plastic that can outgas fumes.

SAFE SOLUTIONS

Cotton shower curtains are becoming very popular nowadays. If you don't find them in your local stores, you can order them by mail from *Allergy Relief Shop, Allergy Resources, American Environmental Health Foundation, Chambers* (they have some unusual fabrics and styles), *Clothcrafters, Janice Corporation, The Natural Choice, Nontoxic Environments, Real Goods, Seventh Generation,* or *Vermont Country Store.*

FOOTWEAR AND SHOE CARE

Most footwear is made from various kinds of plastic, including **acrylic, nylon, polyester, polyurethane,** or **polyvinyl chloride.** Somewhere stamped on the shoe or the box you'll find the material the shoe is made from. "Man-made" generally means "plastic." And they are glued with **formaldehyde**-based adhesives.

Socks and stockings also are made from plastics, generally acrylic or nylon.

SAFE SOLUTIONS

Wear shoes made entirely of leather. To avoid formaldehyde, look for leather shoes that are stitched instead of glued. Most leather shoes are made from dyed leather, but according to leading dermatologists, the dye is so firmly fixed to the leather that reactions to it would be extremely rare. It can be difficult to find all-leather shoes, and even when you do, the price may be high. I'll sometimes compromise by buying shoes with a leather upper and a man-made sole—that way the natural material is near my foot and I can have the cushiony soles that feel so good to walk on.

Another option is cotton espadrilles or "Chinese" rubber-soled cotton shoes. These are much less expensive (but also wear out more quickly). Shoes made from hemp, which should last longer, have just come on the market.

Even if you wear plastic shoes, try natural-fiber socks and stockings. They are much softer than the plastic fibers, and they absorb moisture better, making them much more comfortable. Most clothing stores now carry cotton socks, or you can order them by mail. Here are some mail-order sources that will make your feet happy.

American Environmental Health Foundation: organic-cotton socks for men and women

Barbara Coole Designs: cotton, organic-cotton, wool, and wool/cotton socks for men and women, in natural colors

Castle Gray: hemp shoes and sandals for men and women

The Cordwainer Shop: custom-fitted, hand-sewn leather shoes that are rebuildable and come inscribed with your name (expensive, but a good investment)

The Cotton Place: cotton socks for men and women, and cotton and silk stockings

Janice Corporation: a variety of cotton socks for men and women, including cotton stockings (with cotton garter belt) and tights; women's cotton slippers with suede soles

Karen's Nontoxic Products: cotton canvas espadrilles

Kiwis: handmade custom leather sandals for men and women (with cushion or leather soles) to match your footprint. These sandals can be resoled and cost less than ready-made leather sandals sold in fine shoe stores.

The Natural Choice: natural shoe polish and leather-care products

The Ohio Hempery: "Eco-Dragon" sandals made of 100 percent hemp—even the soles!

Reflections Organic: a dozen different styles of organic-cotton socks and stockings for men and women, in natural, natural brown, and natural green

> *Vermont Country Store:* women's cotton and wool socks, tights, and stockings
>
> *Winter Silks:* silk socks and stockings for men and women

LUGGAGE AND BAGS

Are you starting to get the idea that the problem with all textile products is that they are made from plastic? Here are some more: luggage and handbags and fanny packs and backpacks . . . tote bags, duffle bags, briefcases—all **nylon, polyester,** or **polyvinyl chloride** plastic.

SAFE SOLUTIONS

As with shoes, you can always go with leather. It's expensive, but look around and you may find some bargains, particularly in import shops. I've taken to collecting untreated leather bags that turn a warm honey color as they age. I buy them when I see them, and I know it's a lifetime investment.

More affordable are natural fibers. I've seen some linen luggage and tote bags, and bags made from grasses. Again, shop around.

Here are some mail-order sources for luggage and bags of all sorts made from organic and natural cotton, and hemp.

> *Barbara Coole Designs:* natural-cotton canvas duffle shoulder bags, fanny packs, totes, knapsacks, and others, which can be custom dyed
>
> *Castle Gray:* hemp bags, pouches, wallets, and fanny packs
>
> *Clothcrafters:* tote bags and miscellaneous specialty bags, such as flannel shoe bags
>
> *Janice Corporation:* natural-cotton tote bags
>
> *Karen's Nontoxic Products:* bags of all sizes in brightly colored Guatemalan cottons; and cotton shopping bags and string bags

The Ohio Hempery: a good selection of hemp back-packs, day packs, tool belts, pouches, attachés, wallets, and more

Organic Cottons: organic-cotton reusable canvas lunch bags and grocery tote sacks

Patti Collins Canvas Products: cotton canvas bags—purses, totes, backpacks, duffles, school bags, and more, in more than a dozen colors

Port Canvas Company: handmade cotton canvas bags—hand-stitched cotton canvas luggage with cotton webbing in a variety of styles and sizes, including carry-on and garment bags; duffles; totes; handbags; briefcases; and more, all available with custom monogramming

FABRICS, YARNS, AND NOTIONS

How can I say this another way? Again, more plastics—**acrylic, nylon, polyester,** and **polyvinyl chloride,** and more **formaldehyde**-based no-iron finishes.

SAFE SOLUTIONS

If you knit or sew, you have a wonderful opportunity to be truly creative with the new organic-cotton and hemp fabrics and yarns. I've seen some stunning clothing made by combining the fibers in their own natural shades, or accented with natural-dye threads. You'll love the softness of these fabrics, which get even nicer with repeated washings.

Instead of plastic buttons, look in your local fabric store for buttons made of wood, metal, cloisonné, ceramic, pewter, shell, leather, horn, stone, or tagua nut.

Allergy Relief Shop: organic-cotton batting, and cotton elastic

Barbara Coole Designs: natural-cotton, hemp, and organic-cotton fabrics

Cotton Clouds Mail Order Yarns: cotton and organic-cotton yarns in more than 20 weights and textures and 1,500 colors; weaving looms and equipment, cotton rug warp; wooden crochet hooks; and bamboo knitting needles

The Cotton Place: unbleached-cotton duck, felt padding, sateen, and muslin fabrics; linen and noil silk; cotton/rubber elastic; cotton and silk thread; and a variety of cotton trims and yarns

Green Mountain Spinnery: homemade "Greenspun" organic-wool and organic cotton/wool yarns, spun using canola and coconut oils instead of petroleum-based products

Heart of Vermont: organic-cotton poplin, denim, flannel, canvas, and batting; and organic-wool batting

Hendricksen's Natürlich: hemp canvas and summer cloth, hemp/silk fabric, and cotton/hemp muslin suitable for clothing, upholstery, and draperies

Homespun Fabrics: natural-cotton fabrics up to ten feet wide, with interesting textures; can be used for draperies, upholstery, clothing, wall coverings, tablecloths, and bedspreads

Jamie Harmon: hand-spun wool yarns in natural colors (white, gray, or brown) or dyed with natural dye

Janice Corporation: unbleached-cotton fabrics in several weights, cotton sheeting and flannel, organic cottons, and cotton batting; cotton thread, lace, bias tape, elastic, and zippers; and natural-cotton yarn

The Living Source: cotton felt and muslin, cotton elastic, blue denim

Ocarina Textiles: hand-woven fabrics made from naturally colored organic cottons

Organic Cottons: organic-cotton jersey, pointelle, french terry, ticking, flannel, canvas, chambray, and other fabrics; cotton/rubber elastic; and cotton thread

Organic Interiors: more than 50 organic-cotton upholstery and drapery fabrics, some naturally colored

Sajama Alpaca: alpaca yarns (hand spun) and spinning wool dyed with plants indigenous to the highlands of Bolivia. The wool comes from animals who live on the open range, kept by local people who spin the yarn themselves

Straw Into Gold: alpaca/merino wool, cotton, silk, silk/linen, silk/wool, and wool yarns in natural shades and a wide range of dyed colors; fibers for spinning—angora, camel hair, cashmere, flax, goat hair, ramie, silk, wool, and yak; and spinning and weaving equipment

Sureway Trading Enterprises: good prices on a comprehensive selection of natural and white silk fabrics from corduroy to organza, plus silk/wool blends for suiting (some dyed)

Testfabrics: untreated fabrics ready to dye: linen, silk, wool, and more than 50 varieties of cotton; untreated yarns from natural, scoured, bleached, or mercerized cotton, spun silk, and worsted wool

Thai Silks: nearly 100 silk fabrics—also some linen and wool—many in natural shades

IRONS AND IRONING-BOARD COVERS

Okay, let's face it. If you're going to wear natural fibers, you're going to have to do a certain amount of ironing. So you'll want that to be a safe experience, too.

Nowadays, most irons and ironing-board covers are coated with **tetrafluoroethylene** plastic, better known as **Teflon.** Given that heating plastic makes it outgas its toxic fumes, irons and ironing-board covers seem odd places to put it, particularly since a nonstick finish is not even necessary. Tetrafluoroethylene fumes can be irritating to eyes, nose, and throat, and can cause breathing difficulties.

SAFE SOLUTIONS

First, cover your ironing board with a cotton pad and cover. These are sold in virtually every hardware store, or you can order them by mail from **Clothcrafters, Janice Corporation,** or **The Living Source.** Then, get yourself a *good* iron, not a cheap one. I have a **Rowenta** with a shiny heating surface (no Teflon), and I was surprised the first time I used it what a difference a good iron makes. It's heavy to lift, but it glides along the fabric so smoothly, removing every wrinkle without any pressure on my part.

Yes, it's a drudgery to iron, but the pleasure and health I gain from the natural fibers is more than worth whatever time and effort it takes to maintain them.

KITCHEN AND TABLE LINENS

Kitchen and table linens are a mixed bag of naturals and plastics. Virtually every kitchen towel I've seen is cotton (because it absorbs moisture better, I'm sure), yet try to find a tablecloth that isn't made from **vinyl** or **polyester** with an easy-care **formaldehyde** finish! Old potholders lying around your house or at garage sales may contain **asbestos;** new ones do not.

SAFE SOLUTIONS

You can buy cotton kitchen towels everywhere, and cotton terry-cloth potholders are sold at every hardware store. **Clothcrafters** sells cotton aprons and chef's hats, stuffed cotton potholders, and a Big Oven Glove. **Organic Cottons** has organic-cotton aprons, potholders, and oven mitts.

For the table, **Clothcrafters** makes inexpensive cotton napkins with colored borders, and blue-striped denim placemats. **Vermont Country Store** has sturdy "mountain weave" cotton tablecloths, napkins, and placemats in lots of colors, plus checked cotton-damask table linens in several colors and patterns. **Testfabrics** has plain, untreated-cotton napkins and placemats, and custom-made cotton tablecloths. Your best bet for finding cotton tablelinens in a local store is at an import store.

BATH LINENS

Most bath towels are cotton—again, because cotton is so absorbent, it's the logical choice for a towel—but some are blended with **polyester. Acrylic** is often used for bath rugs and other bathroom accessories.

SAFE SOLUTIONS

All-cotton towels are sold by the pile at department stores, in every color. Virtually all department stores now carry natural cotton; some carry towels made with naturally colored cotton as well. If you need to, you can order cotton bath towels by mail from *Allergy Relief Shop, Clothcrafters, Janice Corporation, Karen's Nontoxic Products,* or *Real Goods.*

Some catalogs are worth noting for their exceptional selection of bath linens. *Chambers* carries luxurious cotton bath linens to go with their luxurious natural-fiber bed linens. *Garnet Hill* has extra-plush Egyptian cotton towels and bath rugs and real Turkish towels (super thick with fringe!), as well as natural-cotton bath linens. *Seventh Generation* offers the biggest selection of natural and naturally colored bath linens, in a number of different styles and patterns.

Chapter 10

HOME OFFICE AND ART SUPPLIES

OST OF US HAVE office and art supplies around the house, especially things like glue, paper, pens, and markers. If you are creatively inclined or have children, you probably have paints and craft supplies around, too. In addition, most people also come into weekly, if nor daily, contact with computers and copy machines.

Although scientific documentation is incomplete, there is significant epidemiological and toxicological evidence that some ingredients in professional art materials and craft supplies may cause human health problems ranging from organ damage to birth defects and cancer. Although these effects have been observed under conditions of more prolonged and higher levels of exposure than would normally occur in your home, there is a legitimate concern about the safety of these materials even at lower levels of exposure.

Common symptoms that have been associated with exposure to art materials and office supplies through ingestion, inhalation, or skin absorption include dizziness, headaches, blurred vision, general fatigue, nausea, nervousness, loss of appetite, chronic cough, skin problems, depression, and shortness of breath.

Labeling

Labels on office supplies carry very little information about their ingredients or dangers. Though it has recently been reformulated, typewriter correction fluid, for example, contained toxic chemicals for many years, with no indication on the label that they were even present in the product.

The labels on art materials, on the other hand, are beginning to improve. There are two types of art materials—the usually less toxic consumer products designed for general use, and the frequently more toxic professional/industrial products intended for use by trained professionals in controlled environments. Since both are widely available to consumers in art- and office-supply stores, it's important to learn how to read the labels in order to choose less toxic products.

The labeling of art materials is supervised by the Consumer Product Safety Commission (CPSC), which administers three laws: the Federal Hazardous Substances Act (1970), the Poison Prevention Packaging Act (1970), and the Consumer Product Safety Act (1972). Under the Federal Hazardous Substances Act, the CPSC may require precautionary labeling of hazardous substances or ban substances for which labeling is determined to be insufficient to protect the public health.

Despite these laws, many art materials have insufficient labeling, which is a result not of inadequate regulations but of lack of enforcement of these laws. California, New York, Massachusetts, Illinois, Tennessee, and Oregon all have more detailed state laws that attempt to improve art-product labels.

Some common problems encountered in choosing art supplies include:

- Unlabeled products. Artists and craftspeople can purchase ceramic chemicals, clays, dyes, pigments, solvents, plastic resins, and other hazardous materials in paper sacks, with no ingredient information.
- Improperly labeled products. Many product labels are missing information such as the manufacturer's address or precautions.

- Foreign product labels. Many products are imported from other countries whose labeling requirements are different from our own.

To avoid the more stringent regulations for consumer-product labeling, some product manufacturers label their products "For professional use only" or "For industrial use only." As a consumer, it is wise to stay away from these products.

Not all products are poorly labeled. At least twenty-nine companies have joined the Arts and Crafts Materials Institute, an industry group that has developed voluntary standards for the safety and quality of both consumer and professional/industrial art supplies. In evaluating the safety of a product, the Institute's toxicologist considers both the concentration and the potential acute and chronic health effects of the ingredients, as well as possible uses and misuses of the products.

Manufacturers of safe products can pay a fee to the Institute for permission to display certain certification seals such as the CP Nontoxic (Certified Product) seal, the AP Nontoxic (Approved Product) seal, and the Health Label. These seals represent that the product has been "certified in a program of toxicological evaluation by a medical expert to contain no materials in sufficient quantities to be toxic or injurious to humans or to cause acute or chronic health problems."

AP and CP Nontoxic labels are used on children's art supplies. CP products additionally meet specific requirements of material, workmanship, working qualities, and color standards. The Health Label is used on adult art materials to assure that they are properly labeled with health and use information, and includes a line that states, "Nontoxic," or "Warning: Contains [name of the hazardous substance]." One drawback to this system is that the toxicologist's assessment of the safety of a product is based on a literature review, not on actual testing of the product itself.

As with any product, read and follow instructions, and follow any precautionary advice. "Use with adequate ventilation" does *not* translate to "Open the window"; it means that sufficient ventilation must be provided to keep airborne concentrations of the product's mist, dust, fumes, or vapors below the levels considered hazardous for the user. Since proper ventilation can be complex to arrange, the average consumer should choose products that don't require such precautions. In case of accidental ingestion of an art material, or if symptoms arise during use, call your local poison-control center immediately. Don't follow the antidote on the label, as many are incorrect. Again, when possible, products should be chosen that will not produce symptoms during use or accidental ingestion.

Last, but not least, don't make the mistake of choosing a product without a warning label over a product with a warning label, assuming that no warning label implies that no warning is necessary. Whenever possible, choose products that list ingredients or give some other clear indication of their safety.

SAFE SOLUTIONS

When I evaluate office and art supplies, I first want to choose supplies that are made from natural materials, if possible. If there are no natural supplies available, I look for the least toxic product that will do the job.

EPOXY, RUBBER CEMENT, AND "SUPER GLUE"

> **DANGER:** Extremely flammable. Vapor harmful. Harmful or fatal if swallowed. Skin and eye irritant. Keep out of reach of children. Bonds skin instantly. Toxic.
>
> **CAUTION:** Do not use near sparks or flame. Do not breathe vapors. Use in well-ventilated room. Keep away from small children.

Adhesives are full of volatile chemicals. **Naphthalene, phenol, ethanol, vinyl chloride, formaldehyde, acrylonitrile,** and **epoxy** are a few of the chemicals more commonly used. All these substances release toxic vapors, and although you probably wouldn't die from breathing them, some are known to cause cancer, birth defects, and genetic changes.

These products also present a secondary danger. Some of

the ingredients, such as phenol, are very easily absorbed through the skin, an exposure we don't usually think about and yet one that is quite likely when applying glues. Our exposure to these chemicals may be small, but we shouldn't underestimate their peril. One book on toxicology describes the skin destruction caused by phenol as follows: "[Phenol] exerts a powerful corrosive action that kills skin tissues with which they come in contact. The top part of the skin then becomes whitish, and the bottom part becomes reddish because of hemorrhaging. Death can result."

SAFE SOLUTIONS

The safest glues on the market are white glues (made from polyvinyl acetate plastic) and yellow woodworking glues (made from aliphatic plastic resin), both widely available at most stores. White glue effectively bonds paper, cloth, wood, pottery, and most other porous and semiporous materials. It is quick-drying, clear, and "nontoxic" (as defined in the Federal Hazardous Substances Act). These glues work for many jobs you wouldn't typically use them for, such as laying hardwood floors, so try them first.

For gluing paper, try a glue stick. These are solid, very-low-odor white glues. I've discovered also a clear liquid nontoxic glue in a squeeze bottle—the one in my desk is called **O'Glue.** It has a very informative label, with the words "nontoxic" and "nonflammable" *and* the CP Nontoxic logo. Look for similar labels, and you'll find adhesives you and your family can use safely.

If you'd like to try your hand at making your own glue, here are some recipes I found in do-it-yourself handbooks.

Blend 4 tablespoons wheat flour and 6 tablespoons cold water to make a smooth paste. Boil 1½ cups water and stir into paste, cooking over very low heat for about 5 minutes. Use when cold.

Blend 3 tablespoons cornstarch and 4 tablespoons cold water to make a smooth paste. Boil 2 cups water and stir into paste, continuing to stir until mixture becomes translucent. Use when cold.

Combine ¼ cup cornstarch, ¾ cup water, 2 tablespoons light corn syrup, and 1 teaspoon white vinegar in a medium saucepan. Cook over medium heat, stirring constantly, until mixture is thick. Remove from heat. In a separate bowl, stir together ¼ cup cornstarch and ¾ cup water until smooth. Add a little at a time to the heated mixture, stirring constantly. Will keep 2 months in a covered container.

If a toxic adhesive is the *only* glue that will do the job, use it in a well-ventilated area (outdoors would be best) and wear a protective mask and gloves. Once completely dry, the adhesives are safe, but you'll want to protect yourself well during application.

TYPEWRITER CORRECTION FLUID

> **WARNING:** Intentional misuse by deliberately concentrating and inhaling the contents can be harmful or fatal. Nonflammable and nonhazardous when used as directed.

Typewriter correction fluids may contain **cresol, ethanol, trichloroethylene,** and **naphthalene,** all toxic chemicals that can be fatal in high doses.

It has always been amusing to me that the label warning states, "Nonhazardous when used as directed." Here are the directions: "Shake well. Touch on. Do not brush. Apply sparingly. Allow 8–10 seconds to dry." Considering the toxicity of the ingredients, more appropriate directions might instruct you to "open all the windows, turn on an exhaust fan, wear a gas mask, and use an eight-foot robotic arm." I know I'm exaggerating, but they might at least instruct you to use it in a well-ventilated area and not breathe the fumes directly.

Note: You might not want to keep typewriter correction fluid around the house; some teenagers use it to get high. A few concentrated whiffs of this stuff can get you high, but it can also cause respiratory arrest, cardiac arrest, and death.

SAFE SOLUTIONS

If you do a lot of typing, you probably have purchased a home computer already, which requires no typewriter correction fluid.

However, if you are like me, you might use this stuff to "white out" other errors, and so still have a bottle around the house.

Water-based typewriter correction fluids are available in most office-supply stores. These are intended for use with copies, rather than typewriters. One coat is rather transparent, but if you let it dry and apply a second coat, it will cover up your errors.

Instead of using a liquid, try the tapes that strike a white powder over the error. If you are typing something that will be printed or copied, you can use adhesive correction tapes to cover whole lines or paragraphs.

ARTISTS' COLORS

The most toxic medium of color likely to be encountered by home artists is acrylic paint, which contains **ammonia, formalde-hyde,** and **acrylonitrile** plastic. The Arts and Crafts Materials Institute has not rated any brand CP. These paints are best avoided by home artists.

Tempera paints and watercolors are not much safer, for they may contain formaldehyde, phenol, and plastics (acrylonitrile, PVC/vinyl chloride). These are considered moderately to very toxic.

The inks used in permanent-ink pens and markers contain **acetone, cresol, ethanol,** phenol, **toluene,** and **xylene,** but I don't know of any studies that have researched the health effects of pens and markers. However, many people, including myself, have reported symptoms associated with using ballpoint pens. I've even seen people's handwriting change! Also, I have had several graphic artists as consulting clients who almost gave up their careers because of the symptoms they were experiencing from the solvents in colored markers. These reactions don't surprise me.

Children's art supplies are a little better. Finger paints generally are made from "nontoxic colors," although formaldehyde often is added as a preservative. Crayons made from **paraffin** generally are considered quite safe. *Clinical Toxicology of Consumer Products* gives them a rating somewhere between "practically nontoxic" and "slightly toxic," which means that a seventy-five-pound child would have to eat between one and two cups of crayons for a toxic effect to occur.

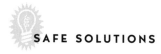

SAFE SOLUTIONS

Here's a natural paint you can make yourself.

Mix ½ cup cornstarch and ¾ cup cold water in a saucepan. Soak 1 envelope gelatin in ¼ cup cold water. Add 2 cups hot water to the cornstarch mixture, and cook over medium heat until it comes to a boil and is clear, stirring constantly. Remove from heat, stir in the gelatin, add ½ cup soap flakes, and stir until thickened and soap is dissolved. Tint with natural colors such as beet juice, blueberry juice, coffee—any food that stains!

You can purchase some beautiful natural art paints, imported from Germany, that are made from resins and oils and are tinted with mineral and plant pigments. **Auro** brand paints can be purchased by mail from ***Sinan Company;*** **Livos** brand paints from ***The Natural Choice*** catalog. (Note: These are not odor free, but are safe to use.) Natural watercolor paints can be ordered by mail from ***Karen's Nontoxic Products, The Natural Baby Company,*** and ***Nova Natural Toys and Crafts.***

There are several brands of water-based markers available in art-supply stores. They come in many colors (the brand I use, **Stabilo,** has about sixty-four different shades) and several tip widths. Ask for water-based-ink markers. They're easy to distinguish from the permanent-ink markers just by smell.

Every stationery and office-supply store sells ballpoint pens with water-based ink. It's not so easy to smell the difference in pens at first, but a water-based ink flows smoothly (and will smudge when wet), while a permanent-ink pen tends to get globs of ink stuck around the point (and won't smudge when wet). **Pilot** pens have water-based ink.

Though crayons made from **paraffin** wax generally are considered nontoxic, as a child I always thought they had a disagreeable odor and I didn't want to use them (perhaps that's why I never developed my drawing talents . . .). Beeswax crayons are a wonderful alternative. The colors are vibrant and they flow smoothly across the paper. I have a set and love to draw with them, even as an adult. You can order beeswax crayons from

Karen's Nontoxic Products, The Natural Baby Company, and *Nova Natural Toys and Crafts.* And, for tiny hands, *Organic Cottons* has beeswax crayons shaped like little stars!

COMPUTERS

There has long been a debate on the safety of sitting in front of a computer screen. Many studies in the past have linked using video display terminals (VDTs) to eye irritation, double vision, rashes on faces, headaches, irritability, stress, and neck and back pains. The FDA, the American Academy of Ophthalmology, the National Institute for Occupational Safety and Health, and the National Academy of Sciences all agree that the amount of radiation given off is too small to pose a threat to health, but recently new studies seem to confirm some risks of being close to a source of electromagnetic radiation.

For example, research reported in 1989 found that there is a higher rate of leukemia in children who live in homes near high-voltage power lines. The pulsed magnetic fields found routinely within a radius of about two feet from the average VDT computer terminal can be as strong or even stronger than the magnetic fields found inside homes near power lines. The evidence against VDTs is inconclusive but caution is worthwhile. (Note: While the liquid crystal display [LCD] screens found on portable computers also produce radiation, it extends out from the computer a shorter distance and operates on a less powerful voltage than VDTs.)

Beyond the radiation issue, there is also a problem with static electricity generated by the high voltages in the air that surround computers and the bodies of the people sitting at keyboards. The positively charged field around a computer neutralizes the negative ions in the air space, creating an area that is high in positive ions. High concentrations of positive ions have been associated with fatigue, metabolic disorders, irritability, headaches, and respiratory problems. In addition, dust, tobacco smoke, and chemical pollutants become positively charged and seek out the nearest grounded or oppositely charged surface, which is usually the operator's face. The particles clinging to your face can cause rashes, itchy eyes, and dry skin. Some people who work at computers get a "sunburn."

Many of the eye problems associated with computer use are caused by glare from improper lighting. Bodily aches and pains are generally the result of poor posture, sitting in one position for too long, and using the wrong furniture.

A study at Columbia University found that women whose jobs involve working with VDTs all day have significantly more physical and mental-health problems than women who use the machines only part of the day, use a typewriter, or use no machines at all. Most of the test subjects experienced increased musculoskeletal problems like wrist and arm pains and neck and finger cramps, increased eye fatigue, and a decreased sense of general well-being.

SAFE SOLUTIONS

Get a laptop computer with an LCD screen. There are hundreds of models on the market now, and prices are coming down fast. The power and portability of the new models make them comparable to desktop models. To make it even safer, use the battery for power while you're working on it, then recharge the battery while you're in another room.

You can block electrical fields with a grounded screen (see Resources) attached to a computer plugged into a properly grounded outlet. Glare screens without grounded wires are worthless from an electrical standpoint. These screens only block the electrical radiation. Right now there is no effective way that I know of to shield magnetic radiation. To protect yourself from magnetic radiation, stay thirty inches from the front and forty inches from the back and sides of the computer. Unplug computers when not in use to completely eliminate magnetic fields.

To eliminate static electricity, put leafy houseplants in your home office and open windows. A negative-ion generator will also work if it is of good quality, proper design, and positioned properly with respect to the computer, the operator, and the air flow in the room. The optimal placement could be overhead or nearby on a table. It is important not to generate too many negative ions, because there is a possibility that your body will absorb negative ions faster than they can be discharged, resulting in a buildup of negative ions on your skin. When this happens, you will begin to attract positive ions, which is just what you don't want. If you want to experiment with this, try a variable-output negative-ion generator and place it in different locations. You should be able to feel the difference as you search for its optimal spot.

For glare control, diffused lighting is best. Make sure sunlight or bare bulbs are not shining directly on your screen. If you need brighter lighting to be able to read text you are inputting, use a small work light that shines on the paper but not on the screen. Use the minimum contrast setting at which you can comfortably see the text; you may be able to work longer with less eyestrain at lower settings. My editor's eye doctor recommends taking an "eye break" every ten minutes: focus on a distant object, or let your eyes wander around the room.

Place your computer equipment on a table that allows you to adjust the screen and keyboard to the proper heights for your body. Sit in a comfortable position and then adjust the screen so you are looking slightly down at it. To adjust keyboard height, sit in a normal position and bend your arms at the elbow to form right angles. Your hands should just fall comfortably onto the keyboard.

Prevent bodily aches and pains by taking frequent breaks. Sitting motionless for long periods slows circulation, reduces muscle tone, and causes fatigue. Take a break every ninety minutes to stretch, walk around, and, if you can, do some other type of work for a short period of time. Hit your "save" key every few paragraphs or at the end of each page. Not only will you have your work protected in case of a power failure, but you can take a few moments to squirm in your chair.

COPY MACHINES, COMPUTER LASER PRINTERS, AND PLAIN PAPER FACSIMILE MACHINES

Most problems associated with copy machines come from older-model "wet-copy" machines, which use a variety of volatile chemical toners—such as **ammonia, ethanol,** and **kerosene**—to produce the copy image. Copied pages continue to smell of these toners for long periods of time. I doubt you can even buy one of these today, but they may be lurking in older offices. Don't buy one at a garage sale!

Nowadays, all new copiers are the "dry-copy" variety, which makes the copy image by electronically fusing odorless carbon powder to the paper. Even these, however, give off fumes—especially ozone, a pungent gas that can cause eye, nose, and throat irritation at low doses, and coughing, chest pains, and fatigue at higher doses. Day-in and day-out exposure to ozone can eventually cause lung disease. Copiers that are well maintained and properly ventilated rarely exceed the safety threshold of 0.1 parts per million (ppm) set by the Occupational Safety and Health Administration and are unlikely to cause health problems. However, the National Institute for Occupational Safety and Health warns that "unnecessary exposure to any concentration, however small, should be avoided." If there is a strong chlorinelike or sulfurlike (or "electric") odor in the room, there is likely to be something wrong with the machine. Toners and other chemicals used in the photocopying process may pose other hazards to workers as respirable vapors and dust particles. Handling copied papers on a regular basis can also produce a skin rash.

New laser computer printers and plain paper facsimile machines use the same internal workings as dry-copy photocopy machines—in fact, one company has combined these three into one machine! So the potential health hazards are the same for these as well.

SAFE SOLUTIONS

Make sure that copy machines, computer laser printers, and plain paper facsimile machines are placed in well-ventilated areas.

PAPER

Generally, paper is considered to be an innocuous product, and it is, relatively speaking. For the most part, the health effects I could find that are associated with paper are various skin problems, the result of various **plastics, acids,** and **formaldehyde** used as coatings on office papers.

Carbonless "carbon" paper contains tiny amounts of **polychlorinated biphenyls (PCBs),** which can enter the body through inhalation or absorption through the skin while handling. PCBs are extremely toxic, causing irritation to eyes, skin, nose, and throat. At high levels they can cause severe liver damage, and they are suspected of causing cancer. The conventional wisdom is that the amount of PCBs used in carbonless "carbon" paper is too small to have ill effects; however, there are at least two cases reported in the *Journal of the American Medical Association* that document contrary information. One woman repeatedly developed itching, reddened, and swollen skin within twenty-four to forty-eight hours after using carbonless "carbon" paper, and another person had an allergic lung response so severe that it was life-threatening.

SAFE SOLUTIONS

Use plain, uncoated papers as much as possible. Many recycled papers have fewer chemical finishes, and using them will help save forests and other natural resources (remember to recycle your office papers, too).

And instead of carbonless "carbon" paper, go back to using real carbon paper, if necessary. In today's computer age, copy paper of any kind may soon become obsolete.

Chapter 11

HOME FURNISHINGS

T HE MAJOR PROBLEM with most home furnishings is that they are made of plastics and good doses of **formaldehyde.** Acrylic plastic carpets, chairs with poly-ester plastic upholstery, and polyurethane plastic foam stuffing all have formaldehyde stain-resistant finishes. The paint on the wall has hundreds of chemicals, including more plastics. And I even see plastic plants here and there in already plastic-filled homes.

SAFE SOLUTIONS

Whenever possible, select home furnishings made from natural materials and nontoxic formulations. Styles have swung to the simple, the authentic, and the real, and it's fairly easy now to find products made from natural materials. Awareness of the health and environmental effects of products *has* spread to the world of interior design, so even though you may not find an all-natural sofa at a discount furniture store, stores such as *Pottery Barn* and *Crate & Barrel* are full of natural furnishings and accessories, and due to concerns about outdoor air pollution, less-toxic paints have reached the mass market.

HOUSEPLANTS

We all are aware that some plants may be poisonous, but we don't often suspect that plants we use in our homes as pleasant decorations may be harmful if they are touched or accidentally eaten by an inquisitive child.

Some plants can be deadly. Azalea, creeping charlie, crocus, hydrangea, lily of the valley, mistletoe, morning glory, oleander, and rhododendron all may cause illness requiring medical attention if eaten.

Other plants contain substances that are irritating to the skin, mouth, and tongue. In some cases, stomach upset and breathing difficulties may occur. Anthurium, Boston ivy, calla lily, dieffenbachia, philodendron, pothos, shamrock, and spathiphyllum are examples of plants that fall into this category.

Amaryllis, buttercup, carnation, cyclamen, daffodil, daisy, ficus benjamina, geranium, holly berry, iris, poinsettia, pyracantha berry, and tulip bulb all can cause skin rashes if contact occurs. If eaten, nausea, vomiting, diarrhea, and abdominal cramps may result.

Contact with the plants themselves is not the only way a poisoning can occur. Accidental ingestion of the water in which poisonous plants have been standing can also have toxic consequences.

Even foods that we commonly eat have some poisonous parts. Avocado, rhubarb, and tomato leaves; apple or pear seeds; apricot, cherry, peach, and plum pits; and the outer green husks of walnuts all can have toxic effects if enough is ingested. However, even a small quantity of green potato sprouts can be very toxic.

SAFE SOLUTIONS

If you have small children in the house, choose decorative plants that have no known toxic effects: African violet, asparagus fern, baby's breath, Boston fern, camellia, coleus, dahlia, dandelion, Easter lily, forget-me-not, fuchsia, gardenia, gloxinia, grape ivy, hibiscus, impatiens, jade plant, jasmine, maidenhair fern, marigold, orchid, pansy, peony, petunia, rose, rubber plant, schefflera, snapdragon, spider plant, violet, wandering Jew, and zinnia. This is not a complete list; if you're not sure about certain plants, call your local poison-control center for information.

If you do have toxic plants in your home, keep them out of reach of children and pets, and wash your hands thoroughly after cutting flowers.

You might want to decorate with edible plants, such as kitchen herbs or small flowers that can be used in salads. Your children may not like the taste of lobelia, nasturtiums, pansies, or violets, but it won't hurt them to nibble on these flowers, and your friends will be impressed with your gourmet cooking!

THE TOXICITY OF PLANTS

Here is an alphabetical list of some of the more common household plants. To see whether or not one of your plants is poisonous (toxic), look it up on this list and check to see which number follows its name. Then read the information that corresponds to that number.

1. **Nontoxic** These plants generally are considered nonpoisonous. Symptoms of illness are unlikely.

2. **Toxic Oxalates** These plants contain irritating substances known as oxalate salts. Eating these plants may cause irritation of the mucous membranes, including pain and/or swelling of the mouth, the lips, and the tongue. Breathing should be observed, since this swelling may interfere with the air passages.

3. **Toxic** These plants may contain any of a wide variety of poisons and may damage the stomach, heart, kidneys, or other organs.

4. **Dermatitic** Touching the sap from these plants may produce a skin rash.

5. **Possibly Toxic or Dermatitic** Information is incomplete, but it does seem to indicate that the plants possibly may cause ill effects.

African Violet (Saintpaulia)	1	Baby Tears (Helxine soleirolii)	1
Agapanthus (Botanical name)	1	Bachelor's Buttons (Centaurea cyanus)	1
Agapanthus (Nerine bowdenii)	3,4	Bear Feet (Cotyledon tomentosa)	1
Aloe (Aloe Barbadensis)	1	Begonia (Species)	1
Aluminum Plant (Pelea cadierei)	1	Bird of Paradise (Strelitzia reginae)	3
Alyssum (Botanical name)	1	Birdnest Sansevieria (Sansevieria Trifasciate)	1
Amaryllis Belladonna (Botanical name)	3	Bird's Nest Fern (Asplenium nidus)	1
Aralia (Fatsia japonica)	1	Bloodleaf (Iresine herbstii)	1
Arrowhead Vine (Wyngonium podophyllum)	2	Bonsai Tree (Pinus pentaphylla)	5
Asparagus Fern (Asparagus plumosus or		Boston Fern (Nephrolepis exalta)	1
Asparagus Densiflorus sprengeri)	4	Boston Ivy (Parthenocissus quinquefolia)	2
Avocado (Persea americana)	5	Bottle Brush (Callistemon species)	1
Azalea (Rhododendron occidentale)	3	Bridal Veil (Tradescantia 'bridal veil')	1

Cactus	I	Goldfish Plant (Columnea leanksi)	I
Pencil cactus	3,4	Gold Toothed Aloe (Aloe nobilis)	3, poss 4
Peyote/mescaline (Lophophora		Grape Ivy (Cissus rhombifolia)	I
Williamsii)	3	Grape Mountain (Berberis mahonia)	I
Candelabra cactus (Euphorbia lactea)	3,4	Heart Ivy (Hedera helix)	3
Caladium (Species)	2	Heartleaf (Philodendron cordatum)	2
Calathea argyraea (Botanical name)	I	Heavenly Bamboo (Nandina domestica)	5
California Poppy (Eschscholzia californica)	5	Hen and Chicks (Escheveria or	
Calla Lilly (Calla palustris)	2	Sempervivum tectorum)	I
Camellia (Botanical name)	I	Hibiscus (Botanical name)	I
Carnation (Dianthus caryophyllus)	3	Holly (Ilex)	3
Castor Beans (Ricinus communis)	3,4	Hyacinth (Hyacinthus orientalis)	3,4
Chinese Evergreen (Aglaonena		Ice Plant (Aptenia cordifolia or	
modestum)	I	Lampranthus)	I
Chrysanthemum (Species)	I–4	Impatiens (Botanical name)	I
Coleus (Species)	I	Indian Hawthorne (Raphiolipos indica)	I
Corn Plant (Dracaena fragrans		Indian Laurel (Ficus nitida)	4
massangeana)	I	Indigo Plant (Indigofera)	3,4
Crape Myrtle (Lagerstroemia indica)	I	Iris (Botanical name)	3,4
Creeping Charlie (Glecona hederacea)	3	Ivy (Hedera helix)	3
Creeping Charlie (Lysimachia nummularia)	I	Jade Plant (Crassula argentea)	I
Creeping Charlie (Pilea nummularifolia)	I	Janet Craig (Dracaena derminesis)	I
Creeping Fig (Ficus)	4	Jerusalem Cherry (Solanum	
Creeping Jenny (Lysimachia)	I	pseudocapsicum)	3
Crown of Thorns (Euphorbia milli)	3	Kalanchoe (Botanical name)	I
Daffodil (Narcissus)	3,4	King Palm (Seaforthia elegans)	I
Dieffenbachia (Species)	2	Lantana (Botanical name)	3
Donkey Tail (Sedum morganianum)	I	Licorice Plant (Glycyrrhizia lepidata)	5
Dracaena Indivisa (Cordyline indivisa)	I	Lilac (Syringa)	I
Dumbcane (Dieffenbachia amoena)	2	Lipstick Plant (Aeschynanthus lobbianus)	I
Emerald Duke (Philodendron hastatum)	2	Madagascar Dragon (Dracaena margiante)	I
Emerald Ripple (Peperomia caperata)	I	Madagascar Jasmine (Stephanotis	
Eucalyptus globulus (Species)	I–3	floribunda)	I
False Aralia (Dizygotheca elegantissima)	I	Madagascar Lace Plant (Aponogeton	
Fiddleleaf Fig (Ficus lyrata)	4	fenestralis)	I
Foxglove (Digitalis purpurea)	3	Majesty (Philodendron hastatum)	2
Fuchsia hybrida (Botanical name)	I	Manzanita (Arctostaphylos)	I
Gardenia (Species)	I	Marble Queen (Scundapsus aureus)	2
Geranium (Pelargonium)	4	Marigold (Calandula or Tagetes)	I
Geranium (Senecio petasitis)	3,4	Maternity or Pregnant Plant (Kalanchoe	
Giant White Inch Plant (Tradescantia		pinnata)	I
albiflora)	I	Mistletoe (Phoradendron flavescens)	3
Glacier Ivy (Hedera graceria)	3	Monkey Plant (Ruella makoyana)	I

Moon Magic (Pilia 'moon magic')   I
Mother-in-Law Tongue (Sansevieria trifasciata)   I
Mother of Pearls (Graptopetalum
    paraguayense)   I
Needlepoint Ivy (Hedera helix 'needlepoint')   3
Nephthytis (Syngonium podophyllum
    albolineatum)   2
Nightshade (Solanum nigrum)   3
Norfolk Island Pine (Araucarica excelsia)   I
Oleander (Nerium oleander)   3
Painted Needle (Coleus)   I
Palm (Species)   I
Pansy (Viola tricolor)   I
Parlor Ivy (Philodendron cordatum)   2
Parlor Palm (Chamaedorea elegans)   I
Peacock Plant (Calathea)   I
Peperomia (Peperomia caperata)   I
Petunia (Species)   I
Philodendron (Species)   2
Philodendron Leaf Peperomia (Peperomia
    scandens variegata)   I
Photinia Arbutifolia (Botanical name)   3
Piggyback Begonia (Begonia hispida
    cucullifera)   I
Piggyback Plant (Tolmiea memziesii)   I
Pilea (Botanical name)   I
Pink Polka Dot Plant (Hypoestes)   I
Plectranthus (Botanical name)   I
Poinsettia (Euphorbia pulcherrima)   3
Ponytail Palm (Beaucarenia recurvata)   I
Pothos (Scindapsus aureus)   2
Pot Mum (Chrysanthemum mortiforium)   3,4
Prayer Plant (Maranta leuconeuna)   I
Privet (Ligustrum species)   3
Purple Velvet or Passion Plant (Gynura
    aurantiaca)   I
Purple Tiger (Calathea)   I
Pyrancanta (Botanical name)   5
Ranunculus (Botanical name)   3,4
Red Princess (Philodendron hastatum)   2
Rhododendron (Rhododendron
    occidentale)   3

Ripple Ivy (Hedera helix 'ripple')   3
Rose (Rosa species)   I-4
Rubber Tree (Ficus elastica decora)   4
Saddle Leaf (Philodendron selloum)   2
Sago Plant (Cycas revoluta)   3
Schefflera (Brassaia actinophylla)   I
Sedum (Botanical name)   I
Sensitive Plant (Mimosa pudica)   I
Silver Tree (Pilea 'silver tree')   I
Snake Plant (Sansevieria trifasciata)   I
Spathiphyllum (Botanical name)   2
Spider Mum (Chrysanthemum
    morifolium)   3,4
Split Leaf Philodendron (Monstera
    deliciosa)   2
Sprengeri Fern (Asparagus densiflorus
    'sprengeri')   4
Stag Horn Fern (Platycerium bifurcatum)   I
Star Jasmine (Trachelospermum
    jasminoides)   I
String of Hearts (Creopegia woodii)   I
String of Pearls (Senecio rowleyanus or
    Senecio herreianus)   3,4
Swedish Ivy (Plectranthus australis)   I
Sweet Pea (Lathyrus odoratus)   3
Tahitian Bridal Veil (Gibasis geneculata)   I
Ti Plant (Cordyline terminalis)   I
Tulip (Botanical name)   4
Umbrella Plant (Cyperus alternifolius)   3
Umbrella Tree (Schefflera actinophylla)   I
Vinca (Species)   3
Wandering Jew (Tradescantia albiflora)   I
Wandering Jew, Red and White
    (Zebrina pendula)   I
Warneckei (Dracaena dermensis)   I
Wax Plant (Hoya exotica)   I
Weeping Fig (Ficus benjamina)   4
Wisteria (Botanical name)   3
Zebra Plant (Aphelandra squarrosa)   I

Source: Regional Poison Control Center,
University of California, Davis

PAINTS AND FINISHES

> **WARNING:** Harmful or fatal if swallowed. May cause slight skin irritation and eye irritation. Vapor and spray mist may be harmful if inhaled.
>
> **CAUTION:** Use with adequate ventilation. Where ventilation is inadequate use a suitable respirator. In case of eye contact, flush eyes immediately with plenty of water for at least 15 minutes. Do not take internally. Keep out of reach of children.

There are many other warnings to be found on paint products depending on their uses and formulas. Generally they are quite lengthy and explain in detail what to do in case of ingestion or overexposure to fumes.

All paint is made from four categories of ingredients: **resins,** for adhesion and durability; **pigments,** for color and hiding power; **additives,** to enhance performance properties; and **solvents,** usually the largest component found in paint, which serve as carriers to dissolve and disperse the other ingredients. Paints generally are classified according to the type of solvent they contain—oil-based paints contain **volatile organic chemical (VOC)** solvents (40 to 60 percent), and water-based paints use water as the primary solvent (though they still generally contain 5 to 10 percent VOC solvents).

In the Los Angeles basin, famous for its smog, one of the larger sources of VOCs is paints for buildings and other structures. According to the California Air Resources Board, more than half (100 million pounds) of the annual 176 million pounds of VOC emissions generated in California come just from paints and coatings. In the Los Angeles area, paints release more VOCs than all of the region's oil refineries and gas stations *combined.* The EPA has estimated that nationally, VOC emissions from architectural paints and coatings exceed 11 billion pounds each year. Southern California has the strictest VOC regulations for paints in the country, requiring emissions of no more than 250 grams per liter.

A Johns Hopkins University study found that more than 300 toxic chemicals and 150 carcinogens may be present in paint. They include **aerosol propellants, ammonia, benzene, ethanol, formaldehyde, glycols, kerosene, lead, pentachlorophenol, phenol, plastics (acrylonitrile, latex, phenolformaldehyde resin, polyester, polyurethane, tetrafluoroethylene), toluene, trichloroethylene,** and **xylene.**

SAFE SOLUTIONS

Because of concerns about the effects of VOCs on air pollution, most solvent-based paints are being phased out. In California, it is illegal to sell solvent-based paints in sizes larger than very small cans. So even major paint manufacturers are providing safer paints.

One of the leaders is Glidden, with their **Spred 2000.** When independently tested at one gram VOC per liter, no VOCs were detected. This paint is available through Glidden dealers across the country (look in the Yellow Pages for one nearest you). My husband painted our kitchen with it. We purchased it at a local store, could have it tinted to any color we wanted, and it was competitively priced. It was easy to spread, dried quickly, didn't smell, and looks great. If you can't find this paint and are limited to buying paint at a local store, at least choose a water-based latex paint over a solvent-based paint.

For years the most popular paint used by people with chemical sensitivities has been the whole line of paints manufactured by **AFM.** Though not sold in stores, they can be ordered by mail from *Allergy Relief Shop, Allergy Resources, American Environmental Health Foundation, The Living Source,* and *Nontoxic Environments.*

Another choice is the natural paints and finishes imported from Germany. **Auro** products (paints, oil finishes, varnishes, and lacquers) are the only plant-based natural paints and finishing products I know of—they contain no petrochemical ingredients of any kind. Colors come from earth pigments. We painted the exterior of our house with Auro paints. While they give a beautiful finish and the colors are gorgeous, they require some patience and new skill to work with (you have to mix your own colors, for instance); they are expensive; and they also have a very strong odor (not toxic, but strong). But I also used Auro clear finish on my desk, and I adore it. It is very soft, and I can feel the wood right through it. There's no hard finish that separates you from the wood. **Auro** products can be ordered by mail from *Earth Studio* or *Sinan Company.*

Livos products (paints, oil finishes, shellac) also are imported from Germany and made from similar natural ingredients, but their paints and some other products contain a nontoxic petrochemical solvent. This doesn't make them less safe (in fact, the company claims their nontoxic petrochemical solvent is safer than Auro's natural solvent). I think the issue between the two is whether or not you want 100 percent natural ingredients. Otherwise, as far as I can tell, they are pretty much the same. Livos products can be ordered by mail from *The Natural Choice.*

Then we come to paints of a completely different sort. **Old-Fashioned Milk Paint** (order from *The Old-Fashioned Milk Paint Company* or *Shaker Workshops West*) is a casein-based paint that is great for furniture, wood, and walls (but may tend to mold in damp locations such as kitchens or bathrooms). It comes in powder form, and you mix it up. It's what our ancestors used before we had plastic paints.

In the wood-finishes department, there are so many new water-based finishes on the market I couldn't begin to list them here. One product I have used with great success is **Flecto Varathane Diamond Finish,** which was recommended to me by the cabinetmaker who built my kitchen cabinets. It gives a hard, waterproof finish that is easy to clean. The can says "low odor," "water cleanup," "2 hour dry"—look for similar indicators on labels of other wood finishes. I had no trouble finding this product at a local store, where other, more toxic finishes by this same manufacturer are sold.

As much as I like to support small businesses, I am making a point here to include paints and finishes made by major manufacturers and to encourage you to use them. These manufacturers sell millions of gallons of products, and if we consumers show them there is a market, they will reduce and eliminate toxic substances in their other products. But if we refuse to buy their good products because they also make toxic products, they have no choice economically but to continue to cater to the market segment that hasn't yet made the switch to safer products.

You can make your own whitewash and milk paint at home. Here are some formulas.

White or Colored Interior Whitewash

Stir 5 pounds hydrated lime into 1 gallon water and let sit overnight. The next morning, add powdered pigment (buy this from the paint store, or natural earth pigments from **Earth Studio, The Natural Choice,** or **Sinan Company**) to the lime water until you reach the desired shade. Remember that the mixture will be further diluted and the paint will dry to a lighter color. Dissolve 1½ pounds salt in 2 quarts warm water and add to the lime mixture. Stir thoroughly and continue to stir every 10 minutes or so while applying the wash. Makes about 2½ gallons. Store leftovers in a tightly closed container.

White or Colored Exterior Whitewash

Stir 5 pounds hydrated lime into 1 gallon water and let sit overnight. The next morning, add powdered pigment to the lime water until you reach the desired shade. Keep in mind that the mixture will be further diluted and that the paint will dry to a lighter color. Dissolve 1½ pounds salt and 1 pound alum in 3 quarts warm water, add to the lime mixture, and place on stove to heat. In a separate pot, melt 1 pound tallow. When both are hot, stir together and apply while still hot. Makes about 3 gallons.

Milk Paint

Pour just enough water in instant nonfat dry milk to reconstitute it into a smooth syrup. Add powdered pigment in small amounts until the desired shade is reached. Apply several coats to raw wood with a brush or rag for a flat finish much like that of latex wall paint.

Another way to make milk paint is to put 6 ounces of hydrated lime into a bucket and add enough milk to make it the thickness of cream (you will need ½ gallon of milk in all). Stir in 4 ounces linseed oil, a little at a time, and add the rest of the milk. Sprinkle 3 pounds finely powdered calcium carbonate over the top and let it sink in before stirring it well into the mixture. Add powdered pigment for color, if desired.

CARPETING AND FLOORING

Synthetic carpet is made from a complex blend of as many as 120 chemicals that can emit many hazardous chemicals. They include **pesticides** (such as **antimicrobials**) **neurotoxic solvents** (such as **toluene** and **xylene**), and the potent carcinogen **benzene. Formaldehyde** also is commonly emitted from carpets, according to reports by the EPA and the Consumer Product Safety Commission (CPSC).

In 1984, I wrote in *Nontoxic & Natural*:

> Avoid synthetic wall-to-wall carpeting. If your floor is laid with it, seriously consider removing it and the padding beneath and installing some type of nontoxic flooring. These carpets not only release minute particles of synthetic materials in the air as they wear, but they and the polyurethane foam padding underneath often outgas vapors of toxic chemicals such as formaldehyde and pentachlorophenol (from the backing), and are treated with mothproofing, soil repellents, moisture repellents, and other finishes. If the subfloor is particleboard, remove it or thoroughly seal it from any living space above and below, because it outgasses formaldehyde heavily.

There were no scientific studies at the time to back this recommendation, but I could see that carpets were making people (including myself) very sick.

It didn't take long for the scientific verification. After a 1988 incident at the offices of the Environmental Protection Agency during which more than 10 percent of the employees reported symptoms after exposure to new carpeting, the EPA, the Consumer Product Safety Commission (CPSC), and other groups began investigating the toxicity of synthetic wall-to-wall carpeting.

Reported symptoms were as diverse as burning eyes, memory problems, chills and fever, sore throats, joint pain, chest tightness, cough, numbness, nausea, dizziness, light-headedness, blurred or double vision, nervousness, depression, and difficulty concentrating. Many reported newly acquired chemical sensitivities after a few days to a few weeks of exposure, and some required hospitalization.

EPA employees made their own analysis of the air-quality data. Based on information from a 1987 University of Arizona study on carpeting which isolated the chemical compound **4-phenylcyclohexene,** they began to monitor for this chemical and found it to be the culprit.

4-phenylcyclohexene is a by-product that is created when **styrene** and **butadiene** are combined to make the latex backing used on almost every carpet for the last thirty to forty years. No one knows how to eliminate its production from the current manufacturing process. Creation of 4-PC is unpredictable; it may be in one sample and not in another.

While industry claims that animal tests show 4-PC to be harmless, an EPA risk-assessment group predicted that it could create nervous system and genetic problems.

Levels of 4-PC to 20 parts per billion (ppb) have been measured in new carpet. This is the chemical that creates "new carpet smell." Four days after installation, levels fall to about 10 ppb, and after about two months, levels decrease to approximately 1 to 2 ppb. You can smell 4-PC down to about .5 ppb. Thus, the EPA has determined that synthetic carpet is a major contributor to indoor air pollution.

In 1991, after the CPSC had received at least 500 complaints about adverse reactions to carpet, New York Attorney General Robert Abrams published a consumer alert. The health effects listed in the alert include flulike symptoms, rashes, worsened respiratory conditions, asthma, and multiple chemical sensitivities. The alert warns also that children are especially at risk, and pregnant women "should also avoid these fumes as they may be harmful to the child." The attorneys general of twenty-six states petitioned the CPSC to require health warnings on new carpet and installation material, but the CPSC refused, saying it was "premature."

Then, in 1992, the alarm about carpets was sounded by **Anderson Laboratories,** a commercial testing lab (they can also test your carpet). Using a standard method that was developed for the U.S. military to test for the presence of nerve gases, researcher Dr. Rosalind Anderson exposed mice to air blown across small samples of carpet both new and up to *twelve* years old, that had caused illness in people. The tests revealed severe neurological, neuromuscular, and respiratory abnormalities in the mice. Some died. This was true even for a sample of carpet as small as seven square inches. Autopsies on the mice showed brain and liver lesions as well as kidney degeneration. Other medical studies have shown a higher incidence of central nervous system damage and lymphocytic leukemia, as well as oral and testicular cancers, in people who lay carpets.

Another concern comes from the ability of carpet to trap and hold airborne household volatile organic compounds (VOCs) as well as lawn-care chemicals tracked in from outside. This is known as the "sink effect." Eventually these chemicals become a hazardous part of house dust, along with particles from the carpet fibers themselves.

Further EPA studies have shown that chemically contaminated carpet dust can be a significant source of chemical exposure for infants and toddlers. Not only are they more susceptible to the unhealthy effects of low-level exposure to chemicals, toddlers also tend to be exposed to a higher level of chemicals from carpet dust because they frequently put their hands in their mouths as they explore the world around them.

Among the many reports I've heard about illness after the installation of synthetic carpeting, perhaps the most dramatic is what happened to Kentucky resident Glenn Beebe after he installed seventy-nine square yards of new carpeting for his home-based business. On the first day, a noticeable pungent odor permeated the rooms. Spiders which had formerly crawled through the house were found immobilized on the new carpeting. After several months, the Beebe family began to experience difficulty in concentrating; headaches; nausea; unquenchable thirst; and burning of the eyes, nose, and sinuses.

In the fall, three office plants were purchased, and within a couple of days the leaves began to turn black. The family's symptoms worsened—they now experienced depression, skin rashes, and insomnia. Finally the carpet was removed and the spiders returned. The Beebes' symptoms lessened, but after nine months of exposure, they found themselves to be hypersensitive to all kinds of irritants.

The Beebes' carpet was tested by the Northern Kentucky Environmental Services and found to release vapors of **ethylbenzene, formaldehyde, methacrylic acid, toluene, amines,** and **styrene.** The Beebes obtained from the carpet manufacturer an additional list of chemicals found in carpeting, which includes **xylene, benzene, acrylic oligomers,** and thirty-two other toxics with such tongue-twisting names as **cyclopentadiene-ethenyl-2-ethylene.**

If you aren't yet convinced to remove your carpet, let me tell you what happened when my husband and I bought the house we currently live in. We had the house inspected for carpenter ants and were given the certification that there were no carpenter ants in our house. After we moved in, we took up the carpet, and underneath it was swarming with carpenter ants, slowly eating away our living room floor. Ugh!

SAFE SOLUTIONS

If you can't take up your carpet, use **AFM Carpet Guard,** a water-soluble siliconate carpet finish that reacts with moisture and carbon monoxide in the air to form an insoluble water- and odor-resistant barrier. I've used this and it really works. Order it by mail from *Allergy Relief Shop, Allergy Resources, American Environmental Health Foundation, The Living Source,* or *Nontoxic Environments.*

AREA RUGS
If you must have carpet, the first choice would be an area rug made of cotton, cotton/wool blend, sheepskin, or unmothproofed wool without jute or latex backing. Some of these rugs have strong-smelling finishes that may or may not be removed. Be sure to check the label on wool rugs to confirm that the rug has not been mothproofed. Many natural-fiber area rugs can be found in

local import and department stores (sometimes they are in the bath department), or try one of these sources.

Allegro Rug Weaving Company: stunning custom handwoven area rugs from 100 percent wool and unbleached linen, dyed with natural dyes

Garnet Hill: beautiful natural-fiber area rugs and natural-rubber underlay pads

Janice Corporation: natural-cotton rag rugs

Sajama Alpaca: area rugs made from alpaca yarns, hand spun and dyed soft colors with plants indigenous to the highlands of Bolivia. The wool comes from animals who live on the open range, kept by local people who spin the yarn themselves.

Seventh Generation: many cotton and jute area rugs

NATURAL FIBER CARPET

Wall-to-wall natural-fiber carpets also can be purchased for covering natural wood or cement subfloors. For carpet padding, use a "rag pad" made of recycled rags and polypropylene felt ("rag pad" is a standard industry term any carpet dealer should recognize). Natural-fiber carpeting is rare in stores, but can be ordered by mail.

Hendricksen's Natürlich: natural carpets made from untreated wool, cotton, seagrass, and sisal; natural latex backing; natural and less-toxic adhesives; wool carpet pads; and natural carpet shampoo and spot remover

Carousel Carpets: a wide selection of natural-fiber carpets; unique hand-loomed natural-color linen and cotton woven rugs, without latex backing, in a wide variety of patterns; and custom-made *anything* (almost). Ask for "Casual Trends" and "Cotton Trends."

Colin Campbell & Sons: "Nature's Carpet" line of carpeting—a "complete absence of chemicals at every stage of the carpet's manufacture and composition"—

made of wool, nontoxic latex from a natural rubber base, and natural jute, in an attractive range of naturally occurring colors; 100 percent natural jute and animal hair undercushions

Dellinger: plush, thick cotton carpet without latex backing, which can be purchased in its natural state or dyed to match any color (ask for style "3333 Linwood")

Sinan Company: untreated, undyed, unmothproofed wool carpet with natural latex backing in three neutral variegated natural colors, imported from Europe

HARDWOOD

If you install new hardwood floors, buy prefinished hardwood floor tiles that have a baked-on finish, of which there are several types on the market (order by mail from **Environmental Home Center**). Choose those that come in six-inch squares and are held together with wire; avoid the twelve-inch squares that are glued together or have foam padding underneath. Remove the tiles from the box and air them outside in the sun for one day before installing. Lay the tiles on a particleboard or cement subfloor with white or yellow glue. Be sure to seal the particleboard subfloor and allow it to dry thoroughly before applying glue: it is not yet known whether dried glue and wood alone form an adequate seal from the formaldehyde gases coming from the particleboard.

Alternatively, you also could install a conventional hardwood strip floor, hammering the nails diagonally in the groove of the tongue-and-groove wood to avoid the need for toxic solvent-based wood filler.

NATURAL LINOLEUM

Natural linoleum is another good choice. Made from linseed oil, pine tree resins, wood flour from deciduous trees, and cork, mixed with chalk, clay, and colored mineral pigments, on a jute backing, it provides an attractive and durable floor covering. Natural linoleum can be ordered from **Hendricksen's Natürlich** or **Environmental Home Center.**

CORK

Cork tiles also are becoming popular natural floor coverings. Durable and economical, they are warm underfoot and provide noise insulation while looking rich and beautiful. Cork tiles can be ordered by mail from **Hendricksen's Natürlich, Environmental Home Center,** and **The Natural Choice.**

OTHER FLOORING

Other types of flooring are much safer to use than synthetic carpet, and easier to find and less expensive to install than natural-fiber carpeting. Use ceramic tile, solid hardwood, brick, marble and other stone tiles, or terrazzo, available at your local flooring and building-supply stores.

FURNITURE

Most home furnishings are made from materials that give off toxic fumes.

Bookcases and desks are often made from particleboard and plywood, which outgas **formaldehyde,** an irritant to eyes, nose, and throat and a suspected carcinogen.

Pillows and padding on stuffed sofas and chairs are generally made from polyurethane foam plastic and can be covered with **acrylic, polyester,** or **polyvinyl chloride** plastic covers. Most upholstery fabrics are coated with a formaldehyde resin to resist stains. One study showed that the addition of furniture to an otherwise empty room tripled formaldehyde levels.

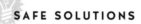

SAFE SOLUTIONS

As much as possible, purchase furniture made from natural materials.

I just realized, as I was thinking about what to write here, that I have very little furniture in my house. My desk is a big old mahogany library table that I bought at a garage sale for twenty dollars, which my husband sanded and refinished for me with **Auro** natural wood finish (order from **Sinan Company**). I'm sitting on an old oak office armchair that I bought at the salvage yard for twenty-five dollars while we were looking for a bathtub—it didn't need refinishing, but I did add two feather pillows for comfort, for which I sewed my own cotton covers. The walls are lined with pine bookcases my husband and I built together, which are now filled with books.

In the living/dining room is a big, yet graceful, old sofa that we purchased at a storage auction for fifty dollars. Last summer we had the spring-filled cushions refurbished with new cotton and the whole thing covered with linen upholstery fabric. At the same time, we re-covered my favorite wing chair—originally from my great-aunt's attic—with an untreated cotton upholstery fabric. I found it relatively easy to identify these untreated natural-fiber upholstery fabrics, because those with formaldehyde finishes are clearly labeled as a positive selling point. We have a few solid-wood end tables that I picked up at Crate & Barrel. After a couple of days in the sun, whatever finish was on them became completely odorless.

Our dining table was another garage-sale find—another library table, this one solid oak, and it didn't even need refinishing. Around it are four Shaker chairs that my husband and I built from kits from **Shaker Workshops.** We applied our own nontoxic finish to the wood pieces, and we wove the cotton-webbing seats (it really is a two-person job).

When purchasing solid-wood furniture, choose unfinished pieces or those protected with natural finishes. Check wood furniture carefully to make sure it is indeed *solid* wood. Often the front will be wood and the backs, sides, inside shelves, and drawer bottoms will be particleboard or plywood. Particleboard can be very convincingly veneered, but it poses no barrier to formaldehyde.

Metal furniture is available in a number of styles: modern, high-tech functional, outdoor, and office. It can be the least-toxic furniture available, if care is taken to avoid such components as synthetic seat pads and soft vinyl finishes. Avoid particleboard in metal furnishings, especially under plastic-laminate desktops.

Consider, too, buying used furniture. There are many attractive and functional pieces that can be recycled for your home or office and inexpensively refinished or recovered. Look in the Yellow Pages under "Furniture Dealers—Used" and "Office Furniture and Equipment—Used," or check at flea markets and storage auctions.

Upholstered furniture should be covered with a prewashed natural-fiber fabric and stuffed with cotton or wool batting or feathers. An economical way to have custom upholstered furniture is to buy used sofas and chairs and have the frames recovered and restuffed.

> *Bright Future Futon:* wood frames and cotton or organic-cotton futons for convertible sofa beds and chairs, with coffee and end tables to match
>
> *Shaker Workshops* and *Shaker Workshops West:* fine Shaker furniture ready-made and in significantly less expensive kits (you can apply your own natural finishes). Each catalog has a different selection, so if you like Shaker furniture, order them both.
>
> *Sofa U Love:* down-filled sofas with natural, finish-free cotton slipcovers and cushion pillows
>
> *Willsboro Wood Products:* rustic, simple furniture made in the Adirondacks from knotty native cedar; unfinished chairs, rockers, tables, loveseats, bed frames, dressers, and desks with dowel-in-hole construction

LIGHT

Most of the information about the biological effects of artificial light has been accumulated only recently. There has been much observation on this subject, but relatively few scientific studies have been conducted. The observations, however, have been interesting enough to call into question the safety of artificial light, and to prompt scientific investigation.

The problem with artificial light sources seems to be that the spectrum of the light produced is not the same as the spectrum produced by natural sunlight. Our bodies need the natural light of the sun, and tend to function somewhat less than optimally when we are forced to spend most of our hours under unnatural light.

Exposure to artificial light has been associated with decreased calcium absorption (making one more susceptible to osteoporosis); dental caries; fatigue; decreased visual acuity; hyperactivity; and changes in heart rate, blood pressure, electrical brain-wave patterns, hormonal secretions, and the body's natural cyclical rhythms. The National Institute of Mental Health has preliminary data that suggest a link between mood and light, with a striking relationship between light and depression.

Fluorescent lights are particularly suspect. Not only is the spectrum incorrect, but the fixtures produce an audible hum that has been connected to increased stress. Fluorescent lights also have a very fast flicker, which produces effects ranging from visual irritation to epileptic seizures. The prestigious British medical journal *Lancet* reported an association between melanoma, a serious form of skin cancer, and fluorescent light, though the study is not definitive. Skin rashes from fluorescent lights also have been noted in medical journals.

SAFE SOLUTIONS

It seems to make sense that the light sources to which we are exposed should be similar to the lighting environment in which we evolved in nature. There also is some evidence that natural light helps the body to process toxic substances, and this action could be inhibited if sufficient natural light were not available to support body functions.

It is important for our bodies to be exposed to natural light on a daily basis—just as important as getting proper nutrition, sleep, and exercise. Spend as much time outdoors as you can. This doesn't mean direct sunlight, or even being in the sun at all. Shaded light is perfectly acceptable; in fact, it's preferable. The only criterion is that it be *natural*. At home you can sit on a screened porch, under a shaded tree, or next to an open window (a closed window blocks the essential ultraviolet rays). At the office, make a point of eating meals outdoors and getting outside during your lunch hour. Taking breaks for walks during the day also will help.

WALLPAPER

This is the first time I've included wallpaper in one of my books, because it's the first time I've had some safer wallpapers to recommend.

Wallpapers generally are either made of **vinyl** plastic or have a plastic finish on the paper, and there are **solvents** in the adhesive.

SAFE SOLUTIONS

Look for wallpapers that are plain papers, without plastic finishes.

One type of wallpaper has the pattern simply pressed into paper made from 90-percent recycled cotton, to give an embossed texture to the walls. This type of wallpaper was common in Victorian homes. You can just paint right over it. It's more interesting than a flat wall and can hide a multitude of flaws. Order by mail from *Crown Corporation* or *Eurotap.*

Pallas Textiles sells "Earth Paper," a densely textured, stuccolike wallpaper made of paper pulp, stone powder, and straw, with a water-based finish.

Pattern People makes custom wallpapers using clay-coated papers and water-based paints. You can choose from stock patterns or create your own.

Looking for nontoxic wallpaper adhesives, I discovered they are becoming commonplace. Even Home Depot sells water-based adhesives.

So here's another victory for safer shoppers. We *are* making a difference!

WINDOW COVERINGS

The problem with window coverings is, once again, plastics.

Polyester fabrics and **vinyl** window shades become even more of a problem when the sun shines on the window, warming the fabric and causing them to outgas even more.

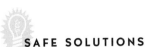

SAFE SOLUTIONS

Choose natural-fiber curtains, drapes, or blinds. I haven't seen them in many stores, but you can order natural-cotton curtains in many styles from *Country Curtains,* and nicely textured thick natural-cotton draperies from *Homespun Fabrics.* These catalogs also carry wooden curtain rods. Other options include aluminum or wood miniblinds.

Chapter 12

BABIES AND CHILDREN

PRODUCTS FOR INFANTS AND CHILDREN carry the same dangers as their adult counterparts—baby food contains the same carcinogenic **pesticides** and crib sheets are saturated with the same **formaldehyde** resins (since formaldehyde can cause insomnia, is it any wonder babies stay awake all night crying?). It is even more important, however, that children be protected from toxics, because they are exposed more often to these hazards. Also, because of children's physiology, every exposure puts them at greater risk.

Children's playing habits cause them to come in more direct contact with toxics. Indoors, children crawl around on carpets, rubbing themselves on formaldehyde-based resins and breathing air close to the floor, where heavier pollutants settle. Outdoors, they roll around on grass and climb trees, coming into contact with pesticides and other toxic hazards in the soil.

In addition, children consume larger amounts of fruit juice and vegetables, which are common vehicles for pesticide exposure unless they are organically grown. Children also drink two to five times more water than adults, giving them an increased ratio of body weight to water pollutants.

Physiologically, children are more vulnerable because of their higher metabolic rate. They require more oxygen, and they breathe in two to three times more air (and therefore pollutants) relative to body size than adults. Children are more physically active than adults, which also increases their breathing rate and intake of pollutants. And, because children suffer more respiratory illness, their frequently blocked nasal passages make them breathe more often through their mouths, which doesn't filter out particles the way nose breathing does. Once ingested, toxic substances can injure lung tissue and be absorbed into the bloodstream.

Once ingested, metals like lead and cadmium—both found in tap water—are absorbed more efficiently through the gastrointestinal tract of the young. Children up to age eight, for example, can absorb up to five times as much lead as adults, and they retain it longer.

Studies indicate also that the young are less capable of binding toxic chemicals to plasma proteins. Protein binding is important because it prevents toxic agents from reaching sites like the brain, where they can do damage.

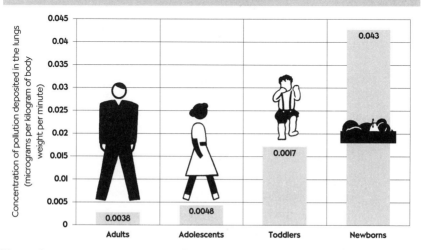

CONCENTRATION OF PARTICLE POLLUTION IN THE LUNGS
CHILDREN VS. ADULTS*

Concentration of pollution deposited in the lungs (micrograms per kilogram of body weight per minute)

Adults	Adolescents	Toddlers	Newborns
0.0038	0.0048	0.0017	0.043

*For particles 1 micron in size at a concentration of 1 milligram per cubic meter

Source: University of California, Irvine, Air Pollution Laboratory

Many of the detoxification systems that normally neutralize and excrete chemicals in the liver and kidneys are immature in young children, and the immune system is not fully functional. Humans do not build up adult levels of certain antibodies until around ten years of age. So, in effect, your child is walking around in the world, being bombarded with the same toxic exposure as adults but without the natural protective armor adults have.

The blood-brain barrier that protects the human brain from some toxic chemicals is not completely formed in the infant, either. Once inside the brain, neurotoxins can have devastating effects. Cells of the developing nervous system are actively growing, dividing, and migrating as well as forming complex networks. Neurotoxic chemicals can interfere with these steps, leading to permanent problems like learning disabilities.

It is especially important that newborns be protected from household toxics, for their bodily systems are the most vulnerable of all. Yet, this is the time when many parents—albeit with good intentions—create very toxic worlds for their babies to live in. A room often is redecorated into a nursery, with new paint, new carpets, washable vinyl wallpaper with little animals, a new crib with a synthetic mattress and brand-new no-iron sheets, new easy-care synthetic clothing, disinfectants (especially disinfectants to protect the baby from germs), scented baby lotions and powders, stuffed animals made from synthetic fibers, plastic rattles. . . . And as the child grows, there is more remodeling, more new toys, more new clothes. I'm not saying here that children shouldn't have or don't need new things, but the constant newness of everything gives children more frequent toxic exposure than adults would have, who tend to use things for a longer period of time.

SAFE SOLUTIONS

All of the safe solutions given in other chapters of this book will serve to protect your little ones as well as you and the rest of your family. In this chapter, I'll focus specifically on providing resources especially for kid-size products.

Your local natural-food store will carry organically grown baby food and natural baby-care products; however, most other items you won't find in a local baby store unless you have one that is exceptionally aware. My best suggestion is to order the *After the Stork, Baby Bunz & Company, Biobottoms, Hanna Anderson, Motherwear,* and *Natural Baby Company* mail-order catalogs and subscribe to *Mothering* magazine—these sources will lead you to most of what you need.

CRIBS

Browsing through some baby catalogs, I came across one that quoted me (!): "No agency is regulating the levels of toluene diisocyanate that are being emitted from your polyurethane, foam-stuffed, polyester-covered, fireproofed mattress." All the same chemicals that come from an adult bed are present in a baby's crib, but your baby gets even more exposure because he spends most of his sleeping and waking hours in the crib, instead of just the one-third of life adults spend in bed.

In addition to the **plastics, flame retardants,** and **formaldehyde** finishes present in beds and bedding, cribs have soft plastics for waterproofing surfaces. All these emit fumes that can be harmful to baby's health.

SAFE SOLUTIONS

The best investment you can make in your child's future is a natural place to sleep. From mattress to receiving blankets, every part of the crib is now available made from natural—even organic—cotton and wool. You probably won't find natural crib components at your local department store or baby outlet, but you can order the pieces easily by mail.

> *Allergy Relief Shop:* cotton mattresses, natural cotton quilted mattress pads, cotton pillows, cotton bed linens and blankets, cotton bumper pads, and cotton flannel waterproof pads
>
> *Bright Future Futon:* natural- and organic-cotton futons and pillows
>
> *Clothcrafters:* cotton flannel sheeting bonded to natural rubber for waterproof bed pads

Garnet Hill: cotton bed linens, blankets, curtains, and quilts, all with whimsical designs

Heart of Vermont: completely organic wool/cotton and all-cotton futons, cotton futon covers, cotton- and wool-filled comforters, cotton "top mattresses" (very thick mattress pads) filled with cotton or wool, washable cotton flannel mattress pads, wool/cotton innerspring mattresses and box springs, cotton and wool pillows, cotton receiving blankets, cotton flannel and chambray crib linens

Janice Corporation: complete cotton crib sets that include mattress, mattress pad, mattress cover, and knit fitted sheets

Karen's Nontoxic Products: organic, cotton and cotton pillows, organic-cotton futons, cotton percale and flannel bed linens; and handmade cotton quilts with custom-embroidered heart designs

The Natural Baby Company: complete cotton crib sets in colors and patterns or natural, cotton crib futons, wool pillows, naturally waterproof wool bed pads, cotton receiving and crib blankets in colors, and wool blankets

The Natural Bedroom: entirely natural crib environments, including cotton/wool innerspring mattresses, wool bumper pads, wool comforters, wool mattress pads, cotton percale or flannel bed linens, and organic-cotton baby blankets

Nontoxic Environments: cotton and cotton/wool crib mattresses, organic-cotton crib and receiving blankets, and organic-cotton "security blankets"

Organic Cottons: organic-cotton flannel or chambray crib linens, organic-cotton receiving blankets, wool comforters, and organic-cotton baby blankets

DIAPERS

Disposable diapers are made from **synthetic fibers** and other **plastics** and unknown **deodorizing chemicals** that are not compatible with a newborn baby's skin. In addition to diaper rash, complaints made to the Consumer Product Safety Commission include chemical burns, noxious chemical and insecticide odors, reports of babies pulling the diapers apart and putting pieces of plastic into their mouths and noses, plastic covers melting on baby's skin, and the chemical dyes on the diapers staining the baby's skin.

In addition, disposable diapers made from bleached white paper contain about 90 parts per trillion **dioxins,** which can cause cancer, birth defects, liver damage, and immune system suppression.

SAFE SOLUTIONS

Use 100 percent cotton cloth diapers with natural-fiber diaper covers. Even if you send the diapers out to a diaper service to be washed, you wind up spending less than you would buying disposables, and your baby will be so much more comfortable.

If you wash the diapers yourself, use the hottest water in your washing machine and wash with a gentle soap and borax (in the laundry-supplies department at your supermarket). Detergent residues can contribute to diaper rash, too. Then run the diapers through the hottest setting on your dryer for forty minutes or longer. This should be sufficient to kill bacteria. Whenever possible, air the diapers outdoors in sunlight, which acts as a natural disinfectant and whitener. Soaking soiled diapers in a mixture of a half cup of borax added to a pail of warm water will reduce odors and staining, and will make diapers more absorbent.

If your local baby store doesn't sell cloth diapers and diaper covers, you can order them by mail from *Baby Bunz & Company, Barbara Coole Designs, Biobottoms, The Living Source, Motherwear,* or *The Natural Baby Company.* Organic-cotton diapers can be ordered from *Allergy Resources, Karen's Nontoxic Products,* and *Organic Cottons.*

BABIES' AND KIDS' CLOTHING

In addition to the dangers from **synthetic fibers** and **formalde-hyde** finishes associated with adult clothing, there is another hazard associated with children's clothing—federal law requires all garments sold as sleepwear for infants and children to be flameproof. In the past, cotton sleepwear was flameproofed with **TRIS.** When TRIS was found to be carcinogenic, other chemicals (which have unknown health effects) were used, or else the sleepwear was made from nonflammable synthetic fibers. While TRIS no longer is used on new sleepwear, secondhand garments may have been treated. (Since the presence of TRIS probably is not on the label, I would steer clear of secondhand sleepwear.)

SAFE SOLUTIONS

Personally, I cannot understand why the government thinks a child needs flameproof sleepwear. I can understand a fire-retardant mattress to protect those who smoke in bed, but in my opinion the possible health effects of flame retardant chemicals, synthetic fibers, and formaldehyde finishes are far worse than the chance that a child will be caught in a fire.

My choice as a parent would be to use any natural-fiber garment as sleepwear—there are many that can be used as such even though they cannot be described as such or recommended for this purpose. Be creative. Oversized cotton T-shirts are a comfortable and inexpensive alternative.

I have had no difficulty finding an abundance of natural-fiber clothing for infants and children in local stores here in northern California. If you can't find what you need close to home, you can outfit your child from head to toe from mail-order catalogs.

> *After the Stork:* a big selection of attractive cotton casual and dress-up clothing for babies and kids, including mother/daughter outfits and real leather and canvas footwear

> *Barbara Coole Designs:* natural-cotton basics that can be dyed to bright colors

Biobottoms: a big selection of colorful playclothes and shoes for babies and kids

Castle Gray: hemp jumpsuits for babies

Garnet Hill: nice cotton clothes for kids

Hanna Anderson: brightly colored, high quality infants' and children's clothes imported from Scandinavia, made from sturdy cotton fabrics; and many "keep warm" items not in other catalogs—even cotton mittens

Karen's Nontoxic Products: organic-cotton and natural-cotton basics, some colored with low impact dyes

The Natural Baby Company: organic-cotton and cotton clothes, and natural-material shoes just for babies

Organic Cottons: organic-cotton basics for babies and kids

BABY FOOD

Like any other processed foods, baby formulas and baby foods may contain **artificial colors, artificial flavors, preservatives** and residues from **pesticides.** And even though they may be fortified with additional nutrients, they are no match for the nutrition provided by the complete whole foods of nature.

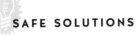

SAFE SOLUTIONS

The best choice for newborns by far is mother's milk. It is endowed with every nutrient your baby needs in the optimum proportions necessary for the perfect growth of your child's body. Breast-fed babies experience fewer illnesses and go to the doctor less often than those who are bottle-fed. Breastfeeding encourages the development of a lifelong bond and sense of security for your baby. And it's only natural—nature has provided mother's milk to feed the baby, so why replace it with anything else?

The **Motherwear** catalog is a complete resource for nursing mothers, filled with attractive natural-fiber fashions for discreet breastfeeding (some with darling matching baby clothes), cotton nursing bras, books on breastfeeding, and other nursing supplies. **Decent Exposures, Garnet Hill,** and **The Natural Baby Company** also have small selections of natural-fiber nursing bras and clothing. **Organic Cottons** has organic-cotton nursing tops and an organic-cotton baby sling.

While breastfeeding is universally accepted as the preferred method for feeding babies (even cans of formula state, "Experts recommend breastfeeding"), there are times when some mothers may prefer, or need, to feed their infants a commercial preparation. To my knowledge, there is no "natural" baby formula on the market (formula is not sold in natural-food stores), nor is it recommended that you make your own out of milk and sugar (particularly do not attempt to feed your baby milk and honey, since infants younger than six months of age cannot digest honey). Some commercial formulas sold in supermarkets are additive-free mixtures of milk, sugar (lactose or corn-based), fat, and nutrients, carefully combined with water to imitate mother's milk. Most major manufacturers also sell a milk-free soy-based formula (I had no trouble finding the soy formula here in northern California, where soy milk is very popular; if it isn't on your supermarket shelves, you can ask your grocer to order it). Read the ingredients and try different brands—though they all are made from the same ingredients, proportions differ (one brand listed sugar as the first ingredient, while another listed milk).

Do not feed unmodified cow's milk to your baby. Nature has designed human mother's milk for human babies; cow's milk is intended to nourish baby calves. Each provides for different nutritional needs. Cow's milk has more than three times the protein of human milk, which, in contrast, contains nearly twice the carbohydrates of cow's milk. The differences put stress on the baby's digestive system and kidneys, which can, in some cases, lead to intestinal bleeding and anemia.

There are a few mix-it-yourself emergency recipes for formula. However, I have not included them here because they require specialized ingredients, such as evaporated milk and corn syrup, that are not on hand in most kitchens. If you are going to keep these specialized ingredients available for emergencies, it's just as easy to keep formula on the shelf.

When your child is old enough to eat solid food, consider making your own baby food or choosing a brand of baby food made from organically grown foods. **Earth's Best** is one brand of organically grown baby food available in many natural-food stores and some supermarkets (and by mail from **Karen's Nontoxic Products**). **The Natural Baby Company** sells a baby-food grinder so you can make your own fresh baby food.

TOYS

A walk down the aisle of any toy store shows the prevalence of **plastics** used to make playthings. Though plastic may be an inexpensive material to make a product your child soon will outgrow, the outgassing of plastics is a major contributor to indoor air pollution, and a roomful of toys (particularly new ones) can easily envelop your child in a toxic cloud.

In one of my old newsletters, I printed a letter from a mother whose child was given a gift of a toy that consisted of a large yellowish clear plastic bowl with three small clear balls that had moving parts inside them. She wrote:

> The small balls were fine, but the large bowl had a terribly putrid odor when we removed it from the plastic bag. When we got home, I put it in the box and then into a closet. I called every store in town that carried it, and had them check their stocks. Each store said theirs also smelled bad.
>
> I decided to write to the company, and found a toll-free number on the box, so I called it. I was told that originally the bowl was made of the same plastic as the balls, but the balls scratched the bowl, so they began using a different plastic that would not scratch the bowl. That new plastic had a foul (but "safe") odor, so they added a vanilla fragrance [probably artificial] to the plastic to cover the foul odor.
>
> I was told that if I put the bowl out in the air for two weeks, the odor would disappear. I also noticed that the bowl had an oily feel to it, and was told that too would dis-

appear. I felt better, but decided the odor was too strong to leave the bowl in the house, so I put it on the patio. After two weeks it smelled the same, and still felt oily. I left it out in the rain and whatever other weather we had for *four months,* before the smell finally left. Still, after *nine months,* the bowl still has a slight smell, so we just don't use it. I am quite disturbed that the bowl is in fact not safe, and wonder how many babies have been and are going to be exposed to it, and what future harm it might cause.

This letter was written to me in 1985, and by 1995, the situation had not changed. Major toy manufacturers in America still are making mountains of plastic toys, even though the dangers of plastics of all kinds are increasingly becoming known.

Just as I was writing this, a copy of *The Green Guide* came in the mail, with a cover story about how Barbie dolls contain **polyvinyl chloride (PVC),** a plastic whose manufacture and disposal creates **dioxins**—the most toxic man-made substances known. While it is unlikely your child will be made ill by direct exposure to a Barbie doll, Barbie is toxic if you consider the entire life cycle of the toy, from its manufacture to disposal. The toxic exposure comes from air pollution caused by the disposal of Barbie, which, though indirect, is related to the product just the same.

SAFE SOLUTIONS

A visit to my local toy store did result in my finding a few wooden toys imported from Europe, but my recommendation to caring parents is to buy toys by mail. From catalogs, you can order all kinds of wooden and stuffed toys made from natural fibers.

The owner of *The Natural Baby Company,* whose catalog is filled with natural toys, has this to say about them:

I have a certain unscientific feeling that natural materials are better for my children's toys. (Scientists just "proved" that loving support during labor is beneficial, that chicken soup is good for colds, and that babies recover from illness quicker if you hold them. In some areas, science is a little slower than mothers.)

Some reasons for natural toys:

1. Kids do eat toys, so I'd prefer that they eat natural ones. A study on wood vs. plastic cutting boards showed significantly higher residual bacteria counts on the plastic ones.

2. Plastic toys break so fast that they end up costing much more!

3. Wild synthetic colors don't seem as peaceful for children as natural ones. Modern toys seem to try to pull the child out of their inner peaceful world and awaken them prematurely to our busy world. What's the rush?

4. The feel and sound of wood, cotton, and wool is ever so much more pleasing than that of plastic, acrylic, and vinyl.

5. Simple basic toys inspire years of inner creativity and fantasy play. Gimmicky toys inspire about 3 hours of noise and then a long, lonely shelf life.

Hearthsong was one of the earlier natural-toy catalogs. I remember when it first started, it was a small catalog created by a mother who lives not far from me. Now it is sixty-eight pages filled with wooden toys and games, natural-fiber dolls, delightful storybooks that connect your child to nature, and natural craft supplies that teach your child practical skills such as weaving, jewelry making, and rolling beeswax candles.

Nova Natural Toys and Crafts has many wooden toys that roll and rattle, natural-fiber stuffed dolls, wood building sets in unusual shapes, a complete set of wooden furniture and appliances to "play house," kid-size musical instruments, wooden dollhouses, lots of story- and songbooks, doll-making supplies, and fantasy dress-up costumes.

For Keeps Friends offers charming homemade natural-fiber dolls with cotton "skin," wool or cotton stuffing, nontoxic painted faces, and plant-dyed cotton or wool hair. Each has unique hair and eye colors and can be custom made to complement your child. Additional clothing, doll beds and cradles, cotton and wool bedtime cuddle bunnies, colorful big block pillows, and wooden Brio toys also are available.

Barbara Coole Designs takes children into the world of

fantasy with custom-made hand puppets, nontoxic face paints, and fantasy capes and hats. Stuffed animals and dolls made of organic cotton can be ordered from **Karen's Nontoxic Products, Nontoxic Environments,** and **Organic Cottons.**

My personal favorite toy catalog is **Ostheimer Wooden Toys.** Their simple, magical wooden toys are designed to awaken the imagination. Made of hardwoods finished with soft-color nontoxic paint, these heirloom quality toys come in the shapes of people, animals, plants, nature spirits, angels, castles . . . make enchanted forests, medieval towns, Indian villages. Each handmade piece has its own spirit.

BABY-CARE PRODUCTS

At the risk of sounding like a broken record, I'll just state for the final time in this chapter that body-care products for baby contain the same kinds of potentially hazardous ingredients as similar products designed for adults—**artificial colors, fragrances,** and **preservatives.** In particular, baby powder usually is made from **talc,** which may be contaminated with carcinogenic **asbestos.**

SAFE SOLUTIONS

Every natural-food store carries natural baby oil, talc-free baby powder and herbal salves—if they don't, ask them to, for these products are easily available through the distributors from which they obtain adult cosmetic products. Two exceptional brands worth mentioning are **Logona** and **Weleda.** Logona products are made from organically grown ingredients, and Weleda products are made from biodynamically grown ingredients whenever possible. Both brands are carried by some natural-food stores, or they can be ordered by mail from the **Logona USA** and **Weleda** catalogs.

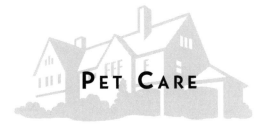

Chapter | 3

PET CARE

JUST AS PRODUCTS FOR KIDS carry the same dangers as their adult counterparts, products for pets have the same hazards as their human counterparts—pet food contains the same carcinogenic **pesticide** residues, and the pesticides used in flea collars are as toxic as the pesticides used to kill any other insects. And just as babies and children are more susceptible to the effects of toxic exposures than adults, so too are animals more susceptible to the effects of toxic exposures than humans.

Animals have long been used in toxicology tests as indicators of potential human dangers because physiologically, most are more sensitive to chemical exposures than we are. Also there is a strong correlation between what is harmful to an animal and what is harmful to humans. Even before animal testing of consumer products began, miners would carry canaries into coal mines—if the birds died, the miners knew harmful gases were present and it was time to leave. Similarly, our awareness of the dangers of pesticides began not because humans were becoming ill, but because of the disappearance of songbirds, who were dying of these toxic chemicals. Only later did we discover that pesticides are harmful to humans, too.

Virtually all substances found to cause cancer in animal studies also cause cancer in humans, so might we extrapolate that a product that causes cancer in humans also could cause cancer in our pets? So I would say that in addition to protecting *ourselves* from the possible exposures to toxins from pet-care products, it is prudent, for our pets' health, to protect *them* from toxic pet-care products (and toxic human products!) as well.

Pets are exposed to toxic substances through different routes than we are. Although both humans and pets inhale toxic pollutants from the air, our pets spend most of their lives on the floor, where fumes can be stronger. Airborne pollutants and dust in carpets and on floor surfaces can land on or be picked up by their fur and then be ingested when pets lick themselves clean. And remember, pets can't read warning labels or learn about toxins on their own (although I think my cats have a sixth sense to stay away from things that are bad for them), so they can't recognize exposures that may be potentially harmful to them.

Anyone who has a pet knows the companionship, devotion, and unconditional love an animal can provide. When we care for our pets with safe products, we give them some of that love in return.

SAFE SOLUTIONS

All of the safe solutions given in other chapters of this book will serve to protect your pets as well as you and the rest of your family. In this chapter, I'll focus on the dangers and alternatives for specific pet products.

Your local natural-food store will probably carry natural pet products, and many pet stores do as well. If you can't find what you are looking for, order **Natural Animal, The Natural Pet Care Company,** and **Shampoo-chez** catalogs. These specialty pet catalogs will provide most of what you need. In addition, **Allergy Resources** and **Karen's Nontoxic Products** carry some pet items.

FLEA CONTROL

IMPREGNATED FLEA COLLARS:

> **CAUTION:** Do not allow children to play with this collar. Dust will form on this collar during storage. Do not get dust or collar in mouth, harmful if swallowed. Do not get dust in eyes, will cause temporary pupillary constriction. In case of contact, flush eyes with water. Wash hands thoroughly with soap and water after handling collar. The dust released by this collar is a cholinesterase inhibitor.

INSECTICIDAL POWDERS AND SHAMPOOS:

> **WARNING:** Causes eye irritation. Do not get in eyes. Harmful if swallowed. While washing pets, avoid getting shampoo in animal's eyes. Do not use on kittens or puppies under six weeks of age.

AEROSOL FLEA BOMBS:

> **CAUTION:** Use only when area to be treated is vacated by humans and pets. Harmful if swallowed or absorbed through skin. Avoid breathing vapors or spray mist. Avoid contact with skin and eyes. Do not apply directly to food. In the home, all food-processing surfaces should be covered during treatment and thoroughly washed before use. Remove pets and cover fish aquariums and delicate plants before spraying. Remove all motor vehicles before use in garages.

Whatever you do, do not use chemical sprays, powders, or collars on your animals. Cats and dogs (and their owners) frequently are poisoned by these pesticides. In fact, most pet poisonings are the result of the **organophosphate** and **carbamate compounds** used to control fleas. Additionally, the active ingredients in flea-control products include the pesticides **DDVP, propoxur, diazinon,** and **carbaryl**—nerve poisons that are toxic to pets and humans and may cause long-term health problems.

Antiflea sprays contain toxic solvents that cause the insecticide to penetrate the skin—both your pet's and yours when you touch the animal.

Flea collars create a toxic cloud around your animal twenty-four hours a day, which you and your children breathe every time you go near your pet. Some flea collars and powders can cause severe conditions such as contact dermatitis on the skin of your pets. Pets breathe the vapors given off by these products, cats lick the material from their fur when they clean themselves, and powders can fall off onto kitchen counters and other surfaces where food is prepared or eaten. Children who pet dogs and cats may pick up the chemicals on their hands.

Flea bombs are particularly dangerous, as they fill your entire house with a poisonous, flammable cloud. In one case reported in the Seattle area, a woman forgot to turn off the pilot light in her stove before using more than a dozen flea bombs. The bombs ignited, blowing out all the windows and shifting the roof—yet the fleas survived.

SAFE SOLUTIONS

Being a cat lover, I've had to deal with the flea problem myself. A dog breeder I once knew told me that healthy animals don't have fleas and she showed me her animals as proof. So I fed my cat well and she got plenty of fresh air and sunshine being outdoors a lot in the forest where we lived, and I never saw a flea.

When my husband and I got another kitten, Zoe, we moved to a rented house in the suburbs that had flea-infested carpets from previous cats. Even though no animals had lived in the house for six months, the fleas were still there. Almost immediately they landed on Zoe, and she scratched and scratched and scratched. We tried everything, but nothing worked for her. Finally, after about a year, we moved to a house out in the country that had hardwood floors, and she was soon flea-free. She had a short bout with fleas sometime later, but we quickly ended it by rubbing diatomaceous earth into her fur (you can get a five-pound bag for practically nothing at a swimming-pool-supply store).

Flea control is an ongoing process. Even though you may kill all the adult fleas, there are still flea larvae waiting to hatch. As with any other insect, it will be impossible to eradicate fleas completely, but you can keep the flea population low enough that they don't bother anyone.

Establish one regular sleeping area for your pet that can be cleaned easily and regularly. Fleas tend to accumulate where animals sleep, so this will make it easier for you to collect them. Bedding materials such as blankets or rugs should be removed and washed frequently.

If you have carpeting, vacuum frequently, daily if necessary, disposing of the vacuum bag after each cleaning. Use the crevice attachment to get in all the corners of floors and upholstery. To speed up the process, have your carpets and upholstery steam-cleaned. Most pest-control places will say this won't work and recommend fumigation, which involves closing up your home and spraying the entire interior with highly toxic chemicals. Before you agree to this expensive procedure, remember: babies, pets, and children will be crawling around on a chemically treated rug, and their defense systems do not easily assimilate these toxic substances.

The easiest way to kill fleas is to heat your home to 122°F for several hours. Just take your pets and plants outside, close the windows and turn up the heat full blast. Take your family on an outing for the afternoon, then come back and vacuum everything.

As a preventive measure, you can try feeding your pet brewer's yeast to make it flea-resistant. The yeast gives an odor to the animal's skin that the fleas find unpleasant. Use twenty-five milligrams per ten pounds of the animal's body weight, beginning in the spring and continuing through the warm season. To prevent intestinal gas, feed the yeast to your pet in small amounts with moist food. If your pet is allergic to yeast, try rice-based B-complex vitamins, available in natural-food stores.

In addition, natural-food stores stock many herbal repellents. Perhaps the easiest approach of all is to rub ground cloves, eucalyptus oil, or strong wormwood tea (wormwood leaves can be purchased from an herbalist or natural-food store) directly into the animal's fur. This seems to work better than the herbal collars available at health-food stores, because the repellent is more evenly distributed around the body.

Another very effective repellent is citrus oil. Studies have shown the citrus oil discourages insects of all types quite effectively. Here's how to turn plain lemons into a powerful flea-repellent:

- Place 4 cut lemons in a saucepan, cover with water, and bring to a boil. Simmer for 45 minutes.
- Cool and strain the liquid, and store in a glass container.
- Apply the liquid liberally to the animal's fur while brushing its coat, so the citrus oil penetrates all the way down to the skin.
- Dry with towels and brush again.

Remember to bathe your pet frequently, and use a flea comb (available at a pet store) at bath time. Run the comb through your pet's fur, and drop the fleas that remain on the comb into a nearby container of soapy water (which should be flushed down the toilet when you're through).

Both **Gardens Alive!** and **The Natural Pet Care Company** are well stocked with natural dietary supplements, repellents, flea killers, shampoos, and other items to safely protect your pet and your home from fleas.

PET FOOD AND NUTRITIONAL SUPPLEMENTS

I used to feed my cat canned or dry pet food, but now I prepare her food from fresh ingredients. She thrives on raw meat. She will eat canned or dry food if it is a natural brand, but if I give her pet food from the supermarket, she paws around it like she's trying to cover up something in her litter box.

Most large corporations that manufacture commercial pet food are concerned about providing an "adequate" product at a low price. They get their protein from cheap **4-D meats**—from animals that are already dead, dying, diseased, or disabled when they're sold. Then they add **sugar** so your pet will like it, and **artificial color** so you'll think it looks fresh. Other additives and contaminants can include **artificial flavors, BHA/BHT, lead, nitrates/nitrosamines,** and **pesticides.**

Many pet foods claim to be "100% nutritionally complete and balanced." This claim legally can be made and printed on commercial products based on information studies using *isolated nutrients* and not whole foods, or by feeding the complete pet food to animals for several weeks to determine whether it prevents obvious disease or malnutrition. Although motivated by an interest to assure quality for the consumer, these tests ignore important nutritional issues and give both producer and consumer a false sense of knowledge and security.

Measuring a food's merit by levels of isolated nutrients tells only a partial story. There are more than forty known, essential nutrients, and more than fifty other nutrients are under investigation. Thus, making sure a food contains appropriate amounts of only a dozen of these nutrients can't possibly assure that a food is "complete."

SAFE SOLUTIONS

Many pet nutritionists recommend adding fresh organic raw meat to your animal's diet. According to Anitra Frazier, author of *The Natural Cat,* "You can't build resistance without some raw food. After three generations on a canned-food diet, the immune system is gone." Proper food combining also is recommended for animals to aid in digestion: feed fruit separately, protein with vegetables, and starch with vegetables.

Studies by Dr. Francis M. Pottenger conducted more than forty years ago showed the superiority of raw food for cats. Dr. Pottenger noticed that cats fed raw meat were healthier, reproduced more easily, and had healthier kittens than cats fed cooked meat. This inspired him to embark on a carefully controlled set of scientific studies that spanned ten years and over nine hundred generations of cats.

In the study of raw versus cooked meat, the raw-meat-fed cats were friendly, even-tempered, well coordinated, and resistant to infections, fleas, and parasites. Miscarriages were rare, and each generation showed striking uniformity in size and skeletal growth. Cause of death was generally old age, and autopsies revealed normal internal organs. The cooked-meat group, in contrast, showed many health problems, which became worse with each successive generation—many of the same problems humans get, such as arthritis and heart problems, from eating refined foods. After the third generation, all the cooked-meat-fed cats had died out.

In *Keep Your Pet Healthy the Natural Way*, Pat Lazarus recommends that one-third to one-half of a dog's daily food should be meat, and that for cats, meat should make up three-fourths of the daily diet. The rest should be fruits, vegetables, and grains, which contain essential nutrients that are not present in meat. Fruits and vegetables should be cut up and eaten raw; use cooked whole grains such as brown rice.

World-famous herbalist-veterinarian Juliette de Bairacle Levy makes food recommendations based on observing what animals eat and how they behave in nature, and then applying these observations to home and kennel care. For adult cats, she suggests two meals a day of milk thickened with uncooked rolled oats or other grains, and one protein meal each day composed of several teaspoons of raw, finely cut meat or lightly steamed, finely cut fish, a pinch of seaweed mineral powder, and a half teaspoon or so of very finely cut herbs such as parsley, mint, dandelion greens, or cress, covered with a teaspoon of light oil. Sprouted grains also are recommended. Five days a week, give meat or fish, one day milk and cereals only, and one day very little food in order to rest the digestive system.

Should you feed your pet a vegetarian diet? All the health and environmental reasons humans should reduce or eliminate their meat intake also hold true for animals. Yet I feel that animals' natural instinct is to eat meat. My cats love mice and flying insects. On the other hand, cats have been reported to be very fond of almonds, sunflower seeds, avocados, peas, corn, spinach, raisins, dried bananas, potatoes, yams, and sweet potatoes. Whether you choose to feed your pet meat or vegetables, the more fresh, unprocessed food you can give them, the better.

Animals have the same need for essential nutrients that humans do, and unless you're feeding your pet homemade meals of organically grown food, your pet's diet may need to be supplemented. You can give your pet the same whole-food-type supplements you use in your own diet, such as brewer's yeast and kelp, or choose nutritional supplements especially formulated for animals.

Anitra Frazier advocates a special vitamin/mineral mix that can be made at home.

Mix together 1½ cups brewer's yeast (for quality of fur), 2 cups bran (to keep intestines healthy), 1 cup lecithin granules (for hair texture and skin quality), ¼ cup kelp (for minerals), and ¾ cup bone meal (for strong bones and nerves). "Add a teaspoon per cat per meal," she says, "and you'll see a difference in a month!"

Finally, give your pet purified water to drink. **Chlorine, fluoride,** and other **water pollutants** are no better for animals than they are for us.

Look for natural pet foods and nutritional supplements at your natural-food or pet store, or order them by mail.

Chapter 14

FINDING A SAFE HOME

THOUGH I'VE PLACED THIS chapter last, it isn't by any means the least important. But moving to a new home to solve toxicity problems is a big change to make, and one I believe should be a last resort.

There are few "perfect" houses. To live in almost any building will require you to make some trade-offs. The good news is that many places with minor toxicity problems can be made safer without much effort or money. There are so many products, so many books, and so many individuals and organizations cataloging the health effects of building materials and safer alternatives (even the American Institute of Architects!), that I must simply refer you to them. If you are considering building or remodeling, it is well worth investigating Recommended Resources before you begin.

Whether you are searching for a new place to live or want to assess the basic structure or safety of your present residence and its surroundings, you will need to identify your priorities, evaluate whether or not an existing building is safe for you to live in or move into, and make your decisions accordingly.

Over the years I've looked at hundreds of dwellings—as potential homes for myself and for clients—and I can tell you that evaluating the safety of a house is both an art and a science. It's more than just getting some air-pollution tests; it's also knowing what to look for.

For example, the most important thing to me when choosing a place to live is clean outdoor air, so I chose to live in a forest in a small rural community, amid dairy and horse ranches and organic farms. The Pacific Ocean is right over a low ridge of hills. I had to replace the carpeting with a wood floor and get rid of an old, leaky gas stove and heating system. Once these improvements were made, the house was fine.

In this chapter, rather than detailing the health effects of each potentially harmful exposure (which are, for the most part, covered elsewhere in the book), I have provided you with the checklist I use when I'm evaluating a dwelling, and some safe solutions to the problems.

The checklist was compiled by Annie Berthold-Bond and me, and originally appeared in a somewhat different form in her magazine, *Green Alternatives* (no longer being published). Use it to help you determine if you live in a safe building, if you need to make improvements in where you live, or if you need to move to another location to protect yourself and your family.

Each checklist question is formatted as follows:

SUBJECT

❏ **The checklist question begins with a check box and is set in boldface type.**

Subquestions below are examples of such a situation; this is not meant to be an exhaustive list, only samples to give you an idea.

THE SAFE SOLUTION

The Safe Solution, as throughout, offers practical means for solving the problem.

GENERAL LOCATION

I believe the most important thing is to have clean outdoor air. If you have to choose between a polluted house in clean air or a clean house in polluted air, choose the polluted house in clean air, because you can fix the house more easily than you can fix the outdoor air quality. I once had a friend who spent considerable time and money fixing his house to be as perfectly nontoxic as he knew how to make it (with my help), but it was in a city with too much outdoor pollution, and finally he had to move out of the city.

Clean air exists in places where there are few pollution sources. Usually, clean air is found around plenty of trees or open space, next to the ocean, up in the mountains, in the desert, or out in the countryside. But these areas are not always perfect. There can be factories, or farms spraying pesticides, or pollutants coming in on prevailing winds. At the same time, clean air can exist in cities, particularly those near oceans. Each place must be evaluated for its own merits.

If you have no choice but to live somewhere with serious outdoor air quality problems, a last resort, yet one that will protect you, is whole-house filtration. With this system, you can continually filter out contaminants, thus provide the home with clean air. Since you won't be opening the windows, it is particularly important that the interior of the house is nontoxic. If you choose to keep the windows closed anyway because you are allergic to pollens and molds that cause serious allergic problems, and you also live in a polluted neighborhood, this could be a helpful system for you.

Wind

❏ **How do the prevailing winds blow?**

The wind can carry clean air or polluted air from locations many miles away. It is important to know what exposures you might have to industrial or agricultural pollutants from different directions and at different times of year.

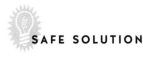

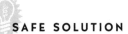

SAFE SOLUTION

Go to your local air-quality office and get their maps and charts on where the most polluted areas are and how the winds blow. Find an area with low pollution measurements to start with, then look to see from which directions the winds blow and how many days per year on average they blow from which direction. Get your own map and mark the cleanest places in the area in which you want to live.

Sun

❑ **Does the dwelling receive adequate sun all year long?**

Is the building in a deep forest?

Is the building in a valley on the north side of a hill?

Do the windows open to the street, gardens, or into the shadow of a light well?

SAFE SOLUTION

Try to have a lot of sun. Check the location for things that might block the sun, particularly other buildings, hills and mountains, and trees. Note the path of the sun across the sky in relation to the building, both through the day (east to west) and through the year (north and south). Ideally, the building would have a morning sun exposure, be shaded in the west, and be situated so that the sun comes in the south-facing windows when it is low in the winter, but not in the summer when it is high in the sky.

Pesticides and Herbicides

❑ **Do you get pesticide or herbicide drift at the dwelling?**

Is the dwelling in a farming community with commercial orchards, croplands, mushroom houses, or other agricultural sites within a mile?

Is there a golf course closer than ¼ mile from the dwelling?

Is the house closer than ½ mile to any other areas that are typically heavily sprayed, such as college campuses, industrial parks, recreation parks, or apartment or condominium complexes?

Drift from agricultural spraying depends on a number of factors. One is the method of spraying. Orchard pesticides, for example, get easily airborne, because they are sprayed up into the air and are carried by the wind. The drift can go three miles. Golf course spraying, on the other hand, is applied very close to the ground, so it is very unlikely that the herbicides will drift as far as three miles. Some crops are sprayed only once a season; others at regular intervals.

SAFE SOLUTION

If the potential for exposure exists, investigate before you buy. You can always close your windows, but the outdoor air will still become contaminated.

Protect yourself against pesticide drift. In some states, individuals are legally protected against pesticides and herbicides drifting onto their property. To find out about your local laws, call your state Department of Environmental Conservation or your state office of the EPA.

❏ Do you get occasional pesticide or herbicide drift?

Are herbicides sprayed along roads near the dwelling?

Are there nearby high-tension power lines, where herbicides are sprayed?

Is the dwelling in a neighborhood where people have their lawns and trees sprayed professionally or privately?

Is the dwelling in a part of town that is sprayed for mosquitoes or other insects?

Is the dwelling next door to a school?

If the wind is blowing your way and you have the windows open, you will have more than a passing exposure—you will have a contaminated home.

SAFE SOLUTION

To prevent pesticides from getting in your home, find out as much as you can about your neighborhood. Whereas it might be difficult to convince people not to spray, if you ask neighbors to alert you as to their spraying plans, at least you can close the windows. Talk to neighbors about organic lawn and garden methods (see chapter 4). It is also worth trying to establish a "toxic-free neighborhood" by joining together with others to approach county and town pesticide decision makers to discuss their spraying plans. In my county, one woman was able to single-handedly convince our road-maintenance department to mow weeds along county roads rather than apply herbicides every spring. Since she did this, other counties in the state have made the change, and you can make your county do it, too.

❏ **Is the dwelling exposed to any low-level yet chronic pesticides or herbicides?**

Is the house located in an old orchard where DDT and other long-lasting pesticides had been used?

Is there a commercial greenhouse on your street, and do they use pesticides and herbicides there?

SAFE SOLUTION

Try to live in a neighborhood without a history of pesticide use. Educate yourself about possible neighborhood pesticide exposures. Find out the history of the surrounding land, and which pesticides nearby businesses might have used or are using. Once you know the specifics, contact one of the pesticide organizations listed in Resources for suggestions.

Electromagnetic Fields

❏ **Is the dwelling exposed to high levels of electromagnetic fields?**

Are there high-tension power lines near the house?

Is the house near a radio tower transmitter?

Is an electric-power station within ⅛ to ¼ mile of the dwelling?

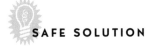

SAFE SOLUTION

Live in an area free of power lines or stations. Use a gauss meter to take accurate measurements of possible exposures (see Electromagnetic Fields in chapter 2).

❏ **Is the dwelling exposed to moderate levels of electromagnetic fields?**

Is the electric transformer on the telephone line, servicing the entire block, within 75 feet of your house?

Do you get a lot of radio interference from cellular phones?

Is the neighborhood electric line within 25 feet of the house?

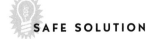

SAFE SOLUTION

Reduce exposures as much as possible. While moderate levels are not dangerous, use a gauss meter to determine exactly where your exposure lies and how much you are being exposed to.

Industrial Pollution

To protect the public, Congress passed the Community Right to Know Act, by which industry is required to report toxic emissions. The results of these reports are printed in the Toxics Release Inventory (TRI), which is available on microfiche in larger libraries. If a visual assessment of your area indicates concern, a trip to your library will help you ascertain if this type of pollution is a problem for you.

❏ **Is the dwelling exposed to chronic, toxic fumes from industrial sources?**

Is the dwelling within 1 mile downwind of a plant that burns hazardous waste or coal?

Is it less than 3 miles downwind of smokestack industries, or less than 2 miles upwind of smokestack industries?

Can you smell industrial chemicals from the dwelling?

SAFE SOLUTION

If you are exposed to chronic fumes and you can't move to an area with clean air, you should seriously consider installing a whole-house filtration system.

❏ **Is the dwelling exposed to intermittent fumes from industrial sources?**

A few times a month, when the wind changes, can you smell fumes from a smokestack industry a number of miles away?

SAFE SOLUTION

Reduce the fumes as much as possible. Use your nose to alert you to unpleasant chemical odors, and close the windows when the wind blows pollutants to the house. Find out as much as you can about local industrial polluters, and join with other neighbors to monitor the industry.

❏ **Is the dwelling near industrial storage of chemicals that are "harmless" except in the case of a fire or accident?**

Are there large amounts of pesticides stored in a nearby barn?

Is the dwelling near a nuclear power plant?

SAFE SOLUTION

An accident could be a health catastrophe for you and your family. Make certain these facilities are maintained properly. Best not to live near such a potential source of danger.

Neighborhood Pollution

❏ **Is the house exposed to chronic, toxic fumes from a neighborhood source?**

Is the dwelling across the street from a dry-cleaning company?

Is there a gas station or diesel truck stop at the end of the block?

Is the person who lives next door a cocaine manufacturer? (This is no joke. The process of making cocaine involves such toxic chemicals that SWAT teams have to put on protective gas masks before entering cocaine manufacturing dens.)

Is the house next to an airport and continually exposed to jet fuel?

SAFE SOLUTION

Move if you can, or install a whole-house air filtration system.

❏ **Is the dwelling exposed to intermittent toxic fumes from the neighborhood?**

Is the dwelling in the suburbs and exposed to chemicals your neighbors might use, such as those in house paint or roof tar?

Do you smell your neighbors' charcoal lighter fluid?

Do the people in the house upwind burn their trash outside? Do they burn plastic as well as paper?

SAFE SOLUTION

Develop friendly relations with your neighbors. Consider beginning a neighborhood chemical alert system so that neighbors call each other to tell them to close their windows when they are using toxic chemicals. Better yet, share copies of this book with your neighbors and work together to create a toxic-free neighborhood. This is worth doing even on a small scale with all your immediate neighbors.

❏ **Is the house exposed to chronic, low-level chemical exposure from a neighborhood source?**

Is the dwelling near a busy street or freeway?

Are there gas stations or any other businesses that use toxic materials nearby?

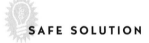

SAFE SOLUTION

Before you start looking for a place to live, get a street map and mark the main arteries and bus routes—don't even bother to look at any houses on those streets. Drive around and look for neighborhoods and streets that are quiet and have little traffic. You won't have zero traffic unless you live at the end of a long private driveway. Remember to note the prevailing winds and whether they carry pollutants from nearby busy streets. Use your nose to track down the sources of other chemicals, and see if you can persuade the persons responsible to change their habits, close their windows, or take whatever measures specific to the situation that would help reduce your exposure.

IMMEDIATE SURROUNDINGS AND BUILDING SHELL

Age of Building

❏ **Was the dwelling built or renovated within the last 5 years?**

SAFE SOLUTION

Unless the building or renovating was done with nontoxic materials, the more time that has passed between construction and your occupation, the better. At the very least, try to avoid living in a structure that has been built or altered in the past year. Dwellings built before the late 1960s are your best bet. Since then, many more toxic products have been routinely used in building structures. Before about 1965, real wood construction and hardwood floors were the norm. After 1965, a lot of particleboard and plywood began to be used in places where it might be difficult to remove and replace. If you are looking for a home with hardwood flooring and all-electric appliances, a suburban tract house or apartment building built in the early 1960s is where you'll find it.

Sharing Walls and Halls in Apartment Buildings

❑ **Do you often smell strong chemicals through the walls or from the halls?**

Are the halls of the building exterminated on a regular basis?

Does your next-door neighbor use a kerosene space heater?

Is there a central ventilation system that moves air between units instead of bringing in fresh air from the outside?

Can you smell chemicals through the walls, such as mothballs or oil paints?

SAFE SOLUTION

A single, detached dwelling is preferable. Speak to your neighbors to identify possible risks. Usually people are very accommodating about removing troublesome chemicals. Sometimes, though, a person's livelihood involves the use of some harmful substances. A furniture maker is one example. Give neighbors real suggestions, such as how to control weeds in their lawn without herbicides, or a gift of an inexpensive chimney-style barbecue starter if charcoal lighter fluid wafts into your backyard.

Garage

❑ **Is all or part of the living space connected to a garage?**

Is your apartment unit or house built directly over the garage?

Do garage vents open into apartment-building hallways?

Is the "fresh air intake" vent for central heating or air-conditioning located in the garage?

Does the garage connect directly to any part of your house (i.e., is there a door leading from your kitchen into the garage)?

SAFE SOLUTION

Do what you can to prevent automobile exhaust fumes from entering your living space. If there is a common door, install weather stripping to prevent exhaust from seeping around and under the door. Or, if you live in an apartment building, keep windows closed during the hours (such as rush hours—7–9 AM and 6–8 PM) when many cars are coming and going.

Pesticide History

❏ **Has the house ever been exterminated?**

Do current or did previous owners hire professionals to apply pesticides?

What kind of pesticide habits do the current owners have? Check in closets and under sinks for cans of household pesticides.

SAFE SOLUTION

Try to find a house that has never been exterminated. Try to track down all the previous owners to ask them about the pesticide history of the house. Then call one of the pesticide organizations listed in the Resources to find out the longevity and toxicity of the specific pesticides. Some organophosphate pesticides, for example, can dissipate after only five years. Others, such as chlordane, a profoundly neurotoxic pesticide that was used on more than 30 million structures in the United States to fumigate for termites and carpenter ants, can last for many years and may contaminate a structure forever. (If you are unsure if chlordane residue is present, have a test done before purchasing a house and making an expensive mistake.)

Be particularly careful about houses that have been bought and resold repeatedly, because each time they were sold, they were probably fumigated. Better to choose a structure that has had one owner for many years.

❏ **Does the house need to be exterminated?**

SAFE SOLUTION

If there are pest problems and extermination is recommended, find the least toxic approach to handling the problem. Better yet, look for a pest-control company that uses nontoxic methods. Many companies now use cold or electricity to kill bugs—look in the Yellow Pages and find the exterminator's general philosophy before paying him to come out for an inspection. If you have difficulty finding someone locally to do the job, contact the pesticide organizations listed in Resources.

❑ **Were mothballs used in closets or furniture?**

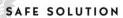

SAFE SOLUTION

Mothballs can leave residues of their toxic fumes for up to five years after they have been removed, so if possible, choose a home where mothballs have not been used. If mothballs are the only (or one of the few) problems in an otherwise perfect dwelling, you can lessen their outgassing by painting the closet or cabinet with **AFM Hard Seal.**

Electromagnetic Fields

❑ **Are there strong electromagnetic fields emanating from within the house?**

SAFE SOLUTION

Interior EMF problems are often easily resolved. Use a gauss meter indoors to check for strong localized fields. The meter may indicate a particular appliance—such as an electric stove, television, or light fixture—which simply can be replaced or moved. If faulty wiring is an EMF source, the gauss meter will show strong fields emanating from the wall. If this is a serious problem, hire an electrician to repair the wiring.

Foundation

❑ **Is the basement or crawl space damp, or does the house smell of mold?**

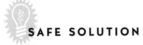

SAFE SOLUTION

A dry house is ideal. Mold, which can cause structural damage as well as allergic reactions, can only grow in conditions that are damp and dark and where the air is still. Anything you can do to make moldy areas dry and light and move the air will help control or even eliminate mold problems. Certain locations lend themselves to chronic mold problems: damp, foggy coastal areas; heavily forested sites; and particularly forested sites with a stream running near the house. If you are very sensitive to mold, choose a house in a sunny location.

❏ **Has the foundation been damp-proofed with an asphalt-based sealant?**

SAFE SOLUTION

Contact **AFM Enterprises** for their recommendations for a low-tox damp-proofing method.

❏ **Is the foundation made of treated wood?**

Is the foundation made of logs treated with creosote?

Was pressure-treated wood used in the foundation?

SAFE SOLUTION

Try to avoid treated wood, and replace it wherever you can. Contact **AFM Enterprises** for appropriate low-tox sealants.

❏ **Is there radon in the house?**

SAFE SOLUTION

Low or nonexistent radon levels are ideal. Especially before you buy a home, use a test kit to confirm that radon is not present (see Radon in chapter 2). If you have to fix a radon problem, it is better to know about it before you buy, and sometimes better to find another house if radon is a problem and not easily resolved.

House Siding

❏ **Has the house siding been treated for insects, as would be common in a log or wood-sided home?**

SAFE SOLUTION

Replace treated siding with wood siding or shingles (left to weather naturally or finished with a low-toxicity paint or finish).

❏ **Is the siding made out of asbestos cement?**

SAFE SOLUTION

Replace siding with wood siding or shingles (left to weather naturally or finished with a low-toxicity paint or finish).

Formaldehyde

❏ **Was urea formaldehyde foam insulation (UFFI) used in the house?**

SAFE SOLUTION

This is mostly a concern with dwellings built in the 1970s. Don't buy a house that has UFFI, and consider moving if you live in a building with this type of insulation. UFFI is very difficult and expensive to remove.

❏ **Was particleboard used in the construction of the house?**

Was particleboard used as a subflooring or in wall construction?

Are there particleboard cabinets in the kitchen or bathroom, or in other "built-in" areas?

Was particleboard used as an underlayment for countertops (look inside cabinets to see if particleboard is exposed)?

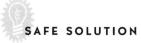

SAFE SOLUTION

The best solution is to avoid houses with a lot of particleboard. If you have it, follow the directions for formaldehyde mitigation in chapter 2.

Asbestos and Fiberglass

❑ **Is asbestos present in the house?**

Is there textured paint or patching compound applied before 1977?

Do the ceiling or walls have a crumbly "cottage cheese" appearance?

Is there visible insulation above stove, furnace, or pipes installed between 1920 and 1972?

SAFE SOLUTION

Not all products containing asbestos pose a health risk. The risk exists only when the fibers are released into the air, so if the insulation or wall texturing is in good condition, it's best to leave it alone. However, if you are considering purchasing a house that contains asbestos, it is better to remove the asbestos before you move in (and consider it to be part of the purchase price) rather than face a costly problem down the road.

❑ **Is fiberglass insulation exposed in any vents, where it could become airborne?**

SAFE SOLUTION

Correct this problem as soon as possible, as inhaling fiberglass fibers can be very harmful to your lungs. This problem should be fixed before you move into a house.

Ventilation

❑ **Does the house have adequate ventilation?**

Are there operable windows, or is air provided by a mechanical ventilation system?

Are there sufficient operable windows, fans, or opening skylights to allow cross ventilation (that is, air coming in one window and going out another on the opposite side of the room or house)?

Is there sufficient air movement outside the window to bring air into the house (windows that open into light wells, for example, don't give much ventilation)?

In areas where temperatures are exceptionally warm or cold and the dwelling is "sealed" for energy efficiency, is there some other form of ventilation other than opening the window, such as an air-to-air heat exchanger?

SAFE SOLUTION

Make sure there is adequate fresh air coming into the house and adequate pathways to vent stale air. If the house needs more ventilation, plan where additional ventilation can be installed before buying the house.

FINISHING

Lighting

❑ **Does the dwelling have sufficient natural light?**

SAFE SOLUTION

The healthiest light source is the natural light of the sun. Look at the placement of windows, the path of the sun throughout the day and the seasons, and any obstacles to determine if you can go through the day inside the dwelling with minimal use of artificial light. If necessary, more sunlight can be brought into the house with the installation of windows and skylights (see Light in chapter 11).

Paints and Finishes

❏ **Is there paint containing lead (all paints applied before 1980)?**

SAFE SOLUTION

If you are considering renovating an old house, be aware that you will probably be stirring up lead paint dust. Take care during renovations to keep children from the area. Wear dust masks when sanding paint, and be sure no paint dust remains (see Lead in chapter 2).

❏ **Was the dwelling recently painted?**

Was an oil-based or water-based paint used?

Will the dwelling need painting on the interior or exterior before or shortly after you move in?

Was a urethane finish applied to the floors?

Was a new coat of stain or finish applied to cabinets or woodwork?

SAFE SOLUTION

If paints or finishes were recently applied, the curing process can be speeded up by use of heat. Close all the doors and windows and leave the heat on at the highest setting for about a week. Oil-based paints may need to be cured longer. Open the windows for ten minutes or so every day to let the fumes out.

If the dwelling needs paint, choose a less-toxic brand (see paint section in chapter 11).

Carpeting

❏ **Is there carpet in the house?**

SAFE SOLUTION

The ideal dwelling has hardwood floors and no carpet. If the house has a carpet, both its age and the material from which it is made affect how hazardous it might be. Older carpets are less harmful than newer ones, and natural-fiber carpets are better than those made from synthetic materials.

Often older buildings will have perfectly good hardwood floors hidden underneath the carpet. If you are buying a home, you can lay any flooring you want. If you are renting, see if you can strike a deal with the landlord to remove the carpet. I have re-moved carpet from several apartments with the promise to rein-stall it before moving out. After several years, each landlord decided to install new carpet instead of using the old when I moved out, and I had no further responsibility (be sure to put all the details about carpet removal and replacement in the rental agreement). For more ideas about carpet and flooring, see the car-pet section in chapter 11.

Plumbing

❏ **What type of pipe does the house have?**

SAFE SOLUTION

Find out what type of pipe is used for the incoming water, both within the house and from the main water line. Copper pipe with all-metal pressure fittings is the best choice. There is no evidence that copper leaches into the water from copper pipe or that any excessive copper that might be present in water is in any way harmful to health.

Lead solder, however, is often used to connect copper pipe and galvanized iron pipe, and it does leach lead into the water. If you have lead-soldered pipes, get a water filter that can remove lead. If you have PVC plastic pipes (which are attached with glues that leach carcinogenic vinyl chloride), get a good activated carbon filter (see Water Filters in chapter 5).

HARMFUL EFFECTS OF COMMON SUBSTANCES

INCLUDED HERE is a representative list of harmful substances most commonly found in consumer products, along with their potential health effects. The list is not meant to suggest that everyone will experience these symptoms upon any amount or type of exposure to these chemicals; it is simply condensed information on the toxicological data available regarding these substances.

Everyone reacts differently, individually, to all things. Some people can tolerate exposure to large amounts of chemicals with no ill effects, while others develop complex symptoms even to small exposures—very much like some people can eat a lot and remain slender, while others gain weight even though they consume less food.

The harmful substances listed here fall into two categories. The first covers those ingredients found in consumer products that are classified as and known to be hazardous. Fourteen of these (indicated with an asterisk) are so dangerous that they are included on the Environmental Protection Agency's list of sixty-five "priority pollutants" recognized as being hazardous to human health. The second category includes substances that may appear safe for many people but that pose a problem to those who are sensitive to petrochemical derivatives or have specific other reactions (such as an allergy to perfume, or hyperactivity related to food additives). Read the descriptions of the possible health effects, and then decide which of these substances you want to avoid.

If you have health problems, avoiding any of these chemicals may make a difference.

Aerosol Propellants

Exposure to aerosol propellants can cause heart problems, birth defects, lung cancer, headaches, nausea, dizziness, shortness of breath, eye and throat irritation, skin rashes, burns, lung inflammation, and liver damage. If misdirected, aerosol sprays can cause chemical burns and eye injury.

The most commonly used aerosol propellant is Freon, a lung irritant and central nervous system depressant. In high concentrations, Freon can cause coma or even death.

Aerosol gases also can turn into other, more toxic gases, including fluorine, chlorine, hydrogen fluoride, hydrogen chloride, and phosgene (military poison gas).

Many aerosol products also contain other toxic ingredients that can get into eyes and lungs more easily than they could were these products dispensed by some other method. This can lead to high particle retention in the lungs and cause respiratory problems.

Ammonia (Including Ammonium Chloride, Ammonium Hydroxide, Benzalkonium Chloride, and Quaternary Ammonium Compounds)

These substances cause irritation of eyes and respiratory tract, conjunctivitis, laryngitis, tracheitis, pulmonary edema, pneumonitis, and skin burn.

Asbestos*

Autopsy reports show that 100 percent of urban dwellers have asbestos in their lung tissue. Asbestos exposure can affect almost every organ of the body. Illnesses caused by asbestos exposure include asbestosis, a chronic lung disease; and mesothelioma, an often fatal form of cancer. Asbestos diseases can result from very brief exposures and even exposure to other people who have been exposed (who may have asbestos fibers in their hair or clothing), and may take up to forty years to appear. The EPA announced in 1972 that there is no safe level of asbestos exposure, as *any* exposure to the fibers involves some health risk.

Aspartame (NutraSweet)

According to a letter from Dr. Richard J. Wurman to the *New England Journal of Medicine,* NutraSweet, an FDA-approved natural sweetener made from amino acids, can change levels of chemicals in the brain that affect behavior. Especially affected are people with underlying brain disorders such as Parkinson's disease and insomnia. Aspartame also may cause brain damage in children suffering from phenylketonuria. Because it has been available to the public for only a relatively short time, its long-term effects are unknown.

Scientific testing to establish aspartame's safety prior to FDA approval resulted in brain tumors and grand mal seizures in rat studies, and depression, menstrual irregularities, constipation, headaches, tiredness, and general swelling in human test groups. Furthermore, during human evaluations, two of the subjects underwent cancer operations. (Aspartame has not yet been tested for carcinogenicity.)

When exposed to heat, aspartame breaks down into toxic methyl alcohol. This may occur even at temperatures reached by diet sodas during regular storage.

Benzene*

Benzene is carcinogenic. It also can cause drunklike behavior, lightheadedness, disorientation, fatigue, and loss of appetite.

Benzyl Alcohol/Sodium Benzoate

Intestinal upsets and allergic reactions can result from exposure. Although these substances usually are considered relatively safe, clinical observation by medical doctors has shown them to cause adverse reactions in people who are sensitive to petrochemical derivatives.

BHA (Butylated Hydroxyanisole)/BHT (Butylated Hydroxytoluene)

BHT is a suspected human carcinogen. Studies show that BHT not only is carcinogenic to mice, but also that it promotes existing tumors. Moreover, animal studies reveal that BHA and BHT cause metabolic stress, depression of growth rate, loss of weight, damage to the liver, baldness, and fetal abnormalities.

Clinical observation by medical doctors has shown that BHA and BHT can cause adverse reactions in those who are sensitive to petrochemical derivatives. The late Dr. Benjamin Feingold of Kaiser-Permanente Medical Center widely publicized BHA and BHT as causes of hyperactivity and behavioral disturbances in children. Although it has been very difficult to substantiate this claim with scientific studies, the observations of parents and doctors for more than fifteen years confirm that avoidance of BHA and BHT has significantly improved their children's condition.

Chlorine (Including Chlorine Dioxide and Sodium Hypochlorite)

Symptoms of chlorine toxicity include pain and inflammation of the mouth, throat, and stomach; erosion of mucous membranes; vomiting; circulatory collapse; confusion; delirium; coma; severe respiratory-tract irritation; pulmonary edema; and skin eruptions. Exposure has been linked to high blood pressure, anemia, diabetes, and heart disease, and causes a 44-percent greater risk of gastrointestinal or urinary-tract cancer.

Clinical observation by medical doctors has shown that reactions to chlorine also can occur from chlorine fumes rising from hot or cold running tap water, including such symptoms as red eyes, sneezing, skin rashes, and fainting or dizziness while taking a shower or washing dishes.

Colors

Colors that can be used in foods, drugs, and cosmetics (and hence are known as FD&C colors), as well as U.S. certified colors and artificial colors, are made from coal tar. There is a great deal of controversy about their use, because animal studies have shown almost all of them to be carcinogenic.

The FDA determines the safety of coal-tar colors by testing

for acute oral toxicity, primary irritation, sensitization, subacute skin toxicity, and carcinogenicity by skin application. There are six coal-tar colors permanently listed as being "safe," and others in current use are on an FDA provisional list awaiting further proof of safety or toxicity. Technical materials on FD&C colors warn: "CAUTION: Consult the latest government regulations before using this dye in foods, drugs, and cosmetics."

Food colors were widely publicized by the late Dr. Feingold as a cause of hyperactivity and behavioral disturbance in children. While it has been very difficult to substantiate this claim with scientific studies, the observations of parents and doctors for more than fifteen years confirm that avoidance of artificial colors has significantly improved their children's conditions.

FD&C Yellow No. 5 causes allergic reactions in those sensitive to aspirin. The World Health Organization estimates that half the aspirin-sensitive people in the world, plus nearly 100,000 others, are sensitive to this color, which can cause many different symptoms, including life-threatening asthma attacks. Because of this, all foods produced after July 1, 1982, must list this color on the label separately from any other artificial colors.

D&C colors are coal-tar colors that can be used only in drugs and cosmetics. "Ext. D&C" on a label before a color listing means that it is approved for exterior use only in drugs and cosmetics and may not be used on the lips or mucous membranes. "Traces of D&C" before a color indicates that a form of aluminum, calcium, barium, potassium, strontium, or zirconium has been added to the coal-tar dye.

There are several different types of D&C colors. Azo dyes are made from phenol and are easily absorbed through the skin. Anthraquinone dyes, which are currently being studied for carcinogenicity, are made from benzene. Aniline dyes cause intoxication, lack of oxygen in the blood, dizziness, headaches, and mental confusion.

HC colors are approved only for hair coloring. They include aniline, azo, and peroxide dyes. Symptoms of toxicity from peroxide dyes include skin rash, eczema, bronchial asthma, gastritis—and occasionally, from complications arising from the above, death.

Colors in cleaning products are regulated by the Consumer Product Safety Commission (CPSC), which oversees the makeup of all cleanup products. All the commission requires is that products display warning labels if they contain "hazardous" ingredients; it is not necessary to list what those ingredients are. According to the CPSC, no laws exist regulating the type of dye that may be used to color cleaning products.

Cresol

Cresol can be absorbed through the skin and mucous membranes to affect the central nervous system, liver, kidneys, lungs, pancreas, and spleen. Symptoms of toxicity include dermatitis, digestive disturbances, faintness, vertigo, mental changes, sweating, pallor, weakness, headache, dizziness, ringing in the ears, shock, delirium, skin numbness and discoloration, and death.

Detergents

Detergents are responsible for more household poisonings than any other substance. Exposure causes dermatitis, flulike and asthmatic conditions, severe eye damage, and severe upper digestive tract damage if ingested.

Dyes

Direct dyes (the do-it-yourself, at-home type) contain highly carcinogenic dichlorobenzidene, which is very easily absorbed through the skin. They can cause anemia; jaundice; damage to the central nervous system, kidneys, and liver; and death. Azo, basic, disperse, fiber-reactive, and vat dyes all can cause allergic reactions, as can fluorescent whitening agents.

Ethanol

Symptoms of ethanol toxicity include central nervous system depression, anesthesia, feelings of exhilaration, excessive talkativeness, impaired motor coordination, double vision, vertigo, flushed face, nausea and vomiting, drowsiness, stupor, coma, dilated pupils, shock, hypothermia, and possibly death.

Flame Retardants

TRIS, a leading flame retardant, has been proved to be both mutagenic and carcinogenic to animals. Studies have shown that TRIS can be absorbed through the skin from garments washed more than fifty times. Materials treated with tetrakis (hydroxymethyl) phosphonium chloride (THPC), another retardant, release formaldehyde when the fabric is wet. Additional flame retardants include tetrakis (hydroxymethyl) phosphonium sulfate (THPS), phenol, polybrominated biphenyls (PBBs), and polychlorinated biphenyls (PCBs).

Flavors

More than fifteen hundred different petrochemical-derivative flavoring agents currently are in use. Usually they are listed as a group as artificial or imitation flavors, although occasionally a particular flavoring, such as vanillin, will be listed separately.

Most artificial flavorings are considered safe, but clinical observation by medical doctors has shown that artificial flavors can cause adverse reactions in those who are sensitive to petrochemical derivatives.

The late Dr. Feingold widely publicized artificial flavors as a cause of hyperactivity and behavioral disturbances in children. While it has been very difficult to substantiate this claim with scientific studies, the observations of parents and doctors for more than fifteen years confirm that avoidance of artificial flavors has significantly improved their children's condition.

Fluoride

Fluoride is carcinogenic. More than ten thousand cancer deaths per year are linked to fluoridated water. Exposure also can cause tiredness and weakness, mottling of the teeth, wrinkled skin, a prickly sensation in the muscles, kidney and bladder disorders, constipation, vomiting, itching after bathing, excessive thirst, headaches, arthritis, gum diseases, nervousness, diarrhea, hair loss, skin disorders, stomach disorders, numbness, brittle nails, sinus problems, mouth ulcers, vision problems, eczema, bronchitis, and asthma. Excessive fluoride also can reduce blood vitamin-C levels, weaken the immune system, and cause birth defects and genetic damage. The use of fluoride has been banned in ten European countries.

Formaldehyde

Formaldehyde is a suspected human carcinogen, has been related to teratogenic and mutagenic changes in bacteriological studies, and may be a contributing factor in sudden infant death syndrome (SIDS). The National Academy of Sciences estimates that 10 to 20 percent of the general population may be susceptible to the irritant properties of formaldehyde at extremely low concentrations. Symptoms from inhalation of vapors include cough, swelling of the throat, watery eyes, respiratory problems, throat irritation, headaches, rashes, tiredness, excessive thirst, nausea, nosebleeds, insomnia, disorientation, bronchoconstriction, and asthma attacks. Symptoms from ingestion include nausea, vomiting, clammy skin and other symptoms of shock, severe abdominal pain, internal bleeding, loss of ability to urinate, vertigo, and coma possibly leading to death. Skin contact can cause skin eruptions. Long-term exposure can cause allergic sensitization.

Fragrance

"Fragrance" on a label can indicate the presence of up to four thousand separate ingredients that are not listed at all. Most or all of them are synthetic. Symptoms reported to the FDA have included headaches, dizziness, rashes, skin discoloration, violent coughing and vomiting, and allergic skin irritation. Clinical observation by medical doctors has shown that exposure to fragrances can affect the central nervous system, causing depression, hyperactivity, irritability, inability to cope, and other behavioral changes.

Hexane

Symptoms of exposure are cough, depression, heart problems, nausea, vomiting, abdominal swelling, and headache.

Hydrogenated Oil

The hydrogenation of oil into hard fat (margarine, vegetable shortening) destroys or deforms the essential fatty acids in the oil. Lack of essential fatty acids can contribute to neurological disease, heart disease, arteriosclerosis, skin diseases, cataracts, arthritis, high blood-cholesterol levels, and cancer.

Kerosene

Exposure to kerosene could result in intoxication; burning sensation in chest; headaches; ringing in the ears; nausea; weakness; uncoordination; restlessness; confusion and disorientation; convulsions; coma; burning in the mouth, throat, and stomach; vomiting and diarrhea; drowsiness; rapid breathing; tachycardia; low-grade fever; and death.

Lead*
Early symptoms of lead poisoning include abdominal pains, loss of appetite, constipation, muscle pains, irritability, metallic taste in the mouth, excessive thirst, nausea and vomiting, shock, muscular weakness, pain and cramps, headache, insomnia, depression, and lethargy. Chronic low-level exposure has been found to produce permanent neuropsychological defects and behavior disorders in children, including low IQ, short attention span, hyperactive behavior, and motor difficulties. In high doses, lead can cause brain damage, nervous-system disorders, and death; can affect the kidney, liver, gastrointestinal system, heart, immune system, nervous system, and blood-forming system; and can cause malformations in sperm and low sperm counts. There is no demonstrably safe level for lead.

Because of the overuse of lead products in the past, virtually all air, water, food, and living beings are contaminated. Lead exposure can be lessened, but not completely avoided.

Methylene Chloride
Methylene chloride is a suspected human carcinogen that may be mutagenic.

Mineral Oil
Mineral oil is a suspected human carcinogen, and its use is forbidden as a food coating in Germany. It interferes with vitamin absorption in the body when ingested or rubbed on skin, though it is less dangerous if inhaled.

MSG (Monosodium Glutamate)
Symptoms of MSG toxicity include "Chinese-restaurant syndrome"—numbness, weakness, heart palpitations, cold sweat, and headache. Animal studies show that MSG can cause brain damage, stunted skeletal development, obesity, and female sterility. It is also on the FDA list of additives that need further study for mutagenic, subacute, and reproductive effects. Pregnant women and people on sodium-restricted diets should not use MSG.

Naphthalene*
A suspected human carcinogen, naphthalene can promote skin irritation, headache, confusion, nausea and vomiting, excessive sweating, and urinary irritation. Exposure to a sufficient quantity can lead to death.

Nitrates/Nitrosamines
Relatively harmless, naturally occurring nitrates are changed within the body to nitrites, which cause a lowering of blood pressure, headache, vertigo, palpitations, visual disturbances, flushed skin, nausea, vomiting, diarrhea, methemoglobinemia in infants, coma, and death. They can also turn into nitrosamines, which are carcinogenic.

Nitrobenzene*
Symptoms of exposure include bluish skin, shallow breathing, vomiting, and death.

Paraffin
Impurities in paraffin are carcinogenic. In addition, clinical observation by medical doctors has shown that paraffin can cause adverse reactions in those who are sensitive to petrochemical derivatives.

Pentachlorophenol*
Pentachlorophenol is a carcinogen that also can cause central nervous system depression, lightheadedness, dizziness, sleepiness, nausea, tremor, loss of appetite, disorientation, and liver damage.

Pesticides, Herbicides, and Fungicides*
More than fifteen hundred pesticides, herbicides, and fungicides are used in consumer products, combined with approximately two thousand other possibly toxic substances to make nearly thirty-five hundred pesticide products. More than one hundred of those commonly used are thought to be carcinogenic, mutagenic, or teratogenic.

Some pesticides are extremely long lasting in the environment. An EPA study detected residues of chlordane inside homes twenty years after application. These pesticides also tend to be stored in the fatty tissue, and can accumulate over time to high levels in the body.

Health effects from exposure to pesticides include paralysis; neuritis; sterility; convulsions; dizziness; weakness; tiny pupils; blurred vision; muscle twitching; slowed heartbeat; aplastic anemia; nausea; cough; diarrhea; tremors; damage to the liver, kidneys, and lungs; headaches; respiratory difficulty; coronary edema; coma; suppression of immune function; depression; irritation to ear, nose, and throat; hyperirritability; brain hemorrhages; central nervous system effects; decreased fertility and sexual function; and altered menstrual periods.

Phenol

Phenol is a suspected human carcinogen that also can cause skin eruptions and peeling, swelling, pimples, hives, burning, gangrene, numbness, vomiting, circulatory collapse, paralysis, convulsions, cold sweats, coma, and death.

Plastics

All plastics present a problem because of "outgassing"—the constant release of sometimes undetectable fumes, especially when heated. A good example of this effect is "new car smell"—caused by the outgassing of the plastic materials used in the interior of the car. As well as smelling it, you can see it in the scum that forms on the inside of the windshield. In a study conducted by the National Aeronautics and Space Administration, polyester was found to be the synthetic material that released the most fumes.

> Acrylonitrile* (Lucite/Plexiglas): suspected human carcinogen. Also can cause breathing difficulties, vomiting, diarrhea, nausea, weakness, headache, fatigue, and increased incidence of cancer in humans
>
> Epoxy resins: suspected human carcinogens
>
> Latex: one of the less toxic plastics. Though usually it is considered relatively safe, clinical observation by medical doctors has shown that latex can cause adverse reactions in those who are sensitive to petrochemical derivatives.
>
> Nylon: usually considered relatively safe, but clinical observation by medical doctors has shown that nylon can cause adverse reactions in those who are sensitive to petrochemicals. Both benzene and phenol are used

to make nylon, and minute amounts of these substances that might still be present in the finished product may account for these adverse reactions.

Phenol-formaldehyde resin ("Bakelite"): releases minute amounts of formaldehyde when new

Polyester: can cause eye and respiratory-tract irritation and acute dermatitis

Polyethylene: suspected human carcinogen

Polyurethane: can cause bronchitis, coughing, and skin and eye problems; also releases toluene diisocyanate, which can produce severe pulmonary effects and sensitization

Polyvinyl chloride (PVC): releases *vinyl chloride,** especially when the product is new. Vinyl chloride is carcinogenic, mutagenic, and teratogenic, and can cause mucous-membrane dryness, numbness in the fingers, stomach pains, hepatitis, indigestion, chronic bronchitis, ulcers, Raynaud's disease, and allergic skin reactions.

Polyvinylpyrrolidone (PVP): carcinogenic and also can cause thesaurosis, a lung disease affecting some users of hair spray, causing enlarged lymph nodes, lung masses, and changes in blood cells. The disease is reversible if hair spray is avoided.

Tetrafluoroethylene (Teflon): can be irritating to eyes, nose, and throat, and can cause breathing difficulty; produces poisonous gases when burned, and also may produce these gases to a lesser degree when heated

Saccharin
Saccharin "cause[s] cancer in laboratory animals"—as mentioned explicitly on labels of products that contain it.

Sucrose (Sugar, Corn Sugar/Syrup, Dextrose, Glucose Syrup, Invert Sugar/Syrup, Maple Sugar/Syrup)
Use of sucrose can lead to nutritional deficiencies, lowered resistance to disease, tooth decay, diabetes, hypoglycemia, coronary

disease, obesity, ulcers, high blood pressure, vaginal yeast infections, and osteoporosis.

Sulfur Compounds (Including Potassium and Sodium Bisulfate and Metabisulfite, Sulfur Dioxide, and Sulfuric Acid)

Sulfur compounds can cause fatal allergic anaphylactic shock and asthma attacks. They destroy vitamin B_1 (thiamin); have mutagenic effects on viruses, bacteria, and yeast; and can act synergistically with carcinogens to make them more potent.

Talc

Products containing talc may be contaminated with carcinogenic asbestos. There is *no* safe level of asbestos exposure.

Toluene*

Nervous-system and mental changes, irritability, disorientation, depression, and damage to liver and kidneys may result from exposure to toluene.

Trichloroethylene*

A suspected human carcinogen, trichloroethylene is mutagenic. Symptoms of exposure include gastrointestinal upsets, central nervous system depression, narcosis, heart and liver malfunctions, paralysis, nausea, dizziness, fatigue, and psychotic behavior.

Xylene

Exposure to xylene may cause nausea, vomiting, excessive salivation, cough, hoarseness, feelings of euphoria, headaches, giddiness, vertigo, ringing in the ears, confusion, coma, and death.

HOUSEHOLD POISONS

ALTHOUGH THE PURPOSE of this book is to discourage you from using household toxics, here are some precautions for preventing accidental poisonings, should you choose to continue using them.

GENERAL PRECAUTIONS FOR USING HOUSEHOLD POISONS

- Keep products in their original containers so the original label is available in case of accidental poisoning, and to prevent confusion. Accidental poisonings often occur when lookalike poisons are stored in food and drink containers.

- Don't use more of a product than the directions call for. Using more hardly ever makes a product more effective and can be harmful.

- Keep containers tightly closed to prevent volatile fumes from escaping.

- Use products in well-ventilated areas, outdoors if possible, to avoid breathing fumes.

- Don't mix chemicals. Some combinations, such as chlorine bleach and ammonia (or products such as scouring powders and all-purpose cleaners, which contain these substances), can produce toxic fumes. If you're not a chemist, you won't know what you'll end up with.

- Wear protective clothing if it is recommended on the label.
- Buy only what you need and use it up, or dispose of it properly.
- Carefully clean up after using toxics. Make sure products are properly stored, spills are wiped up, and rags are properly disposed of.
- Of course, keep toxics out of the reach of children.

EMERGENCY ACTION FOR HOUSEHOLD POISONINGS

If you follow the instructions in this book, you will never need to know what to do in case of an accidental poisoning. But if you have toxics in the house, the American College of Emergency Physicians and the American Association of Poison Control Centers recommend the following emergency procedures.

- *Inhaled Poison:* Immediately get the person to fresh air. Avoid breathing fumes. Open doors and windows wide. If victim is not breathing, start artificial respiration.
- *Poison on the Skin:* Remove contaminated clothing and flood skin with water for 10 minutes. Then wash gently with soap and water, and rinse.
- *Poison in the Eye:* Flood the eye with lukewarm (not hot) water poured from a large glass held 2 or 3 inches from the eye. Repeat for 15 minutes. Have patient blink as much as possible while flooding the eye. Do not force the eyelid open.
- *Swallowed Poison:* Unless patient is unconscious, having convulsions, or cannot swallow, give milk or water immediately, then call for professional advice about whether or not you should make the patient vomit. ALWAYS KEEP ON HAND AT HOME a one-ounce bottle of **syrup of ipecac** for each child in the home. Use only on advice of poison-control center, emergency department, or physician.

I suggest you ignore instructions on the product label and call your local poison-control center immediately! If you have toxics and small children in the house, keep that emergency telephone number next to the telephone, and teach your children when they should use it and why.

RECOMMENDED RESOURCES

Fortunately, far too much information now exists on the dangers of and safe alternatives to household toxics to be covered in one book. My intention in this guide has been to give you an overview of the problems and some first steps you can take. But much, much more valuable information is available that covers each subject in more detail. I've listed resources here, organized by chapter, that I have found to be worthwhile references. I encourage you, though, to think for yourself and do your own research and evaluations. Each author, editor, and organization holds a different perspective, and only you can decide what is right for you. If books are out of print, I suggest you look for them in your local library.

I am available personally for telephone or on-site consultations regarding finding and choosing safe products, natural living, and recovery from environmental illness. For information on consulting services, you may contact me at

PO Box 279, Forest Knolls, CA 94933
phone: 415/488-4614
fax: 415/488-0915
e-mail: debra@worldwise.com/debra
website address: www.worldwise.com/debra

MAGAZINES AND NEWSLETTERS

The Green Guide Mothers & Others for a Livable Planet, 40 W. 20th Street, 9th Floor, New York, NY 10011; 212/242-0010 (send SASE for information). Published twice monthly, each issue has a major article involving health or the environment, along with tips and ads for safe products.

Natural Health PO Box 57329, Boulder, CO 80322-7320; 800/666-8576. The bimonthly "guide to well-being" focuses mainly on natural healing, with natural living a part of overall good health practices.

NewAge Journal PO Box 52375, Boulder, CO 80321-3275, 800/234-4556. Bimonthly magazine that covers everything about the New Age, including natural living and articles on spirituality and personal growth.

Safe Home Resource Guide PO Box 3420, Westport, CT 06880; 203/227-1276. A resource guide for low-toxic products for building, interior design, and home care.

Spectrum Spectrum Universal Corp, 2702-D Camellia Street, Durham, NC 27705; 919/383-6492. A holistic newsmagazine.

Yoga Journal 2054 University Avenue, Suite 600, Berkeley, CA 94704; 415/841-9200. Monthly magazine that includes natural living as part of daily yoga practice.

GOVERNMENT AGENCIES REGULATING CONSUMER PRODUCTS

These government agencies will not give you information on safer alternatives, but they can give you detailed information on the danger of products used in and around your house.

U.S. Consumer Product Safety Commission (CPSC) Washington, DC 20207; 800/638-2772. The CPSC's primary goals are to protect the public against unreasonable risks of injury associated with consumer products; to assist consumers in evaluating the comparative safety of consumer products; to develop uniform safety standards; and to promote research and investigation into the causes and prevention of product-related death, injury, and illness. The CPSC puts out free "Fact Sheets" on hazardous products, which outline problems and give minimum suggestions for reducing risks. Foods, drugs, cosmetics, alcohol, and pesticides are exempted from the Commission's authority.

Food and Drug Administration (FDA) 5600 Fishers Lane, Rockville, MD 20857; 301/443-3170. The FDA enforces the federal Food, Drug, and Cosmetics Act and related laws to ensure the purity and safety of foods, drugs, and cosmetics. Many products that fall into these categories are subject to premarket approval by this agency. They can give you information on the safety of food additives, cosmetic ingredients, and pharmaceuticals.

U.S. Department of Agriculture (USDA) Independence Avenue and 14th Street NW, Washington, DC 20250; 202/720-4323. Meat, poultry, fruits, and vegetables are inspected and approved by the USDA.

Environmental Protection Agency (EPA) 401 M Street SW, Washington, DC 20460; 202/260-2090. The EPA regulates the manufacture and use of pesticides, and has jurisdiction over all indoor and outdoor air pollution, water pollution, and hazardous waste.

CHAPTER 1: HOW SAFE IS YOUR HOME?

Books:

The Clinical Toxicology of Consumer Products, by R. E. Gosslin et al. (Baltimore: The Williams & Wilkins Company, 1984). A big, expensive book that is in the reference section of most libraries. Lists many brand-name products and their toxic ingredients that do not appear on the labels, as well as much toxicological data as to their health effects.

Chemical Exposures: Low Levels and High Stakes, by Nicholas Ashford and Claudia Miller (New York: Van Nostrand Reinhold, 1992). A comprehensive report on the definition, causes, and prevention of multiple chemical sensitivities.

Chemical Sensitivity: A Guide to Coping with Hypersensitivity Syndrome, Sick Building Syndrome and Other Environmental Illnesses, by Bonnye Matthews (Jefferson, NC: McFarland & Company, 1993).

A Consumer's Dictionary of Household, Yard and Office Chemicals, by Ruth Winter (New York: Crown Publishers, 1992). Origins and health effects of chemicals found in a variety of consumer products.

Dying from Dioxin, by Lois Marie Gibbs (East Haven, CT: South End Press, 1995).

Everyday Cancer Risks and How to Avoid Them, by Mary Kerney Levenstein (Garden City Park, NY: Avery Publishing Group, 1992).

Guide to Hazardous Products Around the Home (Household Hazardous Waste Project, 1031 East Battlefield, Suite 214, Springfield, MO 65807; 617/422-0880). A personal-action primer covering disposal, safety, and homemade alternatives for the most toxic products, and an A to Z of hazardous products and substances and their health effects.

Healthy Living in a Toxic World, by Cynthia Fincher (Colorado Springs, CO: Piñon Press, 1996). Contains an excellent explanation of how neurotoxins cause illness, and what you can do.

Hormone-Disrupting Chemicals in Our Environment, by Lisa Lefferts (Mothers & Others for a Livable Planet, 40 W. 20th Street, 9th Floor, New York, NY 10011; 212/242-0010).

Household Hazardous Waste: Solving the Disposal Dilemma (Local Government Commission, 1414 K Street, Suite 250, Sacramento, CA 95814; 916/448-1198). Has practical information on how to set up a household hazardous waste disposal program in your community.

Our Stolen Future: Are We Threatening Our Fertility, Intelligence, and Survival?, by Theo Coburn et al. (New York: Dutton, 1996). A comprehensive report on the health effects of toxic chemicals, including hormone disruption, written in lay language.

Running On Empty: The Complete Guide to Chronic Fatigue Syndrome, by Katrina Berne (Alameda, CA: Hunter House Publishers, 1996).

The Rebellious Body: Reclaim Your Life from Environmental Illness or Chronic Fatigue Syndrome, by Janice Strubbe Wittenberg, R.N. (New York: Insight Books, 1996). A good basic overview of all the factors to consider for a successful recovery.

The Safe Shopper's Bible: A Consumer's Guide to Nontoxic Household Products, Cosmetics and Food, by David Steinman and Samuel Epstein, M.D. (New York, Macmillan, 1995). A thick reference book with copious lists of carcinogens, toxics, and brand-name products rated for their relative safety.

Toxics A to Z: A Guide to Everyday Pollution Hazards, by John Harte et al. (Berkeley: University of California Press, 1991). One of the most complete books I've seen that explains the problems of toxicity in everyday language. Includes detailed health and environmental toxicology information for more than 100 commonly encountered toxics.

Organizations:

American Academy of Environmental Medicine PO Box 16106, Denver, CO 80216; 303/622-9755. Information on and referrals for doctors who treat environmental illness.

American Cancer Society Call 800/227-2345 for a referral to your local chapter.

American Environmental Health Foundation 8345 Walnut Hill Lane, Suite 225, Dallas, TX 75231-4262; 800/428-2343, 214/361-9515. Publishes medical articles and books on environmental illness.

Chemical Injury Information Network PO Box 301, White Sulphur Springs, MT 59645; 406/547-2255. An advocacy organization run by the chemically injured, which provides information on chemical usages and injuries.

Citizens' Clearinghouse for Hazardous Waste PO Box 6806, Falls Church, VA 22040; 703/237-2249. Originally founded by the citizens of Love Canal, they address issues of toxic exposure in the community and help citizens organize grassroots campaigns. Has a newsletter and literature on toxics.

EnviroHealth Hotline 800/643-4794. Gives commonsense answers to environmental-health problems. Run by the National Institutes of Health.

Human Ecology Action League (HEAL) PO Box 29629, Atlanta, GA 30359; 404/248-1898. Information on environmental illness and the health effects of household chemicals. Makes referrals to local support groups for those with multiple chemical sensitivities.

INFORM 120 Wall Street, New York, NY 10005-4001; 212/361-2400; Inform@igc.apc.org. Publishes a number of books on various aspects of household toxics, from consumer use to hazardous wastes in the environment, including *Tackling Toxics in Everyday Products,* which lists 250 organizations working on problems caused by the use and disposal of toxic consumer and building products.

National Center for Environmental Health Strategies, Inc. 1100 Rural Avenue, Voorhees, NJ 08043; 609/429-5358. A nonprofit, tax-exempt organization fostering the development of creative solutions to environmental health problems. Provides a clearinghouse and technical services, educational materials, community outreach, policy development, research, support, and advocacy for the public and those injured by chemical and environmental exposures. Expertise in indoor air issues, school-related exposures, pesticides, access and accommodations in employment, housing, education, and public and commercial buildings and rights-of-way, and the rights of those disabled by environmental exposures. Information and media packages available. Speaker's bureau. Books and publications available at discounted prices for members. Publishes *The Delicate Balance.*

Remote Access Chemical Hazards Electronic Library (RACHEL) Environmental Research Foundation, 707 State Road, Princeton, NJ 08540; 609/683-1087. A computer database of information about hazardous materials, including health and some environmental effects.

Toxics Release Inventory To find the database nearest you, call the EPA hotline at 800/535-0202.

Washington Toxics Coalition 4516 University Way NE, Seattle, WA 98105; 206/632-1545; wtc@igc.apc.org. Does original research into toxic household exposures and sells inexpensive fact sheets, books, and reports on safer alternatives.

CHAPTER 2: INDOOR AIR POLLUTION

Books:

Cross Currents: The Perils of Electropollution, The Promise of Electromedicine, by Robert O. Becker, M.D. (Los Angeles: Jeremy P. Tarcher, 1990). Details the dangers of electromagnetic pollution and how to reduce exposure.

Current Switch: How to Reduce or Eliminate Electromagnetic Pollution in the Home and Office (video), by John Banta (order from ***Electro-Pollution Supply.***) A visual how-to on checking for EMF hazards and how to correct them.

The EMF Book, by Mark Pinsky (New York: Warner Books, 1995). A summary of the current research and understanding of the health effects of EMFs, giving safe levels, standards, and detailed guidelines for self-protection.

EMF Resource Directory (order from PO Box 1799, Grand Central Station, New York, NY 10163; 212/517-2800).

Radon: A Homeowner's Guide to Detection and Control, by Bernard Cohen (Mt. Vernon, NY: Consumer Reports Books, 1987).

Radon: The Invisible Threat, by Michael Lafavore (Emmaus, PA: Rodale Press, 1987).

Organizations:

Action on Smoking and Health 2013 H Street NW, Washington, DC 20006; 202/659-4310).

American Lung Association (1740 Broadway, New York, NY 10019-4374; 800/586-4872.

EPA Public Information Center 820 Quincy Street NW, Washington, DC 20011; 202/260-2090. Has information on electromagnetic fields, radon, formaldehyde, and other indoor pollutants. Sponsors a radon hotline (800/SOS-RADON), Indoor Air Quality Information Line (800/438-4318), and Toxic Substances Control Act Hotline (202/554-1404).

National Electromagnetic Field Testing Association (NEFTA) 628-B Library Place, Evanston, IL 60201; 708/475-3696. Registry of independent companies and individuals involved professionally in EMF testing, consulting, mitigation, and research.

National Lead Information Center 1019 19th Street NW, Suite 401, Washington, DC 20036; 800/532-3394.

Plants for Clean Air Clearinghouse 10210 Bald Hill Road, Mitchellville, MD 20721; 301/459-9625, (for brochure send $1 plus SASE). Funds research and acts as a clearinghouse for information on how plants can relieve indoor air pollution problems.

CHAPTER 3: HOUSEHOLD CLEANING AND LAUNDRY PRODUCTS

Books:

Baking Soda: Over 500 Fabulous, Fun and Frugal Uses You've Probably Never Thought Of, by Vicki Lansky (Deephaven, MN: The Book Peddlers, 1995).

Buy Smart, Buy Safe: A Consumer Guide to Less-Toxic Products (Washington Toxics Coalition, 4516 University Way NE, Seattle, WA 98105; 206/632-1545; wtc@igc.apc.org). Lists supermarket brand-name cleaning products in descending order of relative toxicity, including homemade safer alternatives.

Clean & Green: The Complete Guide to Nontoxic and Environmentally-Safe Household Cleaning, by Annie Berthold-Bond (Woodstock, NY: Ceres Press, 1990). More than 500 recipes for natural, homemade cleaning products.

CHAPTER 4: HOME AND GARDEN PEST CONTROL

Books:

Building a Healthy Lawn, by Stuart Franklin (Pownal, VT: Storey Communications, 1988). Written by a professional landscaper, this book shows how to "achieve the emerald green lawn of the American dream."

The Chemical-Free Lawn, by Warren Schultz (Emmaus, PA: Rodale Press, 1989).

Common Sense Pest Control: Least-toxic Solutions for Your Home, Garden, Pets, and Community, by William Olkowski, Sheila Darr, and Helga Olkowski (Newtown, CT: Taunton Press, 1991). The big, definitive book on safer pest controls—700 pages of information from the most knowledgeable people in the field. Compiles their years of experience at the Bio-Integral Resource Center.

Companion Plants and How to Use Them, by Helen Philbrick and Richard Gregg (Old Greenwich, CT: Devin-Adair, 1966).

Dan's Practical Guide to Least Toxic Home Pest Control, by Dan Stein (Eugene, OR: Hulogosi Communication, 1991). The small, practical book on safer pest controls, featuring the 15 most common household pests. Clear drawings for identification, simple solutions.

Designing and Maintaining Your Edible Landscape Naturally, by Robert Kourick (Santa Rosa, CA: Metamorphic Press, 1986). A complete guide to growing beautiful, edible plants.

The Gardener's Bug Book: Earth Safe Insect Control, by Barbara Pleasant (Pownal, VT: Storey Communications, 1994). Identifies 70

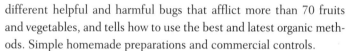

different helpful and harmful bugs that afflict more than 70 fruits and vegetables, and tells how to use the best and latest organic methods. Simple homemade preparations and commercial controls.

Good Bugs for Your Garden, by Allison Mia Starcher (Chapel Hill, NC: Algonquin Books, 1995). Identifies useful garden insects and tells why and how to cultivate them, rather than identifying "pests" and giving instruction for "controlling" them.

Natural Insect Repellents: For Pets, People & Plants, by Janette Grainger and Connie Moore (Austin, TX: The Herb Bar, 1991). Homemade herbal alternatives.

The New Organic Grower: A Master's Manual of Tools and Techniques for the Home and Market Gardener, by Eliot Coleman (White River Junction, VT: Chelsea Green, 1996).

Shepherd's Purse: Organic Pest Control Handbook, by Pest Publications (Summertown, TN: The Book Publishing Company, 1987). A guide to pest identification and control. Includes color illustrations.

Worms Eat My Garbage, by Mary Appelhof (Kalamazoo, MI: Flower Press, 1982). Instructions for setting up and maintaining a worm-based composting system.

Magazines and Newsletters:

Biological Urban Gardening Services (BUGS) PO Box 76, Citrus Heights, CA 95611-0076; 916/726-5377. Quarterly newsletter devoted to reducing the use of agricultural and horticultural chemicals.

Fine Gardening The Taunton Press, PO Box 5506, Newtown, CT 06470-5506; 800/283-7252.

Kitchen Garden The Taunton Press, PO Box 5506, Newtown, CT 06470-5506; 800/283-7252. "The Art of Growing Fine Food" focuses specifically on food from garden to table.

Organic Gardening 33 East Minor Street, Emmaus, PA 18098; 800/666-2206. The classic, practical magazine on the subject.

Organizations

Acres, USA PO Box 8800, Metairie, LA 70011; 504/889-2100. A one-of-a-kind organization that is on the forefront of exploring ecological agriculture, as well as general environmental, political, and health issues. Publishes a monthly newspaper, *Acres USA,* and a catalog of ecogardening books.

Bio-Dynamic Farming and Gardening Association PO Box 550, Kimberton, PA 19442; 610/935-7797. Founded in 1938, this is the oldest group advocating an ecological approach to agriculture, based on the teaching of Rudolph Steiner. Publishes *Biodynamics* (a quarterly magazine) and a catalog of books. Provides an advisory service, training programs, and conferences.

Bio-Integral Resource Center PO Box 7414, Berkeley, CA 94707; 510/524-2567. Practical information on the least toxic methods for managing pests. Publishes the *Common Sense Pest Control Quarterly* and booklets on almost every pest you'll find in your house.

EPA Pesticide Hotline 800/858-7378. A database provides information on health effects and ingredients of pesticides.

National Pediculosis Association PO Box 61089, Newton, MA 02161; 617/449-NITS. Provides information and consultation on head lice problems.

Northwest Coalition for Alternatives to Pesticides PO Box 1393, Eugene, OR 97440; 541/344-5044. Well-documented and scientifically sound information on pesticide hazards, less-toxic alternatives, and strategic community organizing tactics. Publishes the *Journal of Pesticide Reform* and has many programs and publications to reduce pesticide use.

CHAPTER 5: WATER

Books:

Drinking Water Hazards: How to Know If There Are Toxic Chemicals in Your Water and What to Do If There Are, by John Cary Stewart (Hiram, OH: Envirographics, 1990). A comprehensive and well-documented guide to water pollutants, water testing and treatment, and bottled water.

The Sierra Club Guide to Safe Drinking Water (San Francisco: Sierra Club, 1996). Detailed information about 200 municipal systems, bottled water, and home purification devices.

Organizations:

Clean Water Action 31 Pennsylvania Avenue SE, Washington, DC 20003; 202/547-1196. A national citizens' organization working for affordable, clean, and safe water, and controlling toxic chemicals.

EPA Safe Drinking Water Hotline 800/426-4791.

Food & Water RR1 Box 68D, Walden, VT 05873; 800/EAT-SAFE. Nonprofit group dedicated to clean food and water resources.

CHAPTER 6: DRUGS AND MEDICATIONS

Books:

There are more books on natural methods of healing than I could possibly list here, so I've limited my selection to a few basic volumes on home remedies that replace over-the-counter drugs, and a few books in which you can look up the side effects of drugs.

American Medical Association Guide to Prescription and Over-the-Counter Drugs, edited by Charles B. Clayman, M.D. (New York: Random House, 1988). Lists drugs by name and by ailment, including color photos of pills.

Back to Eden, by Jethro Kloss (Loma Linda, CA: Back to Eden Books, 1989). The easy-to-read guide to herbal medicine, natural foods, and home remedies since 1939. Expanded edition contains the original tried-and-true advice, plus new, updated material.

Baking Soda: Over 500 Fabulous, Fun and Frugal Uses You've Probably Never Thought Of, by Vicki Lansky (Deephaven, MN: The Book Peddlers, 1995).

Everybody's Guide to Homeopathic Medicine: Taking Care of Yourself and Your Family with Safe and Effective Remedies, by Stephen Cummings, M.D., and Dana Ullman, M.P.H. (Los Angeles: Jeremy P. Tarcher, 1990). Basic instruction for treating common ailments with homeopathic remedies.

Handbook of Over-the-Counter Drugs and Pharmacy Products, by Max Lebers, R.Ph., et al. (Berkeley, CA: Celestial Arts, 1994). A detailed guide to pharmacy products, their ingredients and health effects, and safe alternatives.

The Home Remedies Handbook: Over 1,000 Ways to Heal Yourself, by the Editors of *Consumer Guide* and Hundreds of Leading Doctors (Publications International, 1994). Emphasis on nutritional and behavioral changes.

The People's Pharmacy, by Joe Graedon (New York: St. Martin's/Griffin, 1996).

Magazines and Newsletters:

Natural Health PO Box 57329, Boulder, CO 80322-7320; 800/666-8576. Covers the wide range of natural healing alternatives, including diet, lifestyle, home remedies, and alternative therapies.

CHAPTER 7: BEAUTY AND HYGIENE

Books:

Baking Soda: Over 500 Fabulous, Fun and Frugal Uses You've Probably Never Thought Of, by Vicki Lansky (Deephaven, MN: The Book Peddlers, 1995).

A Consumer Dictionary of Cosmetic Ingredients, by Ruth Winter (New York: Crown Publishers, 1984). Alphabetical listing of thousands of cosmetic ingredients, how they're used, and their health effects.

The Herbal Body Book: A Natural Approach to Healthier Hair, Skin, and Nails, by Stephanie Tourles (Pownal, VT: Storey Communications, 1994).

The Natural Soap Book: Making Herbal and Vegetable-Based Soaps, by Susan Miller Cavitch (Pownal, VT: Storey Communications, 1995).

Taking Charge of Your Fertility: The Definitive Guide to Natural Birth Control and Pregnancy Achievement, by Toni Weschler, M.P.H. (New York: HarperPerennial, 1996).

Organizations:

Foundation for Toxic-Free Dentistry PO Box 608010, Orlando, FL 32860-8010. Investigates and provides information on the biocompatibility of materials used in dentistry, particularly the health effects of mercury amalgam fillings.

CHAPTER 8: FOOD

Books

The Catalog of Healthy Food, by John Tepper Marlin, Ph.D. (New York: Bantam Books, 1990). A comprehensive guide to healthy food and food hazards, including listings of organic farms, products, and vendors.

Circle of Poison: Pesticides and People in a Hungry World, by David Weir and Mark Shapiro (San Francisco: Institute for Food and Development Policy, 1981). The story of how pesticides banned in the United States are sent to Third World countries, where they are sprayed on foods and then imported back to us.

A Consumer Dictionary of Food Additives, by Ruth Winter (New York: Crown Publishers, 1989). Alphabetical listing of thousands of food additives, how they're used, and their health effects.

Nature's Kitchen: The Complete Guide to the New American Diet, by Fred Rohé (Pownal, VT: Storey Communications, 1986). A practical guide to making the transition to a natural diet.

Pesticide Alert: A Guide to Pesticides in Fruits and Vegetables, by Lawrie Mott and Karen Snyder, of the Natural Resources Defense Council (San Francisco: Sierra Club Books, 1987). Pesticides commonly used on produce, and their health effects.

Pesticides and Your Food: How to Reduce the Risks to Your Health, by Andrew Watterson (London: Green Print, 1991). A food-by-food description of pesticides used on each food worldwide, followed by a dictionary of pesticides used on food and their health effects.

Organizations:

Community Supported Agriculture of North America c/o WTIG, 818 Connecticut Avenue NW, #800, Washington, DC 202/785-5135. Has an annotated directory of CSAs across the country, and a book on how to start a CSA.

Demeter Association for Certification of Bio-Dynamic Agriculture 4214 National Avenue, Burbank, CA 91505; 818/843-5521. Certifies biodynamic food.

Mothers & Others for a Livable Planet 40 W. 20th Street, 9th Floor, New York, NY 10011; 212/242-0010 (send SASE for information). Offers several booklets on organic agriculture and changing your diet.

Natural Organic Farmers Association 411 Sheldon Road, Barre, MA 01005; 508/355-2853. Certifies organically grown food.

Organic Crop Improvement Association 1405 S. Detroit Street, Bellefontaine, OH 43311; 513/592-4983. Certifies organically grown food.

Organic Grapes Into Wine Alliance 1592 Union Street, Suite 350, San Francisco, CA 94123; 800/477-0167.

CHAPTER 9: TEXTILES

Organizations:

Cotton Plus Route 1, Box 120, O'Donnell, TX 79351; 806/439-6646. Consumers can contact Cotton Plus for up-to-date lists of manufacturers and retail distributors of organically grown cotton products.

CHAPTER 10: HOME OFFICE AND ART SUPPLIES

Books:

Artist Beware: The Hazards and Precautions in Working with Art and Craft Materials, by Michael McCann (New York: Watson-

Guptill Publications, 1979). Provides information on toxic substances found in art materials, and how you can set up a nontoxic studio.

Children's Art Hazards, by Lauren Jacobsen (Natural Resources Defense Council, 40 W. 20th Street, New York, NY 10011; 212/727-2700). A basic overview of children's art materials and health hazards, and art precautions for children less than twelve years of age.

Organizations:

The Art and Craft Materials Institute 100 Boylston Street, Suite 1050, Boston, MA 02116; 617/426-6400. Certifies children's and adults' art materials with *CP Nontoxic, AP Nontoxic,* and *Health Label* seals. For a list of approved products, send a self-addressed, stamped envelope.

The Center for Occupational Hazards 5 Beekman Place, Suite 1030, New York, NY 10038; 212/227-6220. A national clearinghouse for information on hazards in the arts. Distributes more than 70 books, pamphlets, articles, and data sheets.

CHAPTER II: HOME FURNISHINGS

Books:

The Natural House Catalog: Everything You Need to Create an Environmentally Friendly Home, by David Pearson (New York: Simon & Schuster, 1996). An excellent overview of the elements of a natural house, plus resources for interior designers, furniture, and home furnishings.

Magazines and Newsletters:

Interior Concerns PO Box 2386, Mill Valley, CA 94942; 415/389-8049. A bimonthly newsletter providing information for designers, architects, builders, and homeowners on environmental products, issues, and industry changes. They also have an *Interior Concerns Resource Guide,* which lists products, manufacturers, consultants, and other resources.

Organizations:

Environmental Protection Agency (EPA) 401 M Street SW, Washington, DC 20460; 202/554-1404. Publishes "Indoor Air Quality and New Carpet: What You Should Know."

CHAPTER 12: BABIES AND CHILDREN

Books:

Baking Soda: Over 500 Fabulous, Fun and Frugal Uses You've Probably Never Thought Of, by Vicki Lansky (Deephaven, MN: The Book Peddlers, 1995).

Blueprint for a Green School, by Jayni Chase (New York: Scholastic, 1995). The definitive book on creating a safe school. Its 688 pages offer easy-to-read and -comprehend explanations of health and environmental problems children encounter in schools, and what you can do about them. Edited by the founder of the Center for Environmental Education.

Healthy Homes, Healthy Kids: Protecting Your Children From Everyday Environmental Hazards, by Joyce M. Schoemaker Ph.D., and Charity Y. Vitale (Washington, DC: Island Press, 1991). A review of common household environmental risks, explaining why children are especially vulnerable and what actions you can take to protect them.

Is This Your Child? Discovering and Treating Unrecognized Allergies, by Doris Rapp, M.D. (New York: William Morrow, 1991). Detailed instructions for determining if your child is being affected physically or behaviorally by chemicals, and what you can do.

The Natural Baby Food Cookbook, by Margaret Elizabeth Kenda and Phyllis S. Williams (New York: Avon Books, 1982).

Poisoning Our Children: Surviving in a Toxic World, by Nancy Sokol Green (Chicago: The Noble Press, 1991). Written by a mother with environmental illness, this book gives a personal perspective to protecting children from household toxics.

WiseWoman Herbal for the Childbearing Years, by Susan S. Weed (Woodstock, NY: Ash Tree Publishing, 1986). Natural remedies for before, during, and after pregnancy.

Magazines and Newsletters:

Mothering PO Box 1690, Santa Fe, NM 87504; 505/984-8116. The most comprehensive, widely distributed magazine on natural mothering. Includes articles written by mothers, and resources for all types of natural products used by babies, children, and mothers. Strong environmental ethic and general natural philosophy.

Organizations:

La Leche League International PO Box 1209, Franklin Park, IL 60131; 800/LA-LECHE. Offers information and support for breastfeeding mothers.

CHAPTER 13: PET CARE

Books:

Are You Poisoning Your Pets? A Guidebook on How Our Lifestyles Affect the Health of Our Pets, by Nina Anderson and Howard Peiper (East Canaan, CT: Safe Goods, 1996). A comprehensive guide to substances that can harm pets, including symptoms of poisoning to watch for, and resources. Guidance is given for keeping your pet healthy.

Baking Soda: Over 500 Fabulous, Fun and Frugal Uses You've Probably Never Thought Of, by Vicki Lansky (Deephaven, MN: The Book Peddlers, 1995).

The Complete Herbal Book for the Dog and Cat, by Juliette de Baïracli Levy (New York: Arco Publishing. 1986). Methods of natural rearing from the internationally renowned pioneer in the field.

Dr. Pitcairn's Complete Guide to Natural Health for Dogs & Cats, by Richard H. Pitcairn, D.V.M., Ph.D., and Susan Hubble Pitcairn (Emmaus, PA: Rodale Books, 1995). The bible of natural pet care; covers diet, natural flea control, and natural remedies.

Keep Your Pet Healthy the Natural Way, by Pat Lazarus (New Canaan, CT: Keats Publishing, 1983).

Natural Insect Repellents: For Pets, People & Plants, by Janette Grainger and Connie Moore (Austin, TX: The Herb Bar, 1991). Homemade herbal alternatives.

The New Natural Cat: A Complete Guide for Finicky Owners, by Anitra Frazier (New York: Penguin Books, 1990). Holistic care for both good health and good behavior. Includes natural treatments for more than 40 common feline health problems.

Your Natural Dog: A Guide to Behavior and Health Care, by Angela Patmore (New York: Carroll & Graf, 1993). An American reprint of a British book, it covers everything from diet and exercise to training, caring for new puppies, and holistic remedies.

Organizations:

American Holistic Veterinary Medical Association 2214 Old Emmorton Road, Bel Air, MD 21015; 410/569-0795. A professional organization of veterinarians who use nontraditional techniques, including alternative nutrition, homeopathy, and acupuncture. Send a self-addressed, stamped envelope for a list of holistic veterinarians in your area.

CHAPTER 14: FINDING A SAFE HOME

Books:

Environmental Resource Guide, by the American Institute of Architects (New York: John Wiley and Sons, 1996). For design professionals, comparative analyses of environmental and health effects of building materials.

Healing Environments: Your Guide to Indoor Well-Being, by Carol Vendia (Berkeley: Celestial Arts, 1995; revised). How the buildings you inhabit can influence your well-being, and what you can do to create a healthy and nurturing home.

Healthful Houses: How to Design and Build Your Own, by Clint Good (Bethesda, MD: Guaranty Press, 1988). Complete architectural specifications for nontoxic building materials.

Healthy House Building: A Design and Construction Guide, by John Bower (Unionville, IN: The Healthy House Institute, 1993). Complete instructions for nontoxic building, including brand-name building materials.

The Natural House Book: Creating a Healthy, Harmonious, and Ecologically Sound Home Environment, by David Pearson (New York: Simon & Schuster, 1989). Designs and ideas for using natural materials in home construction, with beautiful photographs and illustrations.

The Natural House Catalog: Everything You Need to Create an Environmentally Friendly Home, by David Pearson (New York: Simon & Schuster, 1996). An excellent overview of the elements of a natural house, plus resources for architects and building products.

The Smart Kitchen: How to Design a Comfortable, Safe, Energy-Efficient, and Environmentally-Friendly Workspace, by David Goldbeck (Woodstock, NY: Ceres Press, 1989).

The Truth About Where You Live: An Atlas for Action on Toxins and Mortality, by Benjamin Goldman (New York: Times Books/Random House, 1991). A comprehensive picture of communities that have high levels of environmental contamination and illness.

Magazines and Newsletters:

Building with Nature PO Box 4417, Santa Rosa, CA 95402-4417; 707/579-2201. A bimonthly newsletter on the practicalities of natural building. Geared for design professionals, but interesting for anyone to read.

Environmental Building News RR1, Box 161, Brattleboro, VT 05301; 802/257-7300; EBN@sover.net. Detailed analysis of the health and environmental effects of building materials. Reviews resource-efficient building methods and new products. Geared for professionals, but useful to owner-builders.

Organizations:

U.S. Green Building Council 1825 I Street NW, Suite 400, Washington, DC 20006; 202/429-2081. An all-inclusive nonprofit consensus coalition of the building industry, promoting the understanding, development, and accelerated implementation of "green building" policies, programs, technologies, standards, and design practices on a national basis.

MAIL-ORDER SOURCES

FOR BEST RESULTS when dealing with mail-order companies, be specific about what you are interested in. In the world of mail order, catalogs may carry the same items year in and year out, or they may change with every catalog. Sometimes products may be in one catalog, then they are taken out and rotated back into a future catalog. Or, items may appear only seasonally. Therefore items you read about in this book may or may not be in a current catalog, but if you ask specifically for "organic-cotton sweat clothes," then the company can give you an exact reply as to the availability of that product.

On the other hand, I couldn't possibly list every product sold in every catalog, so you are in for some nice surprises. What I tried to do is give you a representative idea of the kinds of products you are likely to find when you order a catalog, rather than be too specific about individual products.

Also be aware that if you just call or write to request a catalog, it could take up to six months for you to receive one. Often companies don't send out catalogs to "inquiries" until they do their next bulk mailing, but if you ask, they will send one right away. When requesting catalogs by mail, *always* write your full name and address legibly on your request letter—don't expect companies to get your address off a letter or a check. Best is to use postcards for requests; they cost less to mail and all the information is on a single card.

While most of the catalogs are free, some companies charge a small fee, often refundable with your first order. Others ask that you enclose a SASE—a self-addressed, stamped, #10 letter-size envelope—with your catalog request to ensure a prompt reply.

Companies designated with an asterisk (*) specially cater to those with chemical sensitivities. These range from having their whole business revolve around serving the chemically sensitive community to having some portion of their business offer special products and services. If you are chemically sensitive, know that if you contact a company so indicated, they will be familiar with your needs and be interested in helping you. If you are not chemically sensitive, these are still good catalogs to shop from, as they carry some of the purest products available (though not necessarily printed in glossy color).

Acres U.S.A.
PO Box 9547
Kansas City, MO 64133
816/737-0064

Garden Pesticides

AFM Enterprises
350 W. Ash Street, Suite 700
San Diego, CA 92101
619/239-0321

Carpeting and Flooring • Paints and Finishes • Wallpaper

After the Stork
PO Box 44321
Rio Rancho, NM 87174-4321
800/441-4775
505/867-7000

Babies' and Kids' Clothing • Sun Protection

agAccess
PO Box 2008
Davis, CA 95617
916/756-7177

Garden Pesticides

Air Check
570 Butler Bridge Road
Fletcher, NC 28732
704/684-0893

Formaldehyde • Lead • Microwave Ovens • Radon

Aireox Research Corporation
PO Box 8523
Riverside, CA 92515
909/689-2781

Air Filters

Alexandra Avery
4717 SE Belmont Street
Portland, OR 97215
800/669-1863
503/236-5926

Beauty and Hygiene

Allegro Rug Weaving Company
802 S. Sherman Drive
Longmont, CO 80501
800/783-1784
303/651-0555

Carpeting and Flooring

Allergy Relief Shop*
3371 Whittle Springs Road
Knoxville, TN 37917
800/626-2810
423/522-2795

Antiperspirants and Deodorants • Bath Linens • Beauty and Hygiene • Beds and Bedding • Cribs • Fabrics, Yarns, and Notions • Hair Color • Mouthwash, Toothpaste, and Toothbrushes • Permanent Waves • Shower Curtains • Tampons and Sanitary Pads

Allergy Resources*
PO Box 444
Guffey, CO 80820
800/USE-FLAX

Air Filters • Baby-Care Products •
Beauty and Hygiene • Beds and Bedding
• Diapers • Fish and Seafood • Food •
Formaldehyde • Household Cleaning
and Laundry Products • Lead • Meat,
Poultry, and Eggs • Pet Care • Radon •
Shower Curtains • Tampons and Sani-
tary Pads • Water

AllerMed Corporation*
31 Steel Road
Wylie, TX 75098
214/442-4898

Air Filters

**American Environmental Health
   Foundation***
8345 Walnut Hill Lane, Suite 225
Dallas, TX 75231-4262
800/428-2343
214/361-9515

Air Filters • Beauty and Hygiene • Beds
and Bedding • Clothing • Electromagnetic Fields • Footwear and Shoe Care •
Household Cleaning and Laundry Products • Shower Curtains • Water Filters

**American Environmental
   Laboratories**
60 Elm Hill Avenue
Leominster, MA 01453
800/522-0094

Water

Anderson Laboratories
PO Box 323
Witartford, VT 05084
802/295-7344

Carpeting and Flooring

Aqua Clean Systems
469 Dougherty Boulevard
Inwood, NY 11096-0338
800/645-2204

Dry Cleaning

Baby Bunz & Company
PO Box 113
Lynden, WA 98264
800/676-4559

Babies and Children • Diapers

Barbara Coole Designs
2631 Piner Road
Santa Rosa, CA 95401
800/992-8924
707/575-8924
73003.1246@Compuserve

Babies' and Kids' Clothing • Beds and
Bedding • Clothing • Diapers • Fabrics,
Yarns, and Notions • Footwear and Shoe
Care • Luggage and Bags • Toys

Biobottoms
PO Box 6009
Petaluma, CA 94953
707/778-7945

Babies' and Kids' Clothing • Diapers

Bountiful Gardens
18001 Schafer Ranch Road
Willits, CA 95490-9626
707/459-6410

Garden Pesticides

Bright Future Futon
3120 Central Avenue SE
Albuquerque, NM 87106
505/268-9738

Beds and Bedding • Cribs • Furniture

Cal Ben Soap Company
9828 Pearmain Street
Oakland, CA 94108
510/638-7092

Household Cleaning and Laundry Products • Dishwater Detergent • Laundry Detergent

Carousel Carpets
1 Carousel Lane
Ukiah, CA 95482
707/485-0333

Carpeting and Flooring

Casco Bay Fine Woolens
34 Danforth Street
Portland, ME 04101
800/788-9842

Clothing

Castle Gray
PO Box 647
Manitou Springs, CO 80829
800/987-3747

Babies' and Kids' Clothing • Clothing • Footwear and Shoe Care • Luggage and Bags

Chambers
PO Box 7841
San Francisco, CA 94120-7841
800/334-9790

Bath Linens • Beds and Bedding • Shower Curtains

ChiPants
120 Rising Road
Mill Valley, CA 94941
415/381-2407
chi@chipants.com
http://www.chipants.com

Clothing

Clothcrafters
PO Box 176
Elkhart Lake, WI 53020
800/876-2009
414/876-2112
http://doorcounty.org/mkt/cl

Bath Linens • Coffee • Cribs • Food Storage • Irons and Ironing-Board Covers • Kitchen and Table Linens • Luggage and Bags • Shower Curtains

Colin Campbell & Sons
1428 West Seventh Avenue
Vancouver BC, Canada V6H1C1
604/734-2758
800/677-5001 (USA)

Carpeting and Flooring

The Cordwainer Shop
67 Candia Road
Deerfield, NH 03037
603/463-7742

Footwear and Shoe Care

Cotton Clouds Mail Order Yarns
5176 S. 14th Avenue, Dept NT
Safford, AZ 85546
800/322-7888

Fabrics, Yarns, and Notions

The Cotton Place*
PO Box 7715
Waco, TX 76714
800/451-8866
817/751-7730

Beds and Bedding • Clothing • Fabrics, Yarns, and Notions • Footwear and Shoe Care

Cotton Threads Clothing
Route 2, Box 90
Halletsville, TX 77964
409/562-2153
micyn@cvtv.net

Clothing

Country Curtains
Red Lion Inn
Stockbridge, MA 01262
800/456-0321

Window Coverings

Crown Corporation
1801 Wynkoop Street
Denver, CO 80202
800/422-2099
303/292-1313

Wallpaper

Cuddle Ewe
10650 County Road 81, Suite U
Maple Grove, MN 55369
800/328-9493

Beds and Bedding

Czimer Foods
13136 W. 159th Street
Lockport, IL 60441
708/301-7152

Meat, Poultry, and Eggs

Decent Exposures
PO Box 27206
Seattle, WA 98125
800/505-4949

Baby Food • Clothing

Deer Valley Farm
RD 1, Box 173
Guilford, NY 13780
607/764-8556

Food • Meat, Poultry, and Eggs

Dellinger
1943 N. Broad
Rome, GA 30161
706/291-7402

Carpeting and Flooring

Diamond Organics
Freedom, CA 95019
800/922-2396

Food

Dutch Mill Cheese Shop
2001 N. State Road 1
Cambridge City, IN 47327
317/478-5847

Milk and Dairy Products

E. L. Foust Company*
Box 105
Elmhurst, IL 60126
800/225-9549

Air Filters

Earth Studio
6761 Sebastopol Avenue, Suite 8
Sebastopol, CA 95472
707/823-2569

Paints and Finishes

Eddie Bauer
PO Box 3700
Seattle, WA 98124-3700
800/426-8020

Clothing

Electro-Pollution Supply
PO Box 3217
Prescott, AZ 86302
520/445-8225

Electromagnetic Fields

Environmental Home Center
1724 4th Avenue
Seattle, WA 98134
800/281-9785
206/682-7332

Beds and Bedding • Carpeting and
Flooring • Paints and Finishes

Eurotap
12228 Venice Boulevard #146
Los Angeles, CA 90066
800/388-9255

Wallpaper

For Keeps Friends
217 SW "C" Avenue #190
Lawton, OK 73501
800/892-9403
405/357-8012

Toys

Gardener's Supply
128 Intervale Road
Burlington, VT 15401-2804
800/863-1700
802/863-1700

Flea Control • Garden Pesticides • Insect Repellents • Lawn Care • Mothballs

Gardens Alive!
5100 Schenley Place
Lawrenceburg, IN 47025
812/537-8650

Flea Control • Garden Pesticides
• Lawn Care

Garnet Hill
Box 262 Main Street
Franconia, NH 03580-0262
800/622-6216
603/823-5545

Babies' and Kids' Clothing • Bath Linens
• Beds and Bedding • Carpeting and
Flooring • Clothing • Cribs • Window
Coverings

Gold Mine Natural Food Company
3419 Hancock Street
San Diego, CA 92110-4307
800/475-FOOD
619/296-8536

Food • Tampons and Sanitary Pads

Granny's Old-Fashioned Products*
PO Box 660037
Arcadia, CA 91066
800/366-1762
818/577-1825

Household Cleaning and Laundry
Products

Grateful Threads
1301 Spruce Street
Boulder, CO 80302
800/317-8122

Beds and Bedding

Great Fermentations
87 Larkspur Street
San Rafael, CA 94901
800/570-2337
415/459-2520
GREATFERM@aol.com

Alcoholic Beverages

Green Ban
PO Box 146
Norway, IA 52318
319/446-7495

Insect Repellents

Green Mountain Spinnery
PO Box 54
Putney, VT 05346
802/587-4528

Fabrics, Yarns, and Notions

Harmony Farm Supply
PO Box 460
Graton, CA 95444
707/823-9125

Garden Pesticides

Heart of Vermont*
PO Box 612
Barre, VT 05641
800/639-4123
802/476-3098

Beds and Bedding • Cribs • Fabrics, Yarns, and Notions

Hearthsong
6519 N. Galena Road
Peoria, IL 61656-1773
800/325-2502

Toys

Hendricksen's Natürlich*
PO Box 1677
Sebastopol, CA 95473
707/824-0914

Carpeting and Flooring • Fabrics, Yarns, and Notions

Home Health
949 Seahawk Circle
Virginia Beach, VA 23452
800/284-9123

Beauty and Hygiene • Drugs and Medications • Water Filters

Homespun Fabrics
PO Box 4315
Thousand Oaks, CA 91359
805/381-0741

Fabrics, Yarns, and Notions • Window Coverings

Hummer Nature Works
Reagan Wells Canyon, Box 122
Uvalde, TX 78801
210/232-6167

Mothballs

Insect Aside
PO Box 7
Farmington, WA 99128
509/287-2200

Household Insecticides

J. Crew
1 Ivy Crescent
Lynchburg, VA 24513-1001
800/562-0258

Clothing

J. Jill
PO Box 3004, Winterbrook Way
Meredith, NH 03253-3004
800/642-9989

Clothing

Jaffe Brothers
PO Box 636
Valley Center, CA 92082-0636
619/749-1133

Food

Jamie Harmon
RD 3, Box 464
Jericho, VT 05465
802/879-0800

Fabrics, Yarns, and Notions

Janice Corporation*
198 Route 46
Budd Lake, NJ 07828
800/526-4237

Antiperspirants and Deodorants • Bath Linens • Beauty and Hygiene • Beds and Bedding • Carpeting and Flooring • Clothing • Cribs • Fabrics, Yarns, and Notions • Food Storage • Footwear and Shoe Care • Household Cleaning and Laundry Products • Irons and Ironing-Board Covers • Kitchen and Table Linens • Luggage and Bags • Mouthwash, Toothpaste, and Toothbrushes • Shower Curtains

Karen's Nontoxic Products*
1839 Dr. Jack Road
Conowingo, MD 21918
410/378-4936
410/378-4621

Artists' Colors • Babies' and Kids' Clothing • Baby Food • Bath Linens • Beauty and Hygiene • Beds and Bedding • Clothing • Coffee • Cribs • Diapers • Dishware • Drugs and Medications • Epoxy, Rubber Cement, and "Super Glue" • Flea Control • Food Storage • Footwear and Shoe Care • Hair Color • Household Cleaning and Laundry Products • Kitchen and Table Linens • Luggage and Bags • Mouthwash, Toothpaste, and Toothbrushes • Permanent Waves • Pet Care • Smoke Detectors • Toys

Kettle Care
710 Trap Road
Columbia Falls, MT 59912
406/892-3294

Beauty and Hygiene

Kiwis
PO Box 763
Lucerne Valley, CA 92356
619/248-7195

Footwear and Shoe Care

L.L. Bean
Freeport, ME 04033
800/221-4221

Beds and Bedding • Clothing • Footwear and Shoe Care • Furniture • Luggage and Bags

Lakon Herbals
RR1, Box 4710 Templeton Road
Montpelier, VT 05602
802/223-5563

Insect Repellents

Land's End
One Land's End Lane
Dodgeville, WI 53595
800/356-4444

Beds and Bedding • Clothing

Lead Check
PO Box 1210
Framingham, MA 01701
800/262-LEAD

Lead

The Living Source*
PO Box 20155
Waco, TX 76702
800/662-8787
817/776-4878

Air Filters • Antiperspirants and Deodorants • Beauty and Hygiene • Beds and Bedding • Cosmetics • Diapers • Fabrics, Yarns and Notions • Flea Control • Food Storage • Household Cleaning and Laundry Products • Irons and Ironing-Board Covers • Kitchen and Table Linens • Laundry Detergent

Logona USA
12 Wall Street
Asheville, NC 28801
800/648-6654
704/252-9630

Baby-Care Products • Beauty and Hygiene • Cosmetics • Hair Color • Household Cleaning and Laundry Products • Sun Protection

Marge Smith
PO Box 30
La Mirada, CA 90638
800/344-9339

Air Fresheners

Motherwear
320 Riverside Drive
Northampton, MA 01060
800/950-2500
413/586-3488

Diapers

National Testing Laboratories
6555 Wilson Mills Road, Suite 102
Cleveland, OH 44143
800/458-3330
216/449-2525

Water

Natural Animal
7000 US 1 North
St. Augustine, FL 32095
800/274-7387

Pet Care

The Natural Baby Company
816 Silvia Street, 800B-S
Trenton, NJ 08628-3299
609/771-9233

Artists' Colors • Babies' and Kids' Clothing • Baby Food • Cribs • Diapers • Tampons and Sanitary Pads • Toys

The Natural Bedroom
175 N. Main Street
Sebastopol, CA 95472
800/365-6563

Beds and Bedding • Cribs

The Natural Choice
1365 Rufina Circle
Santa Fe, NM 87505
800/621-2591

Carpeting and Flooring • Footwear and Shoe Care • Household Cleaning and Laundry Products • Laundry Detergent • Paints and Finishes • Shower Curtains • Water Filters

The Natural Gardening Company
217 San Anselmo Avenue
San Anselmo, CA 94960
415/456-5060

Garden Pesticides

Natural Lifestyle
16 Lookout Drive
Asheville, NC 28804-3330
800/752-2775

Beauty and Hygiene • Beds and Bedding • Clothing • Dry Cleaning • Food • Hair Color • Mouthwash, Toothpaste, and Toothbrushes • Permanent Waves • Smoke Detectors • Tampons and Sanitary Pads • Water Filters

The Natural Pet Care Company
8050 Lake City Way
Seattle, WA 98115
800/962-8266

Flea Control • Pet Care

Nigra Enterprises*
5699 Kanan Road
Agoura, CA 91301
818/889-6877

Air Filters

Nontoxic Environments*
PO Box 384
Newmarket, NH 03857
800/789-4348

Air Filters • Beauty & Hygiene • Beds and Bedding • Cribs • Electromagnetic Fields • Formaldehyde • Household Cleaning and Laundry Products • Insect Repellents • Laundry Detergents • Lead • Radon • Shower Curtains • Tampons and Sanitary Pads • Toys • Water Filters

Nova Natural Toys and Crafts
817 Chestnut Ridge Road
Chestnut Ridge, NY 10977
914/426-3757

Artists' Colors • Toys

Ocarina Textiles
16 Cliff Street
New London, CT 06320
203/437-8189
800/578-4562

Fabrics, Yarns, and Notions

The Ohio Hempery
7002 State Route 329
Guysville, OH 45735
800/BUY-HEMP
614/662-4367

Clothing • Luggage and Bags • Footware
and Shoe Care

Old-Fashioned Milk Paint Company
PO Box 222
Groton, MA 01450
508/448-6336

Paints and Finishes

Organic Cottons
103 Hoffecker Road
Phoenixville, PA 19460
610/495-9986

Artists' Colors • Babies' and Kids' Cloth-
ing • Baby Food • Beds and Bedding •
Clothing • Cribs • Diapers • Fabrics,
Yarns, and Notions • Kitchen and Table
Linens • Luggage and Bags • Tampons
and Sanitary Pads • Toys

Organic Interiors
8 College Avenue
Nanuet, NY 10954
914/623-2114

Fabrics, Yarns, and Notions

The Organic Wine Company
1592 Union Street #350
San Francisco, CA 94123
800/477-0167
415/346-5332

Alcoholic Beverages

Ostheimer Wooden Toys
PO Box 407
Wyoming, RI 02898-0407
800/249-9090

Toys

Pallas Textiles
1330 Bellevue Street
Green Bay, WI 54308-8100
414/468-2600

Wallpaper

Pattern People
10 Floyd Road
Derry, NH 03038-4724
603/432-7180

Wallpaper

Patti Collins Canvas Products
366 Marin Avenue
Mill Valley, CA 94941
415/388-4934

Luggage and Bags

Peaceful Valley Farm Supply
PO Box 2209
Grass Valley, CA 95945
916/272-4769

Garden Pesticides

Port Canvas Company
PO Box H
Kennebunkport, ME 04046
207/985-9767

Luggage and Bags

Pueblo to People
PO Box 2545
Houston, TX 77252-2545
800/843-5257

Clothing

Radon Solutions
PO Box 3309
Allentown, PA 18106
610/481-9555

Radon

Radon Testing Corporation of America
2 Hayes Street
Elmsford, NY 10523
800/457-2366

Radon

Real Goods
555 Leslie Street
Ukiah, CA 95482-5507
800/762-7325
707/468-9214
http://www.realgoods.com

Antiperspirants and Deodorants • Automobiles • Bath Linens • Beds and Bedding • Electromagnetic Fields • Food Storage • Garden Pesticides • Household Cleaning and Laundry Products • Household Insecticides • Laundry Detergents • Lawn Care • Shower Curtains • Smoke Detectors • Water Filters

Reflections Organic
214 N. Lewis Street
Trinity, TX 75862-9801
800/852-9273

Clothing • Footwear and Shoe Care

Royal-Pedic
119 N. Fairfax Avenue
Los Angeles, CA 90036
213/932-6155

Beds and Bedding

S.A.F.E. Home & Office Company
32 S. Main Street, Suite 6
Sebastopol, CA 95472
800/638-3781
707/578-1645

Electromagnetic Fields

The Safety Zone
Hanover, PA 17333-0019
800/338-1635

Combustion By-products • Hair-Removal Products

Sajama Alpaca
PO Box 1209
Ashland, OR 97520
541/488-3949

Beds and Bedding • Carpeting and Flooring • Fabrics, Yarns, and Notions

SelfCare Catalog
2515 E. 43rd Street
Chattanooga, TN 37422
800/345-3371

Drugs and Medications

Seventh Generation
49 Hercules Drive
Colchester, VT 05446-1672
800/456/1177

Antiperspirants and Deodorants • Bath Linens • Beds and Bedding • Carpeting and Flooring • Clothing • Household Cleaning and Laundry Products • Shower Curtains • Tampons and Sanitary Pads

Shaker Workshops
PO Box 8001
Ashburnham, MA 01430-8001
508/827-9900

Furniture

Shaker Workshops West
PO Box 487
Inverness, CA 94937
415/669-7256

Furniture

Shampoo-chez
303 Potrero Street, Building 40-F
Santa Cruz, CA 95060
800/727-PETS

Flea Control • Pet Care

Shelburne Farms
Shelburne, VT 05482
802/985-8686

Milk and Dairy Products

Simmons Handcrafts
42295 N. Highway 36
Bridgeville, CA 95526
707/777-1920

Beauty and Hygiene • Tampons and Sanitary Pads

Sinan Company
PO Box 857
Davis, CA 95617-0857
916/753-3104

Carpeting and Flooring • Paints and Finishes • Wallpaper

Sofa U Love
11948 San Vicente
Brentwood, CA 90049
310/207-2540

Furniture

Soapworks
14450 Griffin Street
San Leandro, CA 94577
800/699-9917
510/357-7300

Household Cleaning and Laundry Products • Dishwater Detergent • Laundry Detergent

Straw Into Gold
3006 San Pablo Avenue
Berkeley, CA 94702
510/548-5247

Fabrics, Yarns, and Notions

Sun Precautions
2815 Wetmore Avenue
Everett, WA 98201
800/882-7860

Sun Protection

Sureway Trading Enterprises
826 Pine Avenue
Niagara Falls, NY 14301-1806
416/596-1887

Fabrics, Yarns, and Notions

Teslatronics
4303 Vineland Road, Suite F8
Orlando, FL 32811
904/462-2010

Electromagnetic Fields

Testfabrics
PO Box 420
Middlesex, NJ 08846
908/469-6446

Fabrics, Yarns, and Notions • Kitchen and Table Linens

Thai Silks
252 State Street
Los Altos, CA 94022
800/722-SILK (in CA: 800/221-SILK)
415/948-8611

Fabrics, Yarns, and Notions

TRA Instruments
2257 S. 1100 East
Salt Lake City, UT 24106
800/582-3537

Electromagnetic Fields

Traditional Products Company
PO Box 564
Creswell, OR 97426
503/895-2957

Mouthwash, Toothpaste, and Tooth-brushes • Shampoos

Tweeds
One Avery Row
Roanoke, VA 24012-8528
800/999-7997

Clothing

Van Cleave & Associates
315 Westbrook Circle
Naperville, IL 60565-3243
800/822-9499

Air Fresheners

Vermont Country Store
PO Box 3000
Manchester Center, VT 05255-3000
802/362-4647

Bath Linens • Beds and Bedding •
Footwear and Shoe Care • Kitchen and
Table Linens • Shower Curtains • Silver
Polish and Other Metal Cleaners

Walnut Acres
Penns Creek, PA 17862
800/433-3998
717/837-0601

Fish and Seafood • Food • Meat, Poultry, and Eggs

Weleda
PO Box 769
Spring Valley, NY 10977
914/352-6145

Baby-Care Products • Beauty and
Hygiene

Whippoorwill Farm
Lakeville, CT 06039-0717
203/435-9657

Meat, Poultry, and Eggs

Willsboro Wood Products
PO Box 509
Keeseville, NY 12944
800/342-3373

Furniture

Winter Silks
PO Box 620130
Middleton, WI 53562
800/648-7455

Clothing • Footwear and Shoe Care

Wolfe's Neck Farm
10 Burnett Road
Freeport, ME 04032
207/865-4469

Meat, Poultry, and Eggs

Womankind
PO Box 1775
Sebastopol, CA 95473
707/522-8662

Tampons and Sanitary Pads

DIRECTORY OF
PRODUCT MANUFACTURERS

AFM coating products (AFM Enterprises, San Diego, CA)

Auro paints and finishes (imported by *Sinan Company*)

Autumn Harp personal-care products (Autumn Harp, Bristol, VT)

Bon Ami Cleaning Powder, Cleaning Cake, and **Polishing Cleanser** (Faultless Starch/Bon Ami, Kansas City, MO)

Brooks Pearwood Toothbrush (*Traditional Products Company,* Creswell, OR)

Coppertone tanning products (Schering-Plough, Memphis, TN)

Bygone Bugs (*Lakon Herbals,* Montpelier, VT)

Dr. Bronner's Pure Castile Soap and **Peppermint Oil Soap** (All-One-God-Faith, Escondido, CA)

Dr. Hauschka cosmetic products (Dr. Hauschka Cosmetics, Wyoming, RI)

Drain King (GT Water Products, Moorpark, CA)

Earth's Best baby food (Earth's Best Baby Food, Middlebury, VT)

Flecto Varathane Diamond Finish (The Flecto Company, Oakland, CA)

FoxFibre (Natural Cotton Colours, Wickenberg, AZ)

Geo cleaning products (Ft. Lauderdale, FL) For a local distributor, call 954/938-9129.

Herbavita hair color (imported by Bioforce of America; Kinderhook, NY)

Lead Check Swabs (Lead Check, Framingham, MA)

Livos paints and finishes (imported by *Natural Choice*)

Logona beauty products (*Logona USA,* Asheville, NC)

Natural World cleaning products (Natural World, Wilton, CT) For a local distributor, call 203/761-0221.

Natracare tampons (Natracare, Boulder, CO)

o.b. tampons (Johnson & Johnson, Racine, WI)

O'Glue (Itoya of America, Torrance, CA)

Old-Fashioned Milk Paint (The Old-Fashioned Milk Paint Company, Groton, MA)

Paul Penders cosmetic products (Paul Penders, Seffner, FL)

Pilot pens (Pilot Corporation of America, Trumbull, CT)

Rain Crystal Glass Distiller (*Scientific Glass,* Albuquerque, NM)

Seagull IV water filter (General Ecology, Lionville, PA)

Spred 2000 paints (The Glidden Company, Huron, OH)

Stabilo pens and markers (Hunt Manufacturing Company, Statesville, NC)

Sucanat Organic Sugar (Pronatec International, Peterborough, NH)

Tampax Naturals and **Tampax Original Regular Tampons** (Tambrands, Lake Success, NY)

Tom's of Maine personal-care products (Tom's of Maine, Kennebunk, ME)

Twinkle Silver Polish (Johnson & Johnson, Racine, WI)

Vitawave Cream Hair Color and **Permanent Waves** (Canoga Park, CA)

Weleda cosmetic products (*Weleda,* Spring Valley, NY)

WorldWise Easy-Clear Sink Trap (WorldWise, San Rafael, CA)

BIBLIOGRAPHY

Alderman, Donna, et al. "How Adequate Are Warnings and First Aid Instructions on Consumer Product Labels: An Investigation." *Veterinary and Human Toxicology*, no. 24, February 1982.

Banik, Dr. Allen E. *Your Water and Your Health*. Rev. ed. New Canaan, CT: Keats Publishing, 1981.

Becker, Robert O., M.D. *Cross Currents: The Perils of Electropollution, The Promise of Electromedicine*. Los Angeles: Jeremy P. Tarcher, 1990.

Becker, Robert O., M.D., and Gary Selden. *The Body Electric: Electromagnetism and the Foundation of Life*. New York: William Morrow, 1985.

Bommersbach, Jane. "The Case Against NutraSweet." *Westword*, January 1983.

Boraiko, Allen A. "Storing Up Trouble . . . Hazardous Waste." *National Geographic*, March 1985.

Brobeck, Stephen, and Anne C. Averyt. *The Product Safety Book: The Ultimate Consumer Guide to Product Hazards*. New York: E. P. Dutton, 1983.

Brown, Halina Szejnwald, et al. "The Role of Skin Absorption as a Route of Exposure for Volatile Organic Compounds in Drinking Water." *American Journal of Public Health*, May 1984.

Calabrese, Edward J., and Michael W. Dorset. *Healthy Living in an Unhealthy World*. New York: Simon & Schuster, 1984.

California State Department of Consumer Affairs. *Clean Your Room! A Compendium Describing a Wide Variety of Indoor Pollutants and Their Health Effects, and Containing Sage Advice to Both Householders and Statespersons in the Matter of Cleaning Up*. Sacramento: California State Department of Consumer Affairs, February 1982.

CIP Bulletin. "Aflatoxin and Food." Carcinogen Information Program, St. Louis, MO.

———. "Broiling and Benzo(a)pyrene." Carcinogen Information Program, St. Louis, MO.

———. "Insecticide Residues in Food." Carcinogen Information Program, St. Louis, MO.

————. "Nitrites and Nitrosamines." Carcinogen Information Program, St. Louis, MO.

Coffel, Steve, and Karyn Feiden. *Indoor Pollution.* New York: Ballantine Books, 1990.

Conry, Tom. *Consumer's Guide to Cosmetics.* Garden City, NY: Anchor Press/Doubleday, 1980.

Consumer Reports. "Are Hair Dyes Safe?" August 1979.

————. "Menstrual Tampons and Pads." March 1978.

————. "Microwave Ovens." March 1981.

————. "The Selling of H_2O." September 1980.

————. "Smoke Detectors." October 1984.

————. "Water Filters." February 1983.

Consumers Union. *Consumer Reports Buying Guide.* Mt. Vernon, NY: Consumers Union, 1981, 1982, 1983.

Cronin, Etain. *Contact Dermatitis,* Edinburgh, Scotland: Churchill Livingstone, 1980.

Donovan, Jennifer. "When You Really Need a Dry Cleaner." *San Francisco Chronicle,* 12 March 1985.

Environmental Action. "Birth Control Blues." May/June 1985.

Fisher, Alexander A. *Contact Dermatitis.* Philadelphia: Lea & Febiger, 1973.

Foster, Douglas. "You Are What They Eat: A Glowing Report on Radioactive Waste in the Sea." *Mother Jones,* July 1981.

Freydberg, Nicholas, Ph.D., and Willis A. Gortner, Ph.D. *The Food Additives Book.* New York: Bantam Books, 1982.

Fritsch, Albert J. (ed.). *The Household Pollutants Guide.* Garden City, NY: Anchor Press/Doubleday, 1978.

Golden Empire Health Planning Center. *Household Hazardous Waste: Solving the Disposal Dilemma.* Sacramento, CA: Golden Empire Health Planning Center, 1984.

Gosselin, R. E., et al. *Clinical Toxicology of Commercial Products.* 4th ed. Baltimore: Williams & Wilkins Co., 1976.

Hawley, G. G. (ed.). *The Condensed Chemical Dictionary.* New York: Van Nostrand Reinhold, 1981.

Heimler, Charles, and Tim Redmond. "Food Irradiation: Will Half-Life Replace Shelf Life?" *San Francisco Bay Guardian,* 27 February 1985.

Higgenbotham, P., and M. E. Pinkham. *Mary Ellen's Best of Helpful Hints.* New York: Warner Books, 1979.

Hunter, Beatrice Trum. *Consumer Beware! Your Food and What's Been Done to It.* New York: Simon & Schuster, 1971.

————. *Beatrice Trum Hunter's Additive Book.* New Canaan, CT: Keats Publishing, 1980.

Keough, Carol. *Water Fit to Drink.* Emmaus, PA: Rodale Press, 1981.

King, Jonathan. *Troubled Water.* Emmaus, PA: Rodale Press, 1981.

————. "VDT: How to Prevent 'Terminal Illness.'" *Medical Self-Care,* Spring 1984.

Kleiner, Art (ed.). "The Health Hazards of Computers: A Guide to Worrying Intelligently." *Whole Earth Review,* Fall 1985.

Lecos, Chris. "Reacting to Sulfites." *FDA Consumer,* December 1985/January 1986.

Lifton, Bernice. *Bugbusters: Getting Rid of Household Pests Without Dangerous Chemicals.* New York: McGraw-Hill Paperbacks, 1985.

Lipske, Michael. *Chemical Additives in Booze.* Washington, DC: Center for Science in the Public Interest, 1982.

Makower, Joel. *Office Hazards.* Washington, DC: Tilden Press, 1981.

Mason, Jim, and Peter Singer. *Animal Factories: An Inside Look at the Manufacturing of Food for Profit.* New York: Crown Publishers, 1980.

Miller, Roger W. "How Onions and a Baked Potato Became Sources of Botulism Poisoning." *FDA Consumer,* October 1984.

Mishell, D. M., and R. Daniel. "Current Status of Intrauterine Devices." *New England Journal of Medicine,* April 1985.

Mott, Lawrie. *Pesticides in Food: What the Public Needs to Know.* San Francisco: Natural Resources Defense Council, 1984.

National Research Council/National Academy of Science. *Indoor Pollutants.* Washington, DC: National Academy Press, 1981.

Nussdorf, M. R., and S. B. Nussdorf. *Dress for Health.* Harrisburg, PA: Stackpole Books, 1980.

Ott, John N. *Health and Light: The Effects of Natural and Artificial Light on Man and Other Living Things.* New York: Pocket Books, 1977.

———. *Light, Radiation & You: How to Stay Healthy.* Greenwich, CT: Devin-Adair, 1985.

Peterson, Iver. "Pollution: The Problem of Heating with Wood." *San Francisco Chronicle,* 7 December 1983.

Pfeiffer, Guy, M.D., et al. *The Household Environment and Chronic Illness: Guidelines for Constructing and Maintaining a Less Polluted Residence.* Springfield, IL: Charles C. Thomas, 1962.

Potter, Morris E., D.V.M., et al. "Unpasteurized Milk: The Hazards of a Health Fetish." *Journal of the American Medical Association,* 19 October 1984.

Regenstein, Lewis. *America the Poisoned.* Washington, DC: Acropolis Books, 1982.

Rinzler, Carol Ann. *The Consumer's Brand-Name Guide to Household Products.* New York: Lippincott and Crowell, 1980.

Roffers, Melanie. "Sweet Seductions." *Medical Self-Care,* January/February 1986.

Saifer, Phyllis, M.D., and Merla Zellerbach. *Detox.* Los Angeles: Jeremy P. Tarcher, 1984.

Samuels, Mike, M.D., and Hal Zina Bennett. *Well Body, Well Earth: The Sierra Club Environmental Health Sourcebook.* San Francisco: Sierra Club Books, 1983.

Shepard, Robin. "Color Your Hair . . . Naturally!" *Mother Earth News,* March/April 1982.

Shuping, Edward R. "Aflatoxin Paranoia: Do You Fit the Mold?" *Vegetarian Times* 46.

Sittig, Marshall. *Handbook of Toxics and Hazardous Chemicals.* Park Ridge, NJ: Noyes Publications, 1981.

Solomon, Stephen. "How Safe Is X-Rayed Food?" *American Health,* March/April 1984.

Stark, N. *The Formula Book.* New York: Avon.

Steele, Gerald L. *Exploring the World of Plastics.* Bloomington, IL: McKnight Publishing, 1977.

Stellman, Jeanne, Ph.D., and Mary Sue Henifin, M.P.H. *Office Work Can Be Dangerous to Your Health: A Handbook of Office Health and Safety Hazards and What You Can Do About Them.* New York: Ballantine Books, 1989.

Stevens, William K. "Scientists Debate Health Hazards of Electromagnetic Fields." *The New York Times,* 11 July 1989.

Swezey, Kenneth M. *Formulas, Methods, Tips & Data for Home & Workshop.* New York: Popular Science Publishing, 1969.

Tortora, P. G. *Understanding Textiles.* New York: Macmillan, 1978.

Twenty Mule Team Borax: The Magic Crystal. Los Angeles: United States Borax & Chemical Corp.

United States Consumer Product Safety Commission. "Asbestos in the Home." Washington, DC: Consumer Product Safety Commission.

———. "Caution! Choosing and Using Your Gas Space Heater." Washington, DC: Consumer Product Safety Commission.

———. "Guide to Fabric Flammability." Washington, DC: Consumer Product Safety Commission.

———. "Fact Sheet #13: Carbon Monoxide." Washington, DC: Consumer Product Safety Commission.

———. "Fact Sheet #17: Flammable Fabrics." Washington, DC: Consumer Product Safety Commission.

———. "Fact Sheet #34: Space Heaters." Washington, DC: Consumer Product Safety Commission.

———. "Fact Sheet #44: Fireplaces." Washington, DC: Consumer Product Safety Commission.

———. "Fact Sheet #55: The Federal Hazardous Substances Act." Washington, DC: Consumer Product Safety Commission.

———. "Fact Sheet #67: Oven Cleaners." Washington, DC: Consumer Product Safety Commission.

———. "Fact Sheet #72: Drain Cleaners." Washington, DC: Consumer Product Safety Commission.

———. "Fact Sheet #79: Furnaces." Washington, DC: Consumer Product Safety Commission.

———. "Fact Sheet #92: Coal and Wood Burning Stoves." Washington, DC: Consumer Product Safety Commission.

———. "Fact Sheet #97: Kerosene Heaters." Washington, DC: Consumer Product Safety Commission.

United States Department of Agriculture and United States Department of Health and Human Services. "Nutrition and Your Health: Dietary Guidelines for Americans." Home and Garden Bulletin, no. 232.

United States Department of Health, Education, and Welfare. "Everything Doesn't Cause Cancer." Washington, DC: National Cancer Institute. NIH Publication, no. 80-2039, April 1980.

United States Environmental Protection Agency. "Pesticide Safety Tips." Washington, DC: Environmental Protection Agency.

United States Food and Drug Administration. "Food Poisoning: The 'Infamous Four.'" An FDA Consumer Memo.

United States Office of the Federal Register. *Code of Federal Regulations*. Washington, DC: U.S. Government Printing Office, 1981.

United States Statutes at Large. *Safe Drinking Water Act*, Vol. 88 Pt. 2, Public Law 93-523. Washington, DC: U.S. Government Printing Office, 1976.

Wallace, Lance A. "Personal Exposures, Outdoor Concentrations, and Breath Levels of Toxic Air Pollutants Measured for 425 Persons in Urban, Suburban and Rural Areas." Unpublished report presented at the annual meeting of the Air Pollution Control Association, 25 June 1984, San Francisco, CA.

Warde, John. "Flower Power." *Organic Gardening*, May 1985.

Waters, Enoc P. "What About Bottled Water?" *FDA Consumer*, May 1974.

Weiss, G. (ed.). *Hazardous Chemicals Data Book*. Park Ridge, NJ: Noyes Data Corporation, 1980.

Winter, Ruth. *A Consumer Dictionary of Cosmetic Ingredients*. New York: Crown Publishers, 1976.

———. *A Consumer Dictionary of Food Additives*. New York: Crown Publishers, 1978.

Woo, Olga, Pharm. D. "Your Guide for Plant Safety." San Francisco: San Francisco Department of Public Health.

Wylie, Harriet. *420 Ways to Clean Everything*. New York: Harmony Books, 1979.

Yiamouyiannis, John, Ph.D. *Lifesavers Guide to Fluoridation*. Delaware, OH: Safe Water Foundation, 1982.

Zamm, Alfred V. *Why Your House May Endanger Your Health*. New York: Simon & Schuster, 1980.

Zimmerman, David R. *The Essential Guide to Nonprescription Drugs*. New York: Harper & Row, 1983.

INDEX

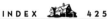